Convergence of Blockchain and Internet of Things in Healthcare

Edited by
Arun Kumar Rana, Vishnu Sharma, Ajay Rana, Maksud Alam and Suman Lata Tripathi

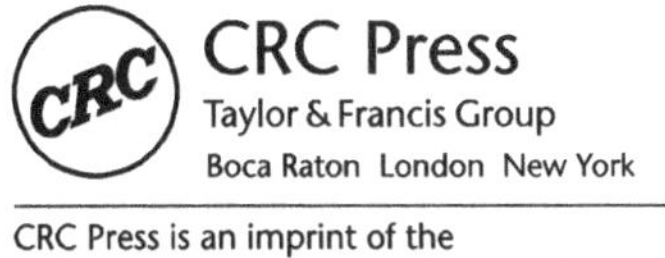

CRC Press
Taylor & Francis Group
Boca Raton London New York

CRC Press is an imprint of the Taylor & Francis Group, an **informa** business

Designed cover image: Shutterstock

First edition published 2024
by CRC Press
2385 NW Executive Center Drive, Suite 320, Boca Raton FL 33431

and by CRC Press
4 Park Square, Milton Park, Abingdon, Oxon, OX14 4RN
CRC Press is an imprint of Taylor & Francis Group, LLC

ISBN: 9781032576619 (hbk)
ISBN: 9781032739588 (pbk)
ISBN: 9781003466949 (ebk)

DOI: 10.1201/9781003466949

Typeset in Sabon
by Deanta Global Publishing Services, Chennai, India

Convergence of Blockchain and Internet of Things in Healthcare

The Internet of Things (IoT) and blockchain are two new technologies that combine elements in many ways. A system where the virtual and physical worlds interact is created by integrating pervasive computing, ubiquitous computing, communication technologies, sensing technologies, Internet Protocol, and embedded devices. A massive number of linked devices and vast amounts of data present new prospects for developing services that can directly benefit the economy, environment, society, and individual residents. Due to the size of IoT and insufficient data security, security breaches may have a huge impact and negative effects. IoT not only connects gadgets but also people and other entities, leaving every IoT component open to a wide variety of assaults. The implementation and application of IoT and blockchain technology in actual scientific, biomedical, and data applications are covered in this book. The book highlights important advancements in health science research and development by applying the distinctive capabilities inherent to distributed ledger systems. Each chapter describes the current uses of blockchain in real-world data collection, medicine development, device tracking, and more meaningful patient interaction. All of these are used to create opportunities for expanding health science research. This paradigm change is studied from the perspectives of pharmaceutical executives, biotechnology entrepreneurs, regulatory bodies, ethical review boards, and blockchain developers.

Key Features:

- Provides a foundation for the implementation process of blockchain and IoT devices based on healthcare-related technology
- Image processing and IoT device researchers can correlate their work with other requirements of advanced technology in the healthcare domain
- Conveys the latest technology, including artificial intelligence and machine learning, in healthcare-related technology
- Useful for the researcher to explore new things like security, cryptography, and privacy in healthcare-related technology
- Tailored for people who want to start in healthcare-related technology with blockchain and IoT

This book is primarily for senior undergraduates, graduate students, and academic researchers in the fields of electrical engineering, electronics and communication engineering, computer science and engineering, and biomedical engineering.

Smart Engineering Systems: Design and Applications

Series Editor- Suman Lata Tripathi

Internet of Things
Robotic and Drone Technology
Edited by Nitin Goyal, Sharad Sharma, Arun Kumar Rana, Suman Lata Tripathi

Smart Electrical Grid System
Design Principle, Modernization, and Techniques
Edited by Krishan Arora, Suman Lata Tripathi and Sanjeevikumar Padmanaban

Artificial Intelligence, Internet of Things (IoT) and Smart Materials for Energy Applications
Edited by Mohan Lal Kolhe, Kailash J. Karande and Sampat G. Deshmukh

Artificial Intelligence for Internet of Things: Design Principle, Modernization, and Techniques
Edited by N. Thillaiarasu, Suman Lata Tripathi and V.Dhinakaran

Machine Learning and Internet of Things in Solar Power Generation
Edited by Prabha Umapathy, Jude Hemanth, Shelej Khera, Abinaya Inbamani and Suman Lata Tripathi

Convergence of Blockchain and Internet of Things in Healthcare
Edited by Arun Kumar Rana, Vishnu Sharma, Ajay Rana, Maksud Alam and Suman Lata Tripathi

For more information about this series, please visit: https://www.routledge.com/

Contents

About the Editors viii
List of Contributors xi

1 Lung Disease Diagnosis Using Machine Learning from a Bibliometric Perspective 1
ANUPAM BONKRA, PUMMY DHIMAN, SUSHIL KAMBOJ, AND SUKHPREET KAUR

2 Industry 4.0 in Manufacturing, Communication, Transportation, and Healthcare 25
KIRAN AHUJA, INDU BALA, AND MAAD M. MIJWI

3 Role and Impact of Blockchain–IoT-Enabled Supply Chain Management Model for Medical Supply 54
INDERPAL SINGH, BALRAJ SINGH, AND ARUN KUMAR RANA

4 The Internet of Things in Healthcare: A Remote Patient Monitoring System 68
DEV GUPTA AND RACHIT JAIN

5 Revolutionizing Industry 4.0 with Blockchain Technology: Opportunities and Challenges 87
RAVI PRAKASH, SHOBHA TYAGI, AND RATNESH LITORIYA

6 Prediction of Breast Cancer Using Machine Learning Techniques for Health Data 116
AARTI, SAURABH KARLING, PUSHPENDRA K RAJPUT, SURBHI, AND PRAVEEN KUMAR MALIK

7 Design and Development of an IoT-Based Smart Medical Device 128

SHAILESH KHAPARKAR, NEETA NATHANI, AND JAGDEESH KUMAR AHIRWAR

8 Revolutionary Finance: Impact of Blockchain and Distributed Ledger Technology on the Financial Industry 146

POOJA JAIN AND RACHIT JAIN

9 Barriers and Benefits of Blockchain Adoption in the Healthcare System 162

KULDEEP PAL AND MUKESH KUMAR

10 Deep Learning-Based Renal Biopsy Image Analysis for Diagnosing Diabetic Kidney Disease 175

SAXENA SACHIN KUMAR, SHRIVASTAVA JITENDRA NATH, AND AGARWAL GAURAV

11 Blockchain: Evolution and Future Scope 196

NAVNEET KAUR, NIDHI CHAHAL, RITU DEWAN, SHIKHA SINGH, GAUTAM BANSAL, DIKSHANT DISHU, AND SANTOSH KUMAR

12 COVID-19 Detection and Pandemic Prevention System Using Data Science 210

ABHIMANYU SINGH NEGI, PRAKHAR GUPTA, RASHI SRIVASTAVA, AND ARUN KUMAR RANA

13 Use of Machine Learning and IoT in Smart Farming: The Future of Agriculture 223

TANUSHREE SANWAL, SANDHYA AVASTHI, MEENAKSHI TYAGI, ANKITA SHARMA, SAPNA YADAV, AND SUMAN LATA TRIPATHI

14 Comprehensive Analysis of Blockchain Frameworks and Their Usability in Various Applications 243

HARISH KUMAR, RAJESH KUMAR KAUSHAL, NAVEEN KUMAR, AND PRAVEEN KUMAR MALIK

15 IoT and Healthcare: Development, Architecture, Security, and Its Applicability in Healthcare 263

MOHIT LALIT, GAURAV BATHLA, SURENDER SINGH, AND SHIRAZ KHURANA

16 Convergence of Blockchain and IoT in Healthcare: Opportunities and Challenges 277

PAWAN WHIG, RASHMI GERA, ASHIMA BHATNAGAR BHATIA, RAHUL REDDY NADIKATTU, AND YUSUF JIBRIN ALKALI

17 From Remote Monitoring to Personalized Care: A Review of IoT-Based Patient Engagement Solutions in Healthcare 297

S. J. SUJI PRASAD, R. MANJULA DEVI, P. KEERTHIKA, P. SURESH, A. REX MACEDO AROKIARAJ, AND M. SANGEETHA

18 Fusion Strategies for Image Processing–Based Multimodal Biometric System 323

NITIN S. NAGORI, KIRAN V. AJETRAO, AND AMEYA K. NAIK

Index 341

About the Editors

Arun Kumar Rana completed his BTech degree at Kurukshetra University, and his MTech and PhD at Maharishi Markandeshwar (Deemed to be University), Mullana, India. His areas of interest include image processing, wireless sensor networks, the Internet of Things, AI, and machine learning and embedded systems. Dr Rana is currently an assistant professor at the Galgotias College of Engineering and Technology, Greater Noida, India, with more than 16 years of experience. Dr Rana is a collaborative researcher and has published more than 110 SCI/ESCI/Scopus/others papers in national and international journals and conference papers. He has also published 10 books with national and international publishers including Taylor & Francis. He has also attended 15 workshops and 12 faculty development programs (FDP). He has guided six MTech candidates. He serves as an editor or reviewer for several international journals and conferences and served as keynote speaker. He is also a member of the Asia Society of Research and SIRG (Scientific Innovation Research Group), Egypt. He has published/granted 10 national and international patents. He has conducted many workshops on IoT and its applications in engineering, wireless networks, and simulators, and teaches the latest techniques related to wireless and IoT technology. He is listed in the world scientist rankings for 2021 and 2022. He was guest editor for the special issue "Routing and Protocols for Energy Efficient Communication," MDPI, SCI, IF-3.004 (Q2).

Vishnu Sharma is a professor and dean of the Department of Computer Science and Engineering at ITS College of Engineering, Greater Noida, India. He earned his BTech, MTech, and PhD from Madhav Institute of Technology & Science (M.I.T.S.), Gwalior, India, in Computer Science and Engineering, and is affiliated with Rajiv Gandhi Technical University, Bhopal. He has published 100-plus papers on MANETs, AI, machine learning, IoT, cryptography and network security, computer networks, and mobile computing in international conferences and international journals/ SCI/Scopus. He has published three books on mobile computing, cyber security and law, and advanced mobile computing, and has been the editor of ten IEEE conference proceedings. He has also organized many IEEE international conferences for the IEEE Uttar Pradesh section. He has 26 years of teaching experience at various reputed engineering institutes and universities, including Jaypee University, Galgotias University, KIET, and Galgotias College.

Ajay Rana has more than 22 years of teaching experience in academia and industry with roles including lecturer, professor, director, dean, and senior vice president (RBEF). His areas of interest include machine learning, Internet of Things (IoT), augmented reality, software engineering, and soft computing. He has 60-plus patents in the fields of IoT, networks, and sensors. He has more than 271 research papers in reputed journals published by ACM, Springer, Elsevier, Taylor & Francis, and others, and from international and national conferences; co-authored 8 books, and co-edited 36 conference proceedings. Rana is chairman of AUN Research Labs, an executive committee member of IEEE Uttar Pradesh Section, a senior member of IEEE, and a life member of the Computer Society of India and ISTE. He is also a member of the editorial boards and review committees of several journals. He has visited many top universities and colleges worldwide, including in Europe, United Arab Emirates, UK, and Asia.

Maksud Alam earned his BTech degree in 2007 from Uttar Pradesh Technical University, Lucknow, India; and his MTech degree in 2012. He earned his PhD from Jamia Millia Islamia, New Delhi, India. He is a recipient of the Visveswaraya PhD Fellowship from the Ministry of Electronics and IT, Government of India, and is currently an assistant professor at Galgotias College of Engineering and Technology, Greater Noida, India. Prior to this, he was a lecturer at the GLA Institute of Technology and Management, Mathura; and Babu Banarasi Das Group of Institutions, Bulandshahr, in 2007 and 2008, respectively. From 2009 to 2016, he served as an assistant professor at the Bharat Institute of Technology, Meerut. He has published more than 12 research papers in reputed journals and conferences such as *IET Microwaves, Antennas & Propagation*, *International Journal of RF and Microwave Computer-Aided Engineering* (Wiley), *Microwave and Optical Technology Letters* (Wiley), *Frequenz*, *Progress in Electromagnetic Research*, and IEEE conferences. His research interests include the Internet of Things and antennas, design and development of electromagnetic band-gap structures, metamaterial antennas, circularly polarized microstrip antennas, reconfigurable antennas, ultrawideband antennas, and defected ground structures.

Suman Lata Tripathi is a professor at Lovely Professional University with more than 21 years of experience in academics and research. She completed her PhD in the area of microelectronics and VLSI design from MNNIT, Allahabad. She earned her MTech in electronics engineering from UP

Technical University, Lucknow, and BTech in electrical engineering from Purvanchal University, Jaunpur. She was also a remote post-doc researcher at Nottingham Trent University, London, in 2022. She has published more than 104 research papers in Springer, Elsevier, IEEE, Wiley, and IOP refereed science journals, conference proceedings, and e-books. She has also published 13 Indian patents and four copyrights. She has guided four PhD scholars and four are in the submission stage. She has organized several workshops, summer internships, and expert lectures for students. She has worked as a session chair, conference steering committee member, editorial board member, and peer reviewer for international/national journals and conferences (IEEE, Springer, Wiley). She received the Research Excellence Award in 2019 and the Research Appreciation Award in 2020 and 2021 at Lovely Professional University, India. She was a recipient of the IGEN Women for Green Technology's Women's Achievers Award on International Women's Day, 8 March 2023. She received the best paper award at IEEE ICICS 2018. She has also received project funding from SERB DST under the scheme TARE in the area of microelectronic devices. She has edited and authored more than 19 books in the areas of electronics and electrical engineering. She has done editing work with top publishers like Elsevier, CRC/Taylor & Francis, Wiley-IEEE, SP Wiley, Nova Science, and Apple Academic Press. She is also book series editor for the series Smart Engineering Systems (CRC Press); Engineering System Design for Sustainable Developments, and Decentralized Systems and Next-Generation Internet (Wiley-Scrivener); and conference series editor for Conference Proceedings Series on Intelligent Systems for Engineering Designs (CRC Press/Taylor & Francis). She serves as academic editor of the *Journal of Electrical and Computer Engineering* (Scopus/WoS, Q2), *International Journal of Reconfigurable Computing* (Scopus, Q3), *Active and Passive Electronic Components* (Scopus, Q4; Hindawi), and special issue guest editor for *Materials: Advances in Nanomaterials and Nanoscale Semiconductor Applications* (MDPI; SCI IF = 3.74, Q2). She is a senior member of IEEE, a fellow of IETE, and a life member of ISC, and is continuously involved in different professional activities along with academic work. Her areas of expertise include microelectronic device modeling and characterization, low-power VLSI circuit design, VLSI design of testing, and advanced FET design for IoT, embedded system design, reconfigurable architecture with FPGAs, and biomedical applications.

Contributors

Aarti
Computer Science and Engineering Department, Lovely Professional University, Punjab, India

Jagdeesh Kumar Ahirwar
Gyan Ganga Institute of Technology & Sciences, Jabalpur, India

Kiran Ahuja
DAV Institute of Engineering and Technology, Jalandhar, India

Kiran V. Ajetrao
Department of Electronics and Telecommunication, K. J. Somaiya College of Engineering, Somaiya Vidyavihar University, Mumbai 400071, India

Yusuf Jibrin Alkali
Federal Inland Revenue Service, Nigeria

A. Rex Macedo Arokiaraj
Department of Information Technology, University of Technology and Applied Sciences (UTAS)-CAS, Ibri, Oman

Sandhya Avasthi
ABES Engineering College, Ghaziabad, India

Indu Bala
School of Electronics and Electrical Engineering, Lovely Professional University, Phagwara, Punjab, India

Gautam Bansal
College of Engineering, Chandigarh Group of Colleges Landran, Mohali, Punjab, India

Gaurav Bathla
Department of Computer Science vand Engineering Chandigarh University, Mohali, Punjab

Ashima Bhatnagar Bhatia
Vivekananda Institute of Professional Studies, New Delhi, India

Anupam Bonkra
Chandigarh Engineering College, Punjab, India

Nidhi Chahal
Assistant Professor, College of Engineering, Chandigarh Group of Colleges Landran, Mohali, Punjab, India

R. Manjula Devi
Department of Computer Science and Engineering, KPR Institute of Engineering and Technology, Coimbatore, Tamil Nadu, India

Ritu Dewan
Computer Science and Engineering, Galgotias College of Engineering and Technology, Greater Noida, India

Pummy Dhiman
Chitkara University Institute of Engineering and Technology, Chitkara University, Punjab, India

Dikshant Dishu
College of Engineering, Chandigarh Group of Colleges Landran, Mohali, Punjab, India

Agarwal Gaurav
Invertis University, Bareilly, Uttar Pradesh, India

Rashmi Gera
Manav Rachna International Institute of Research and Studies, Faridabad, India

Dev Gupta
Department of Electronics and Communication, Institute of Technology & Management, Gwalior, India

Prakhar Gupta
Department of Computer Science and Engineering, Galgotias College of Engineering and Technology, Greater Noida, India

Pooja Jain
Amity Business School, Amity University, Madhya Pradesh, India

Rachit Jain
Department of Electronics Engineering, Madhav Institute of Technology & Science, Gwalior, Madhya Pradesh, India

Sushil Kamboj
Chandigarh Engineering College, Chandigarh Group of Colleges, Punjab, India

Saurabh Karling
Business Administration, Lovely Professional University, Punjab, India

Navneet Kaur
College of Engineering, Chandigarh Group of Colleges Landran, Mohali, Punjab, India

Sukhpreet Kaur
Chandigarh Engineering College, Chandigarh Group of Colleges, Punjab, India

Rajesh Kumar Kaushal
Chitkara University Institute of Engineering and Technology, Chitkara University, Punjab, India

P. Keerthika
School of Computer Science and Engineering, Vellore Institute of Technology, Vellore, Tamil Nadu, India

Shailesh Khaparkar
Gyan Ganga Institute of Technology & Sciences, Jabalpur, M.P., India

Shiraz Khurana
Department of Computer Science & Engineering, Sharda University, Uttar Pradesh, India

Harish Kumar
Chitkara University Institute of Engineering and Technology, Chitkara University, Punjab, India

Mukesh Kumar
Department of Mechanical Engineering, School of Technology, Quantum University, Roorkee, India

Naveen Kumar
Chitkara University Institute of Engineering and Technology, Chitkara University, Punjab, India

Santosh Kumar
Department of Mechanical Engineering, Chandigarh Group of Colleges, Landran, Mohali, Punjab

Saxena Sachin Kumar
Invertis University, Bareilly, Uttar Pradesh, India

Mohit Lalit
Department of Computer Science and Engineering, Chandigarh University, Mohali, Punjab, India

Ratnesh Litoriya
Medi-Caps University, Indore, India

Praveen Kumar Malik
School of Electronics and Electrical Engineering, Lovely Professional University, Phagwara, Punjab, India

Maad M. Mijwil
Computer Techniques Engineering Department, Baghdad College of Economic Sciences University, Baghdad, Iraq

Rahul Reddy Nadikattu
University of the Cumberlands, Williamsburg, Kentucky, USA

Nitin S. Nagori
Department of Electronics and Telecommunication, K. J. Somaiya College of Engineering, Somaiya Vidyavihar University, Mumbai 400071, India

Ameya K. Naik
Department of Electronics and Telecommunication, K. J. Somaiya College of Engineering, Somaiya Vidyavihar University, Mumbai 400071, India

Shrivastava Jitendra Nath
Invertis University, Bareilly, Uttar Pradesh, India

Neeta Nathani
Gyan Ganga Institute of Technology & Sciences, Jabalpur, India

Abhimanyu Singh Negi
Galgotias College of Engineering and Technology, Greater Noida, India

Kuldeep Pal
Department of Computer Application, School of Technology, Quantum University, Roorkee, India

Ravi Prakash
K.C. College of Engineering & Management Studies and Research, Mumbai Maharashtra, India

S. J. Suji Prasad
Department of EIE, Kongu Engineering College, Perundurai, Tamilnadu, India

Pushpendra K Rajput
UPES University, Dehradun, Uttarakhand, India

M. Sangeetha
Department of IT, NGP Institute of Technology, Coimbatore, Tamilnadu, India

Tanushree Sanwal
KIET Group of Institutions, Delhi-NCR, Ghaziabad, India

Ankita Sharma
KIET Group of Institutions, Ghaziabad, India

Balraj Singh
School of Computer Science and Engineering, Lovely Professional University, Phagwara, Punjab, India

Inderpal Singh
School of Computer Science and Engineering, Lovely Professional University, Phagwara, Punjab, India

Shikha Singh
Computer Science and Engineering, Galgotias College of Engineering and Technology, Greater Noid, India

Surender Singh
Head Career Program, Code Quotient Pvt. Ltd. Mohali, Punjab

Rashi Srivastava
Department of Computer Science and Engineering, Galgotias College of Engineering and Technology, Greater Noida, India

Surbhi
Computer Science and Engineering Department, Lovely Professional University, Punjab, India

P. Suresh
School of Computer Science and Engineering, Vellore Institute of Technology, Vellore, Tamil Nadu, India

Meenakshi Tyagi
KIET Group of Institutions, Ghaziabad, India

Shobha Tyagi
K.C. College of Engineering & Management Studies and Research, Mumbai Maharashtra, India

Pawan Whig
Vivekananda Institute of Professional Studies, New Delhi, India

Sapna Yadav
Jaypee Institute of Information Technology, Noida, Uttar Pradesh, India

Chapter 1

Lung Disease Diagnosis Using Machine Learning from a Bibliometric Perspective

Anupam Bonkra, Pummy Dhiman, Sushil Kamboj, and Sukhpreet Kaur

1.1 INTRODUCTION

The wide spectrum of illnesses that affect the lungs and the airways leading to the lungs are referred to as lung diseases [1]. Some common types of lung disease include:

- Asthma: a chronic disease that causes airway inflammation and constriction, which can make breathing challenging and result in coughing and wheezing [2].
- Chronic obstructive pulmonary disease (COPD): a progressive ailment that makes it thorny to breathe, including emphysema and chronic bronchitis [2].
- Pneumonia: an infection of the lungs that causes inflammation and fluid build-up in the air sacs, which can lead to difficulty breathing, chest pain, and fever [3].
- Tuberculosis (TB): a bacterial infection that mostly affects the lungs and can cause chest pain, coughing, and breathing difficulties [4].
- Lung cancer: the uncontrolled escalation of abnormal cells inside the lungs, which can lead to difficulty breathing, chest pain, and coughing up blood [5].
- Pulmonary fibrosis: a syndrome in which the lungs develop scar tissue, which can cause breathing issues and decreased lung function [6].
- Pulmonary embolism: a blockage in one of the lung's blood vessels caused by a blood clot [7].

The symptoms, causes, and treatments for lung diseases vary depending on the specific condition. Many lung diseases can be prevented or managed with lifestyle changes, such as quitting smoking, avoiding exposure to pollution, and getting vaccinated against certain infections. Some lung diseases can be treated with medication, while others may require surgery or other forms of treatment.

Lung illness can be prevented or stopped in its tracks with early detection and treatment, which will enhance your quality of life and increase your

DOI: 10.1201/9781003466949-1

longevity. The SARS-CoV-2 disease that causes COVID-19 [4] predominantly damages the lungs, leaving some patients with serious lung damage. Alveoli, the microscopic air vesicles in the lungs where both carbon dioxide and oxygen are exchanged, are defined by the disease's swelling and damage. In severe circumstances, this may result in acute respiratory distress syndrome, decreased blood oxygen levels, and breathing difficulties (ARDS). Additional lung-related problems can arise in COVID-19 patients.

It's also critical to keep in mind that some COVID-19 survivors may still suffer long-term lung problems known as post-acute sequelae of SARS-CoV-2 infection (PASC) or "long COVID" [3]. Overall, the COVID-19 pandemic has highlighted the huge impact that lung disease may have on people and communities as well as the significance of continued research to enhance lung disease diagnosis, treatment, and management. Machine learning can be used to diagnose lung diseases by analyzing various types of medical data, for example, chest X-rays [8], computed tomography (CT) scans [4], and pulmonary function tests. Deep learning [5, 9, 10, 11], a popular strategy, is a subset of machine learning to facilitate its pedestal on neural networks. In this approach, a large dataset of lung images is used to train a deep learning model to recognize patterns in the images [12] that are characteristic of specific lung diseases. The model can then be used to classify new images as normal or abnormal and even diagnose the specific disease. Another approach is using a combination of various medical data such as clinical reports, lab results, and imaging data to train a machine learning model. These models are known as multimodal [13] models, which help to perk up the accuracy of the diagnosis. There are several studies that have shown that machine learning can improve the accuracy of lung disease diagnosis compared to traditional methods. However, it is important to note that machine learning models need to be trained and validated on large and diverse datasets to ensure their performance and also should be used in conjunction with other diagnostic methods for better results [14].

The structure of this study is as follows: Following the introduction, a discussion of previous research is presented. In the next section, objectives are defined. Afterwards, the study's methodology is defined and the results are discussed. The last section presents the conclusion of our work.

1.2 LITERATURE REVIEW

A particularly severe and elusive form of cancer is lung cancer. It generally results in mortality for both genders, thus it is more important to take care and promptly and accurately inspect nodules. To recognize lung cancer in its early stages, many procedures have been put into practice [6]. The leading cause of disease-related death worldwide, cancer, is estimated to account for 13.9 million cases and 8.29 million fatalities due to early-stage diagnosis [11]. In the United States, there were 1,682,210 new cases and

595,690 fatalities from cancer in 2018; in 2016, 158,080 people died from lung cancer, and there were 224,391 new cases of the disease. Lung cancer is the most lethal of all malignancies [5]. The survival rate for lung cancer cells is much lower than that of other cancer cells as a result of the impact of lung cancer cells or due to the absence of recognition of lung cancer cells at the very early stage. A datasheet from the American Cancer Society, American Lung Association, and World Health Organization states that the endurance rate has grown from 17.7% to 54.4% when cancer cells are detected at the onset and also if they are limited, in which case the percentage is closer to 16% [1, 7].

The ability to capture oxygen is decreased by lung disorders that hinder the lungs from working normally. Viruses, bacteria, and fungi are frequently the causes of lung illnesses [15]. In some cases, other reasons include genetic abnormalities and exposure to harmful, deadly substances. Sneezing and coughing are rarely methods of spreading lung illnesses to other people. The patient recovers more rapidly and there is less chance of infection spreading throughout the body and to those around them when infections are detected early. One of the best and most reliable ways to detect lung disease is now possible with computer-assisted diagnostics, which can evaluate chest X-rays, CT scans, and other medical images [4]. Convolutional neural networks (CNNs) [16] are precise and efficient solutions for computer-assisted diagnostics. To recognize and decipher patterns in pixel images, it is a form of artificial neural network that makes use of deep learning. It is essential to provide accurate results in order to better serve medical staff and professionals.

Asthma, COPD, infections like tuberculosis, influenza, lung cancer [7], pneumonia, and other breathing problems are just a few of the conditions that fall under the umbrella term "lung disease," which also encompasses many other conditions that affect the lungs. The indications and symptoms of various lung diseases can differ. Common symptoms include a persistent cough, coughing up blood or mucus, having trouble breathing in or out, feeling as though you aren't getting enough air, being less able to exercise, and experiencing pain or discomfort [6]. An environment for data access, analysis, processing, revelation, and algorithm development is needed for the analysis and processing of medical images. Medical imaging is the method and technique for producing images of the human body for use in diagnosis, analysis, and other areas of medical science (such as the study of disease in the context of normal anatomy and physiology). Clinical diagnosis has increasingly used medical CT imaging in recent years [4]. It helps doctors find pathogenic alterations more precisely by assisting in their detection. The various gray levels in computed tomography pictures allow for the differentiation of various tissues [17]. Radiologists can make better decisions thanks to the growing usage of artificial intelligence (AI), the Internet of Things (IoT) [18], and cloud computing in the healthcare industry. Figure 1.1 illustrates the healthy human lung.

Infections, occupational exposures, drugs, and a variety of conditions can all contribute to lung ailments. A number of lung disorders are frequently detected and diagnosed using CT and X-ray chest radiography, two popular anatomic imaging modalities. The diagnosis, treatment, surgery, medical reference, and training of patients all depend heavily on medical imagery. The Digital Imaging and Communications in Medicine (DICOM) standard [19] permits the storage of metadata—textual descriptions—alongside the images. It was the most significant development since the invention of X-rays, and CT has been a pillar of diagnostic radiology ever since [20]. Figure 1.2 shows the categorization of lung diseases using CT scan.

A recent study found that it had an impact on a bigger human population regardless of race or gender. It is a common viral condition brought on by the coronavirus-2 associated with severe acute respiratory syndrome (SARS-CoV-2). The COVID-19 infection harms the respiratory system by resulting in life-threatening pneumonia. The World Health Organization has declared it a pandemic due to the disease's severity and rate of spread. Despite the introduction of several controlling and therapeutic measures since December 2019 [3], the fatality rate associated with COVID-19 infection is rapidly increasing.

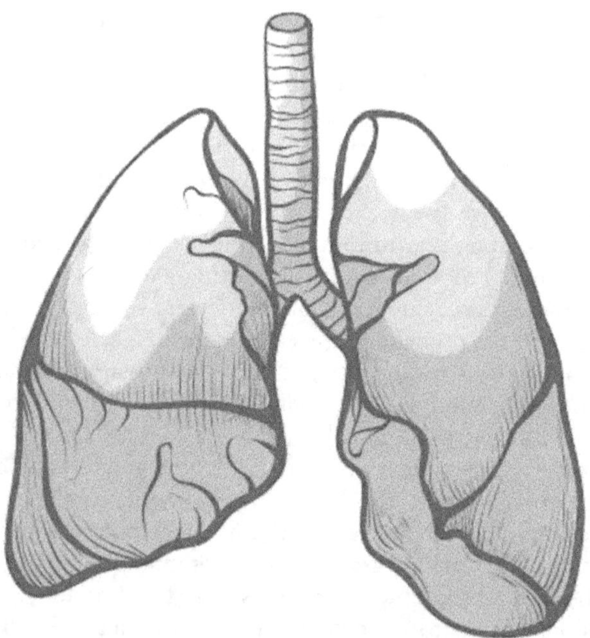

Figure 1.1 Healthy human lung

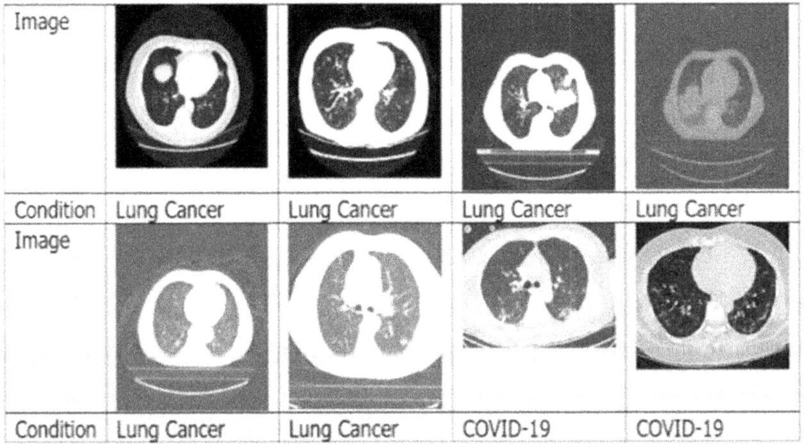

Figure 1.2 Categorization of lung diseases using CT scan

1.3 OBJECTIVE

The following sections present the methodology of the study, and the findings are then discussed. The summary of our effort is given in the final section.

- Growth of the publications and average citations
- Document-wise distribution of publications
- Source impact, author impact
- Most cited countries
- Frequently occurred keywords

1.4 RESEARCH METHODOLOGY

This work makes use of bibliometric analysis. The quantitative method of bibliometric analysis is used to look at bibliographic data [21]. Examples of this approach are science mapping and performance analysis. A piece of software is also utilized to support the bibliometrics analysis [22]. This study examines the sources of publications, the impact factors from both journals and documents, and the most often occurring words in documents. Figure 1.3 displays the procedures used in this study. The Scopus database [23] search was used to locate the data sources. After being retrieved from Scopus, the datasheet was imported into an R data format. After that, Biblioshiny [24] was used to analyze the data, and VOSviewer [25] to visualize the bibliometric networks. The Biblioshiny Bibliometrix tool is

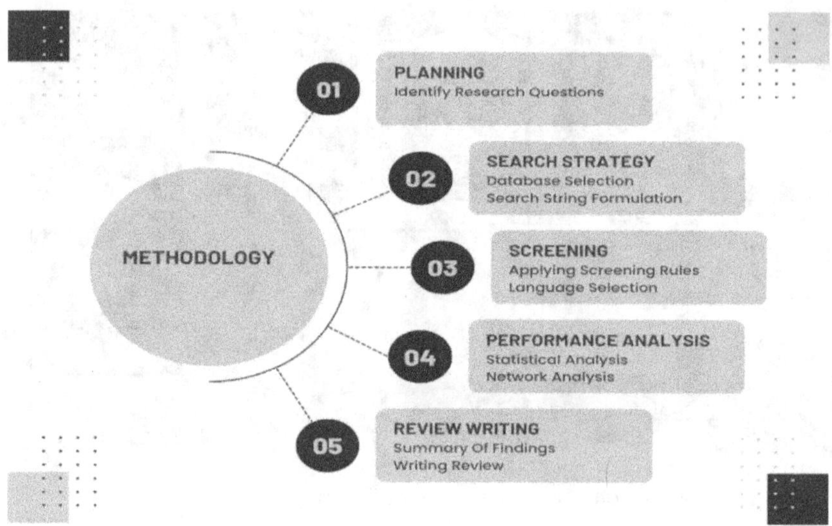

Figure 1.3 Methodology

a component of the R package. In the end, an analysis and judgments are made regarding the results of the software processing.

1.4.1 Data Collection

The most important step when writing a research paper or carrying out any type of research is to review previous literature and research results. A bibliometric study has been chosen for this study. The quantity of academic and scientific books is the focus when analyzing academic literature. As a result, academic research databases are important since they employ reliable sources. A few examples of academic databases are Scopus, Web of Science [26], and PubMed [27]. This investigation made use of Scopus, an Elsevier-owned database that was released in 2004. The largest abstract and citation database as well as one that ranks journals and authors, Scopus is a multidisciplinary database. The database can only be fully accessed with a membership, but it does provide some services for free. For the years 2020 through 2022, data for this study was retrieved from the Scopus repository.

1.4.2 Search Strategy

A search string made up of keywords was created, and the Scopus database was then searched. The search was carried out in the article title, abstract, and keywords by using the Boolean AND operator as demonstrated in the following example:

The search query used for this study is "lung infection" AND "automated diagnosis" AND "machine learning" AND (EXCLUDE (PUBYEAR, 2023)).

After receiving the results, refining was carried out, and some data was exported for examination.

1.4.3 Screening

Using the aforementioned search terms, the quantity of publications received was forwarded for screening. The following list of criteria describes how the articles for this study were bound. There are no limits based on nationality, language, etc. Every publication includes information such as the author, the nation, citations, papers, references, etc.

1.4.4 Performance Scrutiny

Bibliometric analysis [22] is an effective technique for determining how publications affect the scientific community. It is a statistical evaluation of written works, including books, papers, or book chapters, found in accepted scientific publications. This work follows a scientific computer-assisted review technique, therefore certain specialized software has been used to aid in the process [28]. Biblioshiny, the shiny program for Bibliometrix, and VOSviewer (version 1.6.18) were utilized to examine the output csv file from the Scopus database and identify the most significant works, authors, and connections between them.

1.5 RESULTS

1.5.1 Main Information

1.5.1.1 Average Citation per Year

The publication output of our search regarding "Machine Learning for Lung Disease Detection" covered the last three years (Table 1.1). The first publication as per our searched keywords appeared in 2020 and then increased with an increasing rate. Figure 1.4 shows the data overview used

Table 1.1 Average Citations per Year

Year	*Mean TC per Article*	*N*	*Mean TC per Year*	*Citable Years*
2020	26.33	3	6.58	4
2021	18.83	23	6.28	3
2022	2.61	38	1.30	2

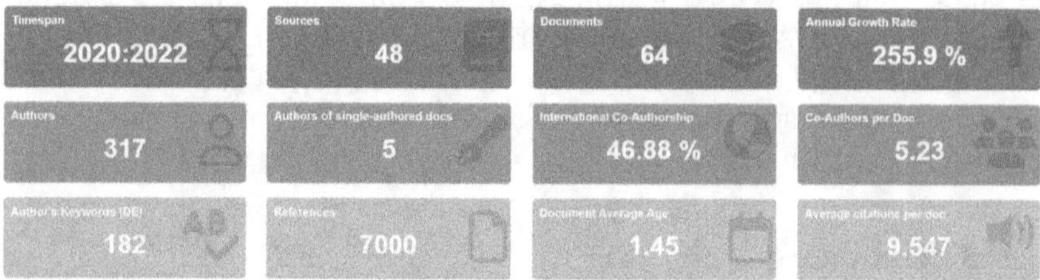

Figure 1.4 Data overview

in this work. The most publications (38) were published in 2022, which was also the highest number ever.

1.5.1.2 Three-Field Plot

The flow of values from one set to another is depicted via Sankey diagrams, a particular sort of visualization [24]. Nodes and links are the terms used to describe the connected objects and relationships, respectively. Every node is represented by a rectangle, and the size of these nodes indicates how frequently the objects they represent occur. The relationship is shown in Figure 1.5 along with the authors' names and keywords in the middle and right fields, respectively, between author, country, and keywords. We have author–country for this graphic. It showed which authors are publishing most on which topic from which countries. From India, S. Agarwal worked mostly using keywords like COVID-19, deep learning, CT scan, and segmentation. Many authors worked using COVID-19 and deep learning. X.

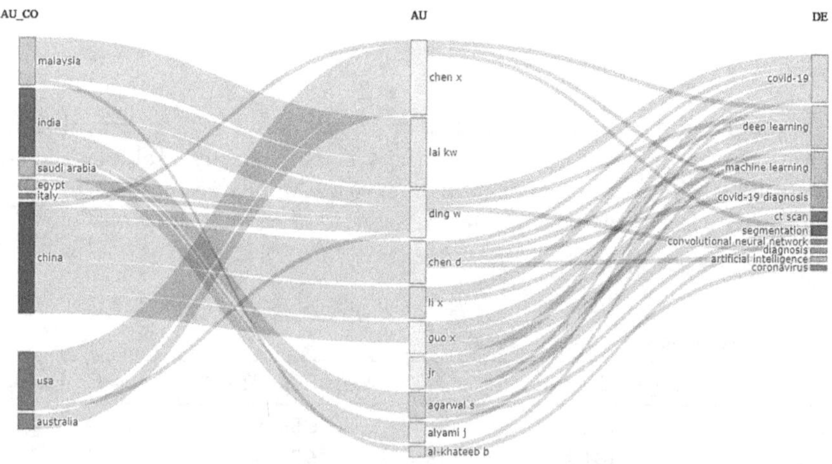

Figure 1.5 Three-field plot

Chen from the USA worked on COVID-19 diagnosis using deep learning (Figure 1.5).

1.5.2 Source Impact

The top ten journals that professionals in the field of lung infection diagnosis favor are listed in Table 1.2. Researchers worldwide rated Elsevier's *Computers in Biology and Medicine* as their top choice for journals. In this journal, four papers with g-indexes were published. With 105 total citations (TC), the Springer Nature publication *Chaos, Solitons & Fractals* was discovered to be one of the most highly cited journals within the stated time.

1.5.2.1 Author's Document Production over Time

Table 1.3 lists the articles that the writers published along with the overall number of citations. To determine the significance of a publication or author, citation analysis counts the instances in which an article is referenced in other writings. Even still, the more citations older papers gain, the better. Citations also show how well the published work was executed.

1.5.2.2 Bradford's Law

Bradford's law is a principle that describes the allotment of articles within a set of journals or a collection of books. The law states that a small number of journals or books will contain a large proportion of the articles or works,

Table 1.2 Source Impact

Source	*h_index*	*g_index*	*m_index*	*TC*	*NP*	*PY_Start*
Computers in Biology and Medicine	3	4	1	24	4	2021
Chaos, Solitons & Fractals	2	2	0.667	105	2	2021
CMES – Computer Modeling in Engineering and Sciences	2	2	0.667	10	2	2021
Computational Intelligence and Neuroscience	2	2	0.667	13	2	2021
2021 1st International Conference on Artificial Intelligence and Data Analytics (CAIDA)	1	1	0.333	10	1	2021
ACM International Conference Proceeding Series	1	1	0.25	3	2	2020
Applied Sciences (Switzerland)	1	1	0.5	1	1	2022
Applied Soft Computing	1	2	0.5	4	2	2022
Archives of Computational Methods in Engineering	1	2	0.5	5	2	2022
Bio Integration	1	1	0:25	11	1	2020

Table 1.3 Author Production over Time

Author	*Year*	*Article Title*	*Source*	*DOI*	*TC*
Agarwal, S.	2022	CHS-NET: A Deep Learning Approach for Hierarchical Segmentation of COVID-19 via CT Images	*Neural Processing Letters*	10.1007/s11063-022-10785-x	3
Agarwal, S.	2022	Modality Specific U-NET Variants for Biomedical Image Segmentation: A Survey	*Artificial Intelligence Review*	10.1007/s10462-022-10152-1	12
Li, X.	2022	Explainable Multi-Instance and Multi-Task Learning for COVID-19 Diagnosis and Lesion Segmentation in CT Images	*Knowledge-Based Systems*	10.1016/j_knosys.2022.109278	0
Chen, X.	2022	Recent Advances and Clinical Applications of Deep Learning in Medical Image Analysis	*Medical Image Analysis*	10.1016/j-.media.2022.102444	29
Chen, D.	2022	Let AI Perform Better Next Time—A Systematic Review of Medical Imaging-Based Automated Diagnosis of COVID-19: 2020-2022	*Applied Sciences (Switzerland)*	10.3390/app12083895	1
Al-Khateeb, B.	2022	An Extensive Review of State-of-the-Art Transfer Learning Techniques Used in Medical Imaging: Open Issues and Challenges	*Journal of Intelligent Systems*	10.1515/jisys-2022-0198	1
Al-Khateeb, B.	2022	Novel Crow Swarm Optimization Algorithm and Selection Approach for Optimal Deep Learning COVID-19 Diagnostic Model	*Computational Intelligence and Neuroscience*	10.1155/2022/1307944	5
Alyami, J.	2022	Computer Vision-Based Prognostic Modelling Of COVID-19 from Medical Imaging	*Studies in Big Data*	10.1007/978-981-19-2057-8 2	0
Alyami, J.	2022	Deep Learning-Based Lung Infection Detection Using Radiology Modalities and Comparisons on Benchmark Datasets in COVID-19 Pandemic	*Studies in Big Data*	10.1007/978-981-19-2057-8 18	0
Lai, K.W.	2022	Radiological Analysis of COVID-19 Using Computational Intelligence: A Broad Gauge Study	*Journal of Health Care Engineering*	10.1155/2022/5998042	2

(Continued)

Table 1.3 (Continued) Author Production over Time

Author	*Year*	*Article Title*	*Source*	*DOI*	*TC*
Guo, X.	2022	A Survey on Machine Learning in COVID-19 Diagnosis	*CMES – Computer Modeling in Engineering and Sciences*	10.32604/cmes.2022.017679	7
Ding, W.	2021	RCTE: A Reliable and Consistent Temporal-Ensembling Framework For Semi-Supervised Segmentation of COVID-19 Lesions	*Information Sciences*	10.1016/j.ins.2021.07.059	3
Ding, W.	2021	Fusion of Intelligent Learning for COVID-19: A State-of-the-Art Review and Analysis on Real Medical Data	*Neurocomputing*	10.1016/j.neucom.2021.06.024	6
Li, X.	2021	AI-Empowered Computational Examination of Chest Imaging for COVID-19 Treatment: A Review	*Frontiers in Artificial Intelligence*	10.3389/frai.2021.612914	3
Chen, X.	2021	Momentum Contrastive Learning for Few-Shot COVID-19 Diagnosis from Chest CT Images	*Pattern Recognition*	10.1016/}.patcog.2021.107826	53
Lai, K.W.	2021	An Overview of Deep Learning Techniques on Chest X-Ray and CT Scan Identification of COVID-19	*Computational and Mathematical Methods in Medicine*	10.1155/2021/5528144	16
Chen, D.	2020	A Review of Automated Diagnosis of COVID-19 Based on Scanning Images	*ACM International*	10.1145/3449301.3449778	3

while a large number of journals or books will contain a small proportion of the articles or works. This principle is often used in library science and information science to help organize and categorize large collections of materials. In bibliometrics, it's used to analyze the productivity of journals, authors, and research fields. Biblioshiny generates a per-zone publication distribution by applying Bradford's law, as seen in Figure 1.6. According to Table 1.4, Zone 1 included 10 sources, Zone 2 contained 17, and Zone 3 contained 21 sources. The division of the available information into three zones demonstrates the clustering of the sources, with Zone 1's resources serving as the main sources for information on machine learning–based themes for lung disease diagnosis.

1.5.3 Author's Impact

1.5.3.1 Author's Document Publication in 2022

The author's document publication refers to the specific papers, articles, or other scholarly works that an author has published. Table 1.5 shows the article title, source, DOI, total citations received by that article, and total citations per year. X. Chen received the highest number of citations (29) for his article "Recent Advances and Clinical Applications of Deep Learning in Medical Image Analysis."

1.5.3.2 Most Relevant Affiliation

In a bibliometric study, the most relevant affiliation is the institution or organization that a researcher is associated with when they publish a paper

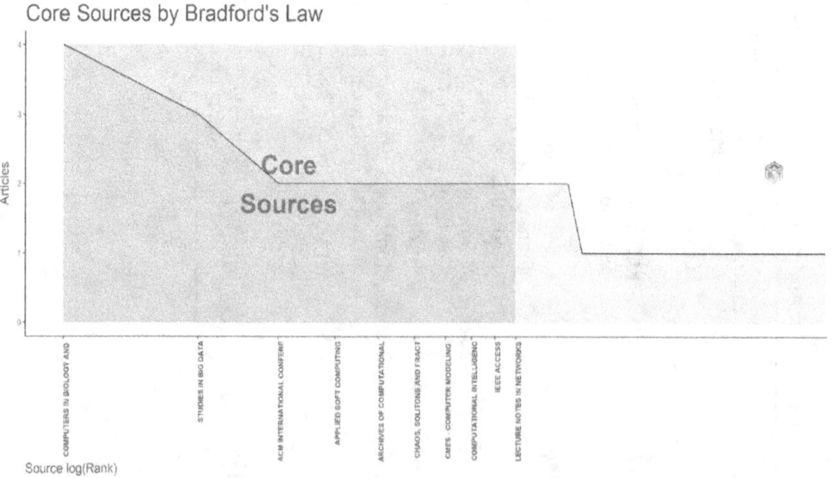

Figure 1.6 Bradford's law

Table 1.4 Tabular Presentation of Bradford's Law

Source Rank	*Freq*	*cumFreq*	*Zone (Source Rank)*	*Zone*	*Source Rank*	*Freq*	*cumFreq*	*Zone (Source Rank)*	*Zone*
Computer in Biology and Medicine	1	4	4	Zone 1	*Diagnostics*	25	1	41	Zone 2
Studies in Big Data	2	3	7	Zone 1	*Intelligence*	26	1	42	Zone 2
ACM International Conference Proceeding Series	3	2	9	Zone 1	*Frontiers In Bioscience-Landmark*	27	1	43	Zone 2
Applied Soft Computing	4	2	11	Zone 1	*Frontiers in Public Health*	28	1	44	Zone 3
Archives of Computational Methods in Engineering	5	2	13	Zone 1	*Information Sciences*	29	1	45	Zone 3
Chaos, Solitons & Fractals	6	2	15	Zone 1	*Intelligent Decision Technologies*	30	1	46	Zone 3
CMES – Computer Modeling in Engineering and Sciences	7	2	17	Zone 1	*Interdisciplinary Sciences Journal—*	31	1	47	Zone 3
Computational Intelligence and Neuroscience	8	2	19	Zone 1	*International Journal of computer science*	32	1	48	Zone 3
IEEE Access	9	2	21	Zone 1	*International Journal of Imaging Systems and Technology*	33	1	49	Zone 3

(*Continued*)

Table 1.4 (Continued) Tabular Presentation of Bradford's Law

Source Rank	*Freq*	*cumFreq*	*Zone (Source Rank)*	*Zone*	*Source Rank*	*Freq*	*cumFreq*	*Zone (Source Rank)*	*Zone*
Lecture Notes in Networks and Systems	10	2	23	Zone 1	*International Series in science*	34	1	50	Zone 3
Physical and Engineering Sciences in Medicine	11	2	25	Zone 2	*IRBM*	35	1	51	Zone 3
Scientific Reports	12	2	27	Zone 2	*Journal of Healthcare Engineering*	36	1	52	Zone 3
Sensors	13	2	29	Zone 2	*Journal of Intelligent Systems*	37	1	53	Zone 3
2021 1st *International Conference on Artificial Intelligence and Data Analytics (CAIDA)*	14	1	30	Zone 2	*Journal of Physics: Conference Series*	38	1	54	Zone 3
2022 2nd *International Conference On Artificial Intelligence and Signal Processing* (AISP)	15	1	31	Zone 2	*Knowledge-Based Systems*	39	1	55	Zone 3

(Continued)

Table 1.4 (Continued) Tabular Presentation of Bradford's Law

Source Rank	*Freq*	*cumFreq*	*Zone (Source Rank)*	*Zone*	*Source Rank*	*Freq*	*cumFreq*	*Zone (Source Rank)*	*Zone*
Applied Sciences (Switzerland)	16	1	32	Zone 2	*Mathematics*	40	1	56	Zone 3
Artificial Intelligence Review	17	1	33	Zone 2	*Medical Image Analysis*	41	1	57	Zone 3
Bio Integration	18	1	34	Zone 2	*Neural Processing Letters*	42	1	58	Zone 3
Cognitive Computation	19	1	35	Zone 2	*Neurocomputing*	43	1	59	Zone 3
Complex and Intelligent Systems	20	1	36	Zone 2	*Pattern Recognition*	44	1	60	Zone 3
Computational and Mathematical	21	1	37	Zone 2	*Radiology: Artificial Intelligence*	45	1	61	Zone 3
Computerized Medical Imaging and Graphics	22	1	38	Zone 2	*SN Computer Science*	46	1	62	Zone 3
Computers, Materials and Continua	23	1	39	Zone 2	*Soft Computing*	47	1	63	Zone 3
Current Medical Imaging	24	4	40	Zone 2	*Traitement du Signal*	48	1	64	Zone 3

Table 1.5 Author Publications in 2022

Author	*Year*	*Title*	*Source*	*DOI*	*TC*	*TCpY*
Chen, X.	2022	Recent Advances and Clinical Applications of Deep Learning in Medical Image Analysis	*Medical Image Analysis*	10.1016/j.media.2022.102444	29	14.5
Agarwal, S.	2022	Modality Specific U-Net Variants for Biomedical Image Segmentation: A Survey	*Artificial Intelligence Review*	10.1007/s10462-022-10152-1	12	6
Al-Khateeb, B.	2022	Novel Crow Swarm Optimization Algorithm and Selection Approach for Optimal Deep Learning Covid-19 Diagnostic Model	*Computational Intelligence and Neuroscience*	10.1155/2022/1307944	5	2.5
Agarwal, S.	2022	CHS-NET: A Deep Learning Approach for Hierarchical Segmentation of Covid-19 via CT Images	*Neural Processing Letters*	10.1007/s11063-022-10785-x	3	1.5
Chen, D.	2022	Let AI Perform Better Next Time—A Systematic Review of Medical Imaging-Based Automated Diagnosis of Covid-19: 2020–2022	*Applied Science (Switzerland)*	10.3390/app12083895	1	0.5
Al-Khateeb, B.	2022	An Extensive Review of State-of-the-Art Transfer Learning Techniques Used in Medical Imaging: Open Issues and Challenges	*Journal of Intelligent Systems*	10.1515/jisys-2022-0198	1	0.5
JR	2022	Covid-19 Detection on Chest X-Ray and CT scan: A Review of the Top-100 Most Cited Papers	*Sensors*	10.3390/s22197303	0	0
Li, X.	2022	Explainable Multi-Instance and Multi-task Learning for COVID-19 Diagnosis and Lesion Segmentation in CT Images	*Knowledge-Based Systems*	10.1016/j.knosys.2022.109278	0	0
Alyami, J.	2022	Computer Vision-Based Prognostic Modelling of COVID-19 from Medical Imaging	*Studies in Big Data*	10.1007/978-981-19-2057-8	0	0

or other scholarly work. This can be their place of employment, the organization that funded their research, or any other group with which they have a professional association. In this study, Ahsanullah University of Science and Technology, Hohai University, and the University of Malaya had nine publications each (Table 1.6).

Figure 1.7 shows the most cited countries in lung disease diagnosis using machine learning during the reported period. India is a developing country but still ranked second in highly cited countries after Canada having 119 citations. Among Asian countries, India secured the top position.

1.5.4 Keyword Network Visualization

Network visualization is the process of creating graphical representations of network data. These visualizations can aid in finding patterns, trends, and connections within the data that might not be immediately obvious from the raw data alone.

Common techniques include node-link diagrams, adjacency matrices, and force-directed layouts. Popular tools for creating network visualizations include Gephi [21], Cytoscape, and NodeXL. A network analysis of keyword co-occurrences, which examines the connections between keywords [29], is a method for mapping the study domain in a certain topic. The term "keywords" refers to a group of words used in computerized databases to enable correct indexing and to maximize the sourcing of scientific papers. The intensity of the link between two keywords indicates how frequently one term and another term appear in an article together. The overall number of appearances in a document can be determined by counting all the links. In this study, we used the VOSviewer software, and we set six as the minimum occurrence of author keywords, which means that words

Table 1.6 Most Prominent Affiliations

Affiliation	*Articles*
Ahsanullah University of Science and Technology	9
Hohat University	9
University of Malaya	9
Dongguk University	8
Sun Yat-Sen University	8
Shenzhen Technology University	7
Geneva University Hospital	6
Islamic Azad University	6
University of Electronic Science and Technology of China	6
Commonwealth Scientific and Industrial Research Organisation	5
Harbin Institute of Technology	5
Humanitas Research Hospital	5

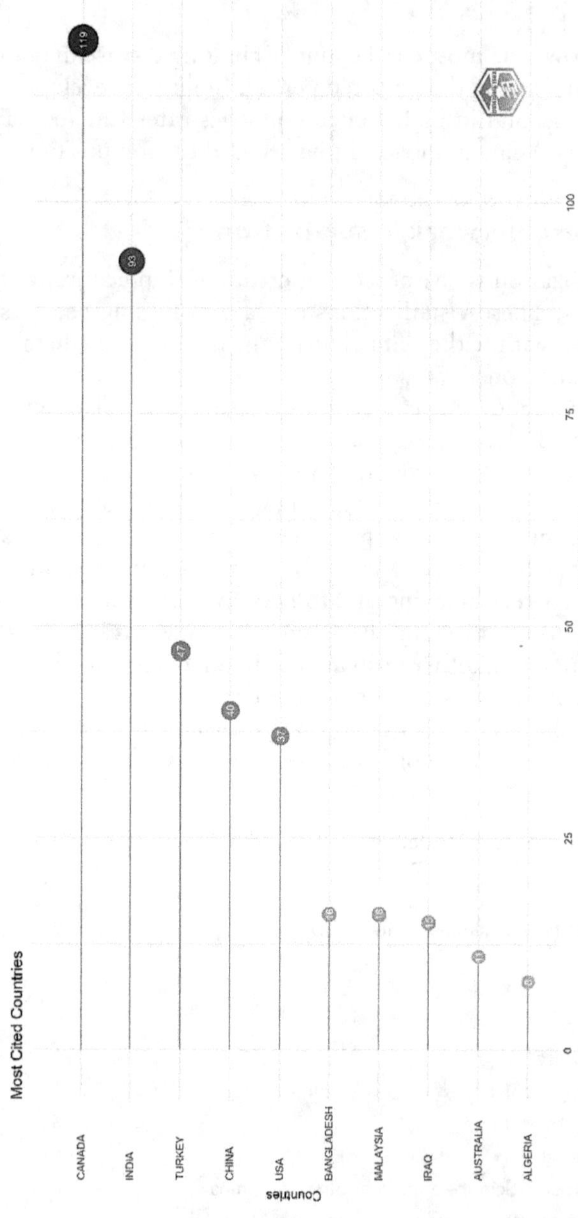

Figure 1.7 Most cited countries

must appear on the bibliometric map at least six times between them when they occur in the same document with each other.

Figure 1.8 shows the total 41 keywords from the title and abstract divided into four clusters—Red, Green, Blue, and Yellow—having 615 links and a total link strength of 1387. The red cluster (n = 17) includes deep learning used to diagnose lung infection. The blue cluster (n = 6) had the keywords automated diagnosis, chest, x-ray, rt pcr, world health organization. The green cluster (n = 13) shows the challenges in disease identification and the use of artificial intelligence to combat this issue. The yellow cluster (n = 4) shows the significance of CNN in lung infection disease.

1.5.4.1 Most Frequently Used Keywords

Table 1.7 shows the most frequent keyword used by the researchers in this study. Here we set the minimum occurrence to ten.

A word cloud is a graphical depiction of the frequency of terms in a particular text. It is also referred to as a tag cloud or text cloud [14]. The size of each word in the cloud is proportional to its frequency, and the cloud can be arranged in different ways, such as alphabetically or by frequency. Word clouds are often used to quickly identify the most important words in a text, such as the keywords in a research paper or the main topics of a news article. They can also be used to visualize the content of social media posts or the sentiment of customer reviews. Many online tools and software programs are available to create word clouds, including Wordle, Tagxedo, and

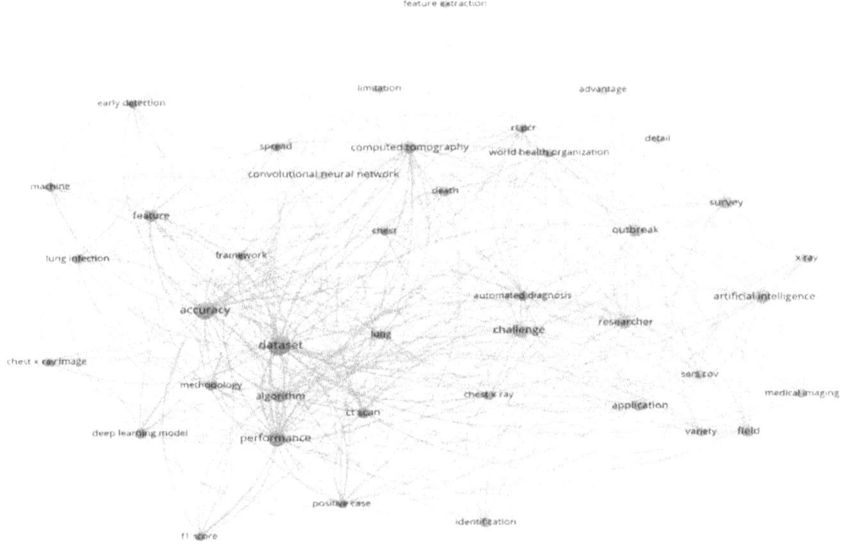

Figure 1.8 Keyword network visualization

Table 1.7 Top Ten Most Frequently Used Keywords

Keyword	*Occurrences*
Deep Learning	58
COVID-19	33
Computerized Tomography	26
Diagnosis	25
Human	23
Medical Imaging	22
Artificial Intelligence	21
Humans	20
Coronaviruses	17
Diagnostic Imaging	16

Word Cloud Generator. The word cloud in Figure 1.9 was produced using the Biblioshiny app of the Bibliometrix program. For the graphics parameters, author keywords were employed. Choosing author keywords has the major advantage of providing insight into significant topics and emerging research trends. Only 25 different keywords were permitted.

1.5.4.2 Bibliographic Coupling

If two works quote the same third work, they are said to be bibliographically connected. In other terms, bibliographic coupling refers to the similarity between two publications' reference lists. The stronger the relationship between two publications' bibliographies, the more references they have

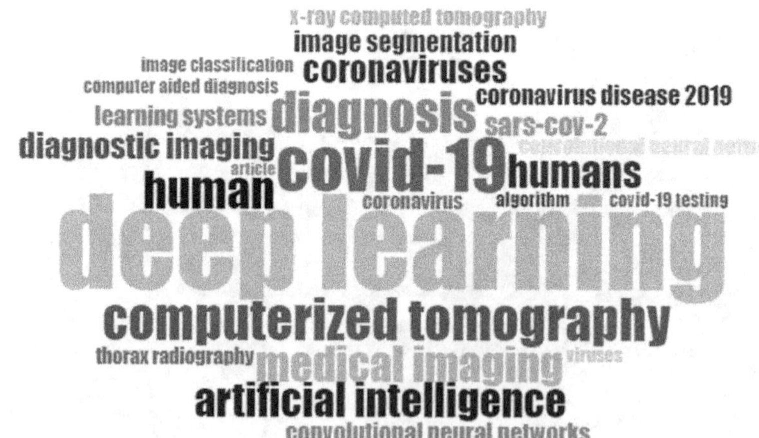

Figure 1.9 Keyword tag cloud

in common. Bibliographic coupling is a method used to analyze the relationship between scientific papers by looking at the references cited within the papers. Country-wise bibliographic coupling refers to the analysis of the relationship between scientific papers from different countries [24]. In this approach, the papers are categorized according to their countries of origin, and the connections between the publications are examined within each country group. This can be used to determine which nations are more productive in a particular area of research, which nations collaborate more frequently, and which nations' citizens are most frequently mentioned for their work. Researchers can better comprehend the global distribution of scientific research, international cooperation trends, and national research productivity by using this kind of study. To create maps of the country-level bibliographic coupling, a program called VOSviewer is employed.

In Figure 1.10, which shows country-by-country bibliographic coupling, the minimum number of documents per country and the minimum number of citations for a country were both set to three. Out of 39 countries, 12 satisfied this standard. The overall strength of the bibliographic coupling ties with the other nations will be computed for each of the 12 countries. The nations chosen will have the strongest overall linkage.

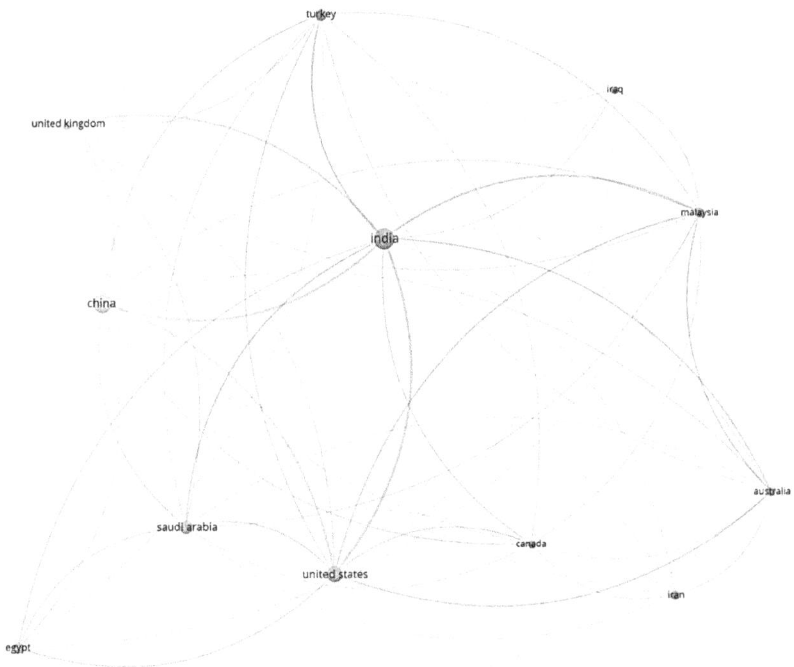

Figure 1.10 Country-wise bibliographic coupling

1.6 CONCLUSION

The research output on applying artificial intelligence to diagnose lung diseases from 2020 to 2022 was examined in the current study. The publications are seen to be steadily expanding. Journal papers were discovered to be the researchers' preferred format for publishing their research. In this study, Canada was revealed to be the most productive nation. India held the top spot among Asian nations. According to the overall number of citations, X. Chen and S. Agarwal are the authors of this subject who are the most pertinent. The journals *Computers in Biology and Medicine* and *Chaos Solitons & Fractals* are the most popular sources for publications, according to the bibliometric criteria of publications count, citations, and h-index. The COVID-19 virus, which is brought on by the SARS-CoV-2 virus, mostly damages the lungs, inflicting significant lung damage in certain individuals. The study's conclusions state that the terms now under investigation in this field include deep learning, COVID-19, computerized tomography, diagnosis, human, and medical imaging. It is difficult or impossible to describe how black box models came to a specific conclusion or prediction since they are thought to be opaque. By making models more transparent, interpretable, and therefore more reliable, XAI, or explainable artificial intelligence, seeks to overcome this problem. The idea is to raise the quality of publications in this sector by conducting more research on the application of XAI in lung disease detection.

REFERENCES

1. S. Mukherjee and S. U. Bohra, "Lung cancer disease diagnosis using machine learning approach," *Proceedings 3rd International Conference on Intelligent Sustainable Systems ICISS, 2020*, pp. 207–211, 2020, doi: 10.1109/ICISS49785.2020.9315909.
2. A. M. Antoniadi et al., "Current challenges and future opportunities for XAI in machine learning-based clinical decision support systems: A systematic review," *Appl. Sci.*, vol. 11, no. 11, pp. 1–23, 2021, doi: 10.3390/app11115088.
3. N. Heidari, M. Jafari Navimipour, M. Unal, S. Toumaj Unal, and S. Toumaj, "The COVID-19 epidemic analysis and diagnosis using deep learning: A systematic literature review and future directions," *Comput. Biol. Med.*, vol. 141, no. November 2021, p. 105141, 2022, doi: 10.1016/j.compbiomed.2021.105141.
4. D. N. Gumble and R. D. Ghongade, "Machine learning system to detect lung infection using CT scan," *IJSCE*, vol. 9, no. 6, pp. 394–401, 2021.
5. S. S. Raoof, M. A. Jabbar, and S. A. Fathima, "Lung cancer prediction using machine learning: A comprehensive approach," *2nd International Conference on Innovative Mechanisms for Industry Applications - Conference Proceedings*, pp. 108–115, 2020, doi: 10.1109/ICIMIA48430.2020.9074947.

6. S. Tripathi, S. Shetty, S. Jain, and V. Sharma, "Lung disease detection," no. 8, pp. 1–7, 2021, doi: 10.35940/ijitee.H9259.0610821.
7. B. Alsinglawi et al., "An explainable machine learning framework for lung cancer hospital length of stay prediction," *Sci. Rep.*, vol. 12, no. 1, pp. 1–10, 2022, doi: 10.1038/s41598-021-04608-7.
8. K. Prajapati, J. Patel, and K. Pathak, "Lung diseases using deep learning: A review paper," *Int. Res. J.*, pp. 1694–1699, 2018 [Online]. Available: https://www.academia.edu/download/58145940/IRJET-V5I12316.pdf.
9. A. Mathew, P. Amudha, and S. Sivakumari, "Deep learning techniques: An overview," *Adv. Intell. Syst. Comput.*, vol. 1141, no. January, pp. 599–608, 2021, doi: 10.1007/978-981-15-3383-9_54.
10. P. Dhiman, A. Kaur, and A. Bonkra, "Fake information detection using deep learning methods: A survey," *2023 International Conference, on Artificial Intelligence and Smart Communication (AISC)*, 2023, pp. 858–863, doi: 10.1109/AISC56616.2023.10085519.
11. S. Bharathy, R. Pavithra, and B. Akshaya, "Lung cancer detection using machine learning," *Proceedings – IEEE International Conference on Artificial Intelligence and Computer Applications ICAAIC 2022*, vol. 7, no. 01, pp. 539–543, 2022, doi: 10.1109/ICAAIC53929.2022.9793061.
12. A. Bonkra, A. Noonia, and A. Kaur, "Apple leaf diseases detection system: A review of the different segmentation and deep learning methods," *Artificial Intelligence and Data Science*, 2022, pp. 263–278.
13. A. Jangra, A. Jatowt, S. Saha, and M. Hasanuzzaman, "A survey on multimodal summarization," *J. ACM*, vol. 37, no. 4, 2021 [Online]. Available: http://arxiv.org/abs/2109.05199.
14. A. Bonkra, P. K. Bhatt J. Rosak Szyrocka, K. Mudul, L. Pilař, A. Kaur N. Chahal and A. K. Rana, "Apple leave disease detection using collaborative ML/DL and artificial intelligence methods: Scientometric analysis," *Int. J. Environ. Res. Public Health*, vol. 20, no. 4, p. 3222, 2023, doi: 10.3390/ijerph20043222.
15. J. Zhu, B. Shen, A. Abbasi, M. Hoshmand-Kochi, H. Li, and T. Q. Duong, "Deep transfer learning artificial intelligence accurately stages COVID-19 lung disease severity on portable chest radiographs," *PLOS One*, vol. 15, no. 7 July, pp. 1–11, 2020, doi: 10.1371/journal.pone.0236621.
16. L. Alzubaidi et al., "Review of deep learning: Concepts, CNN architectures, challenges, applications, future directions," *J. Big Data*, vol. 8, no. 1, December, 2021, doi: 10.1186/s40537-021-00444-8.
17. A. B. Salem Salamh, A. A. Salamah, and H. I. Akyüz, "A study of a new technique of the CT scan view and disease classification protocol based on level challenges in cases of coronavirus disease," *Radiol. Res. Pract.*, vol. 2021, p. 5554408, 2021, doi: 10.1155/2021/5554408.
18. A. Bonkra and P. Dhiman, "IoT security challenges in cloud environment," *Proceedings – 2021 2nd International Conference on Computational Methods in Science & Technology ICCMST 2021*, pp. 30–34, 2021, doi: 10.1109/ICCMST54943.2021.00018.

19. C.-C. Lai, T.-P. Shih, W.-C. Ko, H.-J. Tang, and P.-R. Hsueh, "Severe acute respiratory syndrome coronavirus 2 (SARS-CoV-2) and coronavirus disease-2019 (COVID-19): The epidemic and the challenges," *Int. J. Antimicrob. Agents*, vol. 55, no. 3, p. 105924, March 2020, doi: 10.1016/j.ijantimicag.2020.105924.
20. Z. T. Al-Sharify, T. A. Al-Sharify, N. T. Al-Sharify, and H. Y. Naser, "A critical review on medical imaging techniques (CT and PET scans) in the medical field," *IOP Conf. Ser. Mater. Sci. Eng.*, vol. 870, no. 1, 2020, doi: 10.1088/1757-899X/870/1/012043.
21. V. Osinska and R. Klimas, "Mapping science: Tools for bibliometric and altmetric studies," *Inf. Res. Int. Electron. J.*, vol. 26, no. 4, pp. 1–18, 2021, doi: 10.47989/irpaper909.
22. M. Aria and C. Cuccurullo, "Bibliometrix: An R-tool for comprehensive science mapping analysis," *J. Informetr.*, vol. 11, no. 4, pp. 959–975, November 2017, doi: 10.1016/j.joi.2017.08.007.
23. A. R. Michiel Schotten, M. Aisati, W. J. N. Meester, and S. Steiginga, "A brief history of Scopus: The world's largest abstract and citation database of scientific literature," *Research Analytics*, 1st ed., F. J. Cantu-Ortiz, Ed. New York: Auerbach Publications, 2017, p. 28, doi: 10.1201/9781315155890.
24. P. Dhiman, A. Kaur, C. Iwendi, and S. K. Mohan, "A scientometric analysis of deep learning approaches for detecting fake news," *Electronics*, vol. 12, no. 4, 2023, doi: 10.3390/electronics12040948.
25. N. J. van Eck and L. Waltman, "Software survey: VOSviewer, a computer program for bibliometric mapping," *Scientometrics*, vol. 84, no. 2, pp. 523–538, 2010, doi: 10.1007/s11192-009-0146-3.
26. R. Pranckutė, "Web of Science (WoS) and Scopus: The titans of bibliographic information in today's academic world," *Publications*, vol. 9, no. 1, 2021, doi: 10.3390/publications9010012.
27. S. A. S. Alryalat, L. W. Malkawi, and S. M. Momani, "Comparing bibliometric analysis using PubMed, Scopus, and web of science databases," *J. Vis. Exp.*, vol. 2019, no. 152, 2019, doi: 10.3791/58494.
28. F. Fusco, M. Marsilio, and C. Guglielmetti, "Co-production in health policy and management: A comprehensive bibliometric review," *BMC Health Serv. Res.*, vol. 20, no. 1, pp. 1–17, 2020, doi: 10.1186/s12913-020-05241-2.
29. A. Bonkra, P. K. Bhatt, A. Kaur, and S. Kamboj, "Scientific landscape and the road ahead for deep learning: Apple leaves disease detection," *2023 International Conference on Artificial Intelligence and Smart Communication (AISC)*, 2023, pp. 869–873, doi: 10.1109/AISC56616.2023.10085221.

Chapter 2

Industry 4.0 in Manufacturing, Communication, Transportation, and Healthcare

Kiran Ahuja, Indu Bala, and Maad M. Mijwi

2.1 INTRODUCTION

Industry 4.0, also known as the Fourth Industrial Revolution, represents a transformative era characterized by the convergence of advanced technologies, connectivity, and data-driven innovation across various industries. This revolution is reshaping traditional manufacturing, communication, transportation, and healthcare sectors, ushering in a new era of automation, digitization, and interconnectedness [1–2].

In the manufacturing sector, Industry 4.0 encompasses the integration of technologies such as the Internet of Things (IoT), artificial intelligence (AI), robotics, and big data analytics. These technologies enable the creation of smart factories that leverage real time data, seamless communication between machines, and autonomous systems to optimize production processes, improve efficiency, and reduce costs. With increased automation and connectivity, manufacturers can achieve higher levels of productivity, customization, and responsiveness to market demands.

In the communication industry, Industry 4.0 revolutionizes the way information is transmitted, accessed, and shared. The emergence of 5G networks, IoT devices, and advanced communication technologies enables a hyperconnected environment. It facilitates faster and more reliable data transmission, seamless connectivity between devices, and the integration of various communication channels. This enables businesses and individuals to communicate and collaborate in real time, opening new opportunities for remote work, virtual collaboration, and innovative digital services.

Transportation is undergoing a significant transformation in the Industry 4.0 era. The integration of advanced technologies, such as autonomous vehicles, intelligent transportation systems, and predictive analytics, revolutionizes the way goods and people are transported. Smart logistics management, real-time tracking, and optimization of supply chains enhance efficiency, reduce costs, and improve safety. Additionally, connected

DOI: 10.1201/9781003466949-2

vehicles and smart infrastructure enable the development of autonomous transportation systems, offering the potential for safer, more sustainable, and more efficient transportation solutions.

In the healthcare sector, Industry 4.0 brings about a paradigm shift in healthcare delivery and patient care. The integration of IoT devices, wearables, electronic health records, and AI-driven analytics enables the collection and analysis of vast amounts of patient data. This facilitates personalized medicine, remote patient monitoring, predictive diagnostics, and improved treatment outcomes. Healthcare providers can leverage advanced technologies to enhance patient engagement, optimize resource allocation, and drive preventive and proactive healthcare approaches.

Overall, Industry 4.0 represents a transformative force across manufacturing, communication, transportation, and healthcare. It promises increased productivity, efficiency, and innovation by leveraging the power of advanced technologies, data-driven insights, and interconnected systems. However, it also presents challenges related to cybersecurity, data privacy, workforce transitions, and ethical considerations that must be addressed to fully realize the potential of Industry 4.0 in these industries.

2.1.1 Chapter Contributions

The main contributions of the chapter are highlighted as follows:

1. A detailed SWOT (strengths, weaknesses, opportunities, threats) analysis of Industry 4.0 is presented for the manufacturing industry.
2. A detailed SWOT analysis of Industry 4.0 is presented for the telecommunication industry.
3. A detailed SWOT analysis of Industry 4.0 is presented for the transportation sector.
4. A detailed SWOT analysis of Industry 4.0 is presented for the healthcare sector.

2.1.2 Chapter Organization

This chapter delves into the benefits and challenges that come with Industry 4.0. Section 2.1 explains how businesses can take advantage of these advancements to increase efficiency, lower expenses, and improve customer satisfaction. In Section 2.2, background related to different fields where Industry 4.0 implementation is presented. SWOT analysis in manufacturing, communication, transportation, and healthcare influenced by the continued evolution of Industry 4.0 and the advancements in technology are described in Section 2.3. The benefits of SWOT analysis are presented in Section 2.4. The conclusion is drawn in Section 2.5.

2.2 BACKGROUND

In this section, we will explore the background of Industry 4.0 implementation in each of the sectors (manufacturing, communication, transportation, and healthcare), highlighting key drivers, challenges, and transformative impacts.

2.2.1 Manufacturing Sector

The implementation of Industry 4.0 in manufacturing has been driven by several factors. One of the primary drivers is the need for increased efficiency and productivity to remain competitive in the global market. Manufacturers seek to optimize production processes, reduce costs, and improve product quality. Additionally, rising customer demand for customization and shorter lead times have fueled the adoption of Industry 4.0 technologies [3–5].

The key technologies driving the implementation of Industry 4.0 in manufacturing include the IoT, AI, robotics, and big data analytics. IoT enables the connection and communication of machines, sensors, and devices, facilitating real-time data collection and analysis. AI and robotics enhance automation and intelligent decision-making, improving operational efficiency and quality control. Big data analytics provides insights for predictive maintenance, supply chain optimization, and demand forecasting.

However, implementing Industry 4.0 in manufacturing is not without challenges. Manufacturers face hurdles such as high initial investment costs, legacy system integration, and workforce upskilling. Additionally, concerns related to data security, privacy, and intellectual property protection arise with the increased connectivity and reliance on digital systems.

Despite these challenges, the benefits of Industry 4.0 implementation in manufacturing are significant. Industry 4.0 enables smart factories with interconnected systems, real-time data analytics, and adaptive production capabilities. Manufacturers can achieve greater flexibility, agility, and responsiveness to market demands. The use of digital technologies streamlines operations reduces downtime, and improves resource allocation. Moreover, Industry 4.0 enables improved product quality, customization, and the development of new business models [6].

2.2.2 Communication Sector

Industry 4.0 has also brought significant changes to the communication sector. The increased connectivity, advanced communication networks, and digital transformation have revolutionized the way information is transmitted, accessed, and shared. One of the primary drivers of Industry 4.0 implementation in communication is the demand for faster, more reliable, and seamless connectivity [7].

The deployment of 5G networks is a key enabler of Industry 4.0 in communication. It offers significantly higher data transfer speeds, reduced latency, and increased network capacity. This supports the proliferation of IoT devices, autonomous systems, and real-time communication across various sectors.

The integration of Industry 4.0 technologies in communication enables improved customer experiences, enhanced productivity, and innovative services. For example, smart homes and smart cities leverage IoT devices, sensors, and AI-driven systems to automate processes, optimize resource usage, and enhance quality of life. Virtual reality (VR) and augmented reality (AR) technologies transform the way we interact with digital content, creating immersive experiences in areas like gaming, education, and remote collaboration [7–8].

However, the implementation of Industry 4.0 in communication faces challenges such as infrastructure requirements, interoperability, and cybersecurity. Building robust communication networks and ensuring compatibility between different technologies and devices is crucial. Additionally, securing data and protecting privacy in a hyperconnected environment is a major concern.

The benefits of Industry 4.0 implementation in communication are substantial. It enables faster and more reliable communication, seamless connectivity between devices, and integration across different communication channels. Businesses and individuals can communicate and collaborate in real time, irrespective of geographic distances. This opens new opportunities for remote work, virtual collaboration, and innovative digital services.

2.2.3 Transportation Sector

Industry 4.0 is reshaping the transportation sector by leveraging advanced technologies to enhance efficiency, safety, and sustainability. One of the key drivers of Industry 4.0 implementation in transportation is the need for optimized logistics and supply chain management. The integration of IoT devices, real-time data analytics, and intelligent transportation systems enables efficient tracking, routing, and resource allocation [9].

Autonomous vehicles are a significant aspect of Industry 4.0 implementation in transportation. Self-driving cars, trucks, and drones are being developed to reduce human error, improve road safety, and increase fuel efficiency. These vehicles rely on sensors, AI algorithms, and connectivity to navigate and interact with their surroundings.

The adoption of Industry 4.0 technologies in transportation also enables predictive maintenance, real-time monitoring, and optimization of fleet management. Data-driven insights support better route planning, fuel efficiency, and vehicle performance. Additionally, connected vehicles and smart infrastructure facilitate the development of intelligent transportation systems, enabling vehicles to communicate with each other and with the infrastructure to prevent accidents and congestion [10].

Challenges in implementing Industry 4.0 in transportation include regulatory frameworks, infrastructure requirements, and societal acceptance of autonomous vehicles. Overcoming these challenges requires collaboration between governments, industry stakeholders, and the public to establish standards, invest in infrastructure, and address safety concerns [11].

The benefits of Industry 4.0 implementation in transportation are transformative. It improves operational efficiency, reduces fuel consumption and emissions, and enhances safety through advanced driver-assistance systems. Intelligent transportation systems enable seamless mobility, optimized traffic flow, and reduced congestion. Moreover, Industry 4.0 technologies support the development of sustainable transportation solutions, such as electric vehicles and shared mobility services.

2.2.4 Healthcare

In the healthcare sector, Industry 4.0 is revolutionizing patient care, treatment outcomes, and healthcare delivery. The need for personalized medicine, remote patient monitoring, and efficient healthcare processes has driven the implementation of Industry 4.0 technologies.

The integration of IoT devices, wearables, electronic health records (EHRs), and AI-driven analytics enables the collection and analysis of vast amounts of patient data. Real-time monitoring of vital signs, medication adherence, and disease progression supports proactive healthcare interventions. AI algorithms and machine learning techniques enable predictive diagnostics, drug discovery, and treatment planning.

Telemedicine is a significant application of Industry 4.0 in healthcare. It enables remote consultations, virtual care, and telemonitoring, reducing the need for in-person visits and increasing access to healthcare services. Patients can receive quality care from the comfort of their homes, while healthcare providers can optimize resource allocation and improve patient outcomes.

Implementing Industry 4.0 in healthcare faces challenges related to data privacy, security, interoperability, and regulatory compliance. Protecting patient data, ensuring secure communication channels, and addressing legal and ethical concerns are critical for successful implementation [12–13].

The benefits of Industry 4.0 implementation in healthcare are numerous. It enables personalized and proactive healthcare, improves treatment outcomes, and reduces healthcare costs. Patients have access to remote monitoring, virtual consultations, and self-management tools. Healthcare providers can optimize care delivery, streamline administrative processes, and leverage data-driven insights for research and population health management.

The implementation of Industry 4.0 in manufacturing, communication, transportation, and healthcare represents a transformative shift in these sectors. The integration of advanced technologies, connectivity, and data-driven systems enables increased efficiency, productivity, and innovation.

While challenges exist, the benefits of Industry 4.0 implementation are substantial, ranging from improved operational processes and customer experiences to enhanced safety, sustainability, and personalized care. Continued research, collaboration, and investment are necessary to fully realize the potential of Industry 4.0 across the aforementioned sectors [14–16]. In the next section, a SWOT analysis will be conducted to find the potential opportunities and challenges in various fields.

2.3 SWOT ANALYSIS

The implementation of Industry 4.0 in manufacturing, communication, transportation, and healthcare offers numerous strengths, such as increased efficiency, automation, and improved decision-making. However, challenges such as high implementation costs, cybersecurity risks, and workforce upskilling need to be overcome. By addressing these weaknesses and leveraging the opportunities presented by Industry 4.0, these sectors can embrace transformative changes and unlock the full potential of advanced technologies.

2.3.1 Manufacturing Sector

In manufacturing, the implementation of Industry 4.0 brings both strengths and weaknesses. The strengths include increased automation and robotics, enabling improved efficiency and productivity. Data-driven decision-making is another strength, as manufacturers can leverage the vast amount of data collected to optimize operations. Additionally, Industry 4.0 allows for customization and flexibility, meeting the changing demands of customers. Supply chain optimization is also a strength, as real-time data and connectivity enable better visibility and management. On the other hand, weaknesses include high implementation costs, as adopting Industry 4.0 technologies requires significant investments. Cybersecurity risks are also a concern, given the increased connectivity and reliance on digital systems [17]. Workforce upskilling is another challenge, as manufacturers need to train employees to operate and maintain these advanced technologies. Integration challenges may arise when existing legacy systems need to be integrated with new Industry 4.0 technologies. Lastly, manufacturers may become overly dependent on technology, which can be a weakness during system failures or disruptions. The detailed SWOT analysis is presented in Table 2.1 and the main factors influencing the analysis are provided in Figure 2.1.

Overall, the SWOT analysis of manufacturing based on Industry 4.0 provides valuable insights to manufacturers, enabling them to make informed

Table 2.1 SWOT Analysis of Industry 4.0 Implementation in the Manufacturing Sector

Manufacturing			
Strengths	*Weaknesses*	*Opportunities*	*Threats*
Industry 4.0 enables advanced automation through the use of robotics, AI, and machine learning, leading to increased productivity, efficiency, and cost savings.	Adopting Industry 4.0 technologies requires significant upfront investments in infrastructure, equipment, and training, which can be a barrier for small and medium-sized enterprises (SMEs).	Industry 4.0 enables better visibility and coordination across the supply chain, leading to optimized inventory management, reduced lead times, and improved customer satisfaction.	With increased connectivity and data exchange, the manufacturing industry becomes vulnerable to cyber threats, such as data breaches, intellectual property theft, and system disruptions.
The integration of sensors, IoT devices, and data analytics allows manufacturers to gather real-time information, enabling more informed decision-making and optimization of processes.	The implementation of automation may lead to workforce displacement or require reskilling/upskilling of existing employees to adapt to the changing technological landscape.	IoT-enabled sensors and data analytics can be utilized to monitor machine health and predict maintenance requirements, reducing unplanned downtime and optimizing maintenance schedules.	The rapid pace of technological advancements in Industry 4.0 may result in the risk of investments becoming outdated or being replaced by newer technologies.
Industry 4.0 facilitates the implementation of flexible manufacturing systems, enabling customization and personalization of products to meet individual customer needs.	The increased connectivity and data exchange in Industry 4.0 can introduce cybersecurity risks, including data breaches and potential intellectual property theft.	Industry 4.0 enables manufacturers to offer customized and on-demand manufacturing, catering to individual customer preferences and increasing competitiveness.	The transition to Industry 4.0 may require new skill sets and competencies, creating challenges in upskilling the existing workforce or attracting and retaining skilled talent.

(*Continued*)

Table 2.1 (Continued) SWOT Analysis of Industry 4.0 Implementation in the Manufacturing Sector

Manufacturing			
Strengths	*Weaknesses*	*Opportunities*	*Threats*
The use of advanced sensors and AI-powered analytics enables real-time monitoring and quality control, reducing defects and improving product quality.	Industry 4.0 relies on robust and uninterrupted internet connectivity, and any disruptions or outages can impact manufacturing operations.	Connected systems and real-time data exchange allow for seamless collaboration between manufacturers, suppliers, and customers, fostering innovation and improved supply chain relationships.	The increased collection and utilization of data in Industry 4.0 raise concerns about privacy and the responsible use of personal and sensitive information.
Industry 4.0 enables better coordination and visibility across the supply chain, leading to optimized inventory management, reduced lead times, and improved customer satisfaction.	Integrating diverse Industry 4.0 technologies and legacy systems can be complex, requiring expertise and resources to ensure seamless operations and compatibility.	Industry 4.0 technologies can support sustainable manufacturing practices by optimizing energy consumption, reducing waste, and enabling resource-efficient production.	The implementation of Industry 4.0 technologies may face regulatory hurdles and compliance requirements, particularly related to data privacy, intellectual property, and safety standards.

Sources: From [18–20].

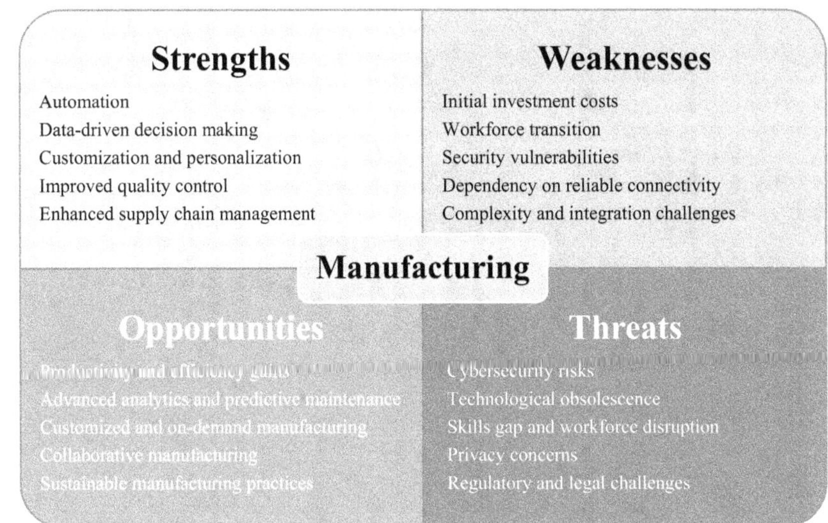

Figure 2.1 Major factors that affect the manufacturing sector while performing SWOT analysis

decisions, capitalize on opportunities, mitigate risks, and optimize their operations in the context of the Fourth Industrial Revolution.

2.3.2 Communication Sector

In the field of communication, Industry 4.0 presents opportunities and threats. The strengths include faster and more reliable communication, seamless connectivity between devices, and integration across different communication channels. Businesses and individuals can communicate and collaborate in real time, regardless of geographic distances. This opens new opportunities for remote work, virtual collaboration, and innovative digital services [21–24]. However, challenges exist, such as infrastructure requirements, interoperability, and cybersecurity [17]. Building robust communication networks and ensuring compatibility between different technologies and devices is crucial. Additionally, securing data and protecting privacy in a hyperconnected environment is a major concern. The detailed SWOT analysis of the communication field is presented in Table 2.2 and the main factors influencing the analysis are provided in Figure 2.2.

Overall, the SWOT analysis of communication based on Industry 4.0 provides valuable insights to organizations, guiding their communication strategies and decision-making processes. It allows organizations to capitalize on strengths and opportunities while addressing weaknesses and mitigating threats. By integrating the analysis findings into their communication

Table 2.2 SWOT Analysis of Industry 4.0 Implementation in the Communication Sector

Communication			
Strengths	*Weaknesses*	*Opportunities*	*Threats*
Industry 4.0 enables seamless connectivity between devices, machines, and systems, facilitating real-time communication and data exchange.	The implementation of Industry 4.0 in communication relies heavily on robust and widespread infrastructure, including high-speed internet connectivity and network coverage, which may not be available in all regions.	Industry 4.0 communication technologies enable real-time collaboration between teams and departments, facilitating faster decision-making and problem-solving.	With increased connectivity and data exchange, the communication domain becomes vulnerable to cyber threats, such as data breaches, hacking, and system disruptions.
Advanced communication technologies, such as 5G, enable faster and more reliable data transmission, reducing latency and enhancing overall communication efficiency.	The integration of new communication technologies may require training and upskilling of employees to effectively utilize and leverage these tools.	Virtual meeting platforms and teleconferencing technologies allow for remote participation and reduce the need for physical travel, saving time and costs.	The rapid pace of technological advancements in Industry 4.0 means that communication technologies can quickly become outdated, requiring ongoing updates and adaptation to remain relevant.
Industry 4.0 technologies enable remote work and virtual collaboration, allowing for increased flexibility and cost savings in communication-intensive industries.	With increased connectivity and data exchange, there is an increased risk of privacy breaches and unauthorized access to sensitive information.	Industry 4.0 communication technologies generate vast amounts of data, providing opportunities for data analytics and deriving actionable insights for improved communication strategies.	Industry 4.0 communication technologies may face regulatory hurdles and compliance requirements, particularly regarding data privacy, security, and international data transfers.

(*Continued*)

Table 2.2 (Continued) SWOT Analysis of Industry 4.0 Implementation in the Communication Sector

Communication			
Strengths	*Weaknesses*	*Opportunities*	*Threats*
AI-powered chatbots and virtual assistants can enhance customer service and support by providing personalized and efficient communication channels.	Integrating legacy communication systems with Industry 4.0 technologies can be challenging, requiring careful planning and investment.	Advanced communication technologies enable personalized customer interactions, leading to improved customer satisfaction and loyalty.	Overreliance on technology and automated communication processes may lead to a loss of personal touch and human interaction, impacting customer relationships and satisfaction.
Industry 4.0 enables real-time sharing of information across the organization, allowing for quicker decision-making and improved coordination.	Unequal access to technology and connectivity may create a digital divide, limiting the benefits of Industry 4.0 communication advancements for certain regions or demographics.	Industry 4.0 facilitates better communication and coordination across the supply chain, enabling seamless information exchange and improved efficiency.	Constant connectivity and communication can lead to digital fatigue and information overload, potentially impacting productivity and employee well-being.

Sources: From [21–24].

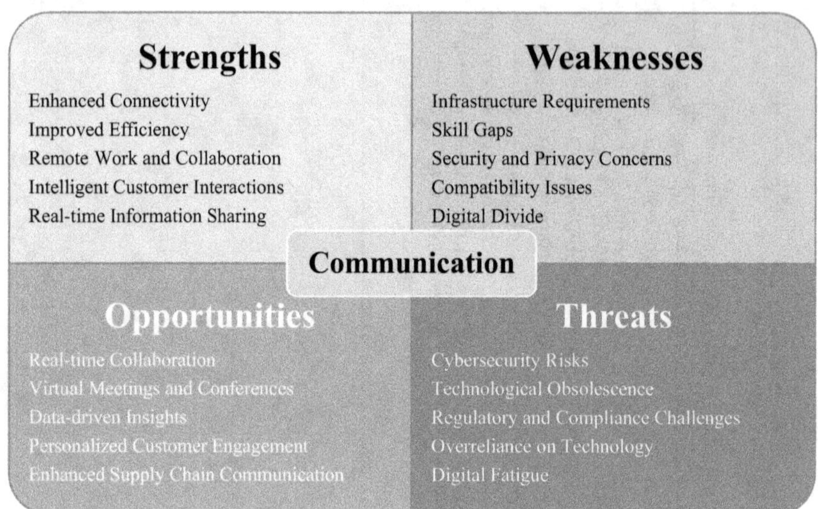

Figure 2.2 Major factors that affect the communication sector while performing SWOT analysis

planning, organizations can enhance their competitive advantage, customer engagement, and operational efficiency in the Industry 4.0 era.

2.3.3 Transportation Sector

Transportation experiences strengths and weaknesses with the implementation of Industry 4.0. The strengths include optimized logistics and supply chain management, efficient tracking, routing, and resource allocation. The integration of IoT devices and real-time data analytics enables these improvements. Autonomous vehicles, a significant aspect of Industry 4.0, have the potential to reduce human errors, enhance road safety, and increase fuel efficiency. However, challenges such as regulatory frameworks, infrastructure requirements, and societal acceptance of autonomous vehicles need to be addressed [25–27]. Overcoming these challenges requires collaboration and establishing standards. Benefits of Industry 4.0 implementation in transportation include improved operational efficiency, reduced fuel consumption and emissions, and enhanced safety through advanced driver-assistance systems. The detailed SWOT analysis of the transportation sector is presented in Table 2.3 and the main factors influencing the analysis are provided in Figure 2.3.

Overall, the SWOT analysis of transportation based on Industry 4.0 provides valuable insights to transportation companies, guiding their strategic planning, operational improvements, and risk management. It enables them to harness the benefits of Industry 4.0 technologies, optimize their

Table 2.3 SWOT Analysis of Industry 4.0 Implementation in the Transportation Sector

Transportation			
Strengths	*Weaknesses*	*Opportunities*	*Threats*
Industry 4.0 technologies enable the optimization of transportation operations, such as route planning, vehicle utilization, and fuel efficiency, leading to reduced costs and improved overall efficiency.	Implementing Industry 4.0 technologies in transportation requires significant upfront investments in infrastructure, equipment, and training, which may be a barrier for smaller transportation companies.	Industry 4.0 paves the way for the development and adoption of autonomous vehicles, leading to increased safety, reduced labor costs, and improved transportation efficiency.	The interconnected nature of Industry 4.0 in transportation introduces vulnerabilities to cyber threats, including data breaches, unauthorized access to sensitive information, and potential system disruptions.
Advanced sensors, GPS, and IoT devices allow for real-time tracking and monitoring of vehicles, shipments, and assets, enabling better logistics management and supply chain visibility.	Adopting Industry 4.0 technologies may require reskilling or upskilling the existing workforce to operate and manage advanced transportation systems, which can be challenging and time-consuming.	IoT-based sensors and data analytics enable smart traffic management systems, optimizing traffic flow, reducing congestion, and improving overall transportation efficiency.	The rapid pace of technological advancements in Industry 4.0 means that transportation companies must continuously update and adapt their systems to remain competitive or risk becoming obsolete.
Industry 4.0 introduces technologies like autonomous vehicles, collision avoidance systems, and driver-assistance tools, enhancing safety in transportation and reducing the risk of accidents.	With increased connectivity and data exchange, transportation systems become vulnerable to cyber threats, such as hacking, data breaches, and system disruptions, necessitating robust cybersecurity measures.	Industry 4.0 technologies, such as delivery drones and intelligent route planning algorithms, present opportunities to optimize last-mile delivery processes, enhancing speed and efficiency.	The adoption of autonomous vehicles and AI-powered transportation systems raises ethical and social concerns regarding job displacement, privacy, liability, and public acceptance, which can pose widespread challenges.

(*Continued*)

Table 2.3 (Continued) SWOT Analysis of Industry 4.0 Implementation in the Transportation Sector

Transportation			
Strengths	*Weaknesses*	*Opportunities*	*Threats*
The integration of data analytics and AI in transportation enables data-driven decision-making, such as demand forecasting, predictive maintenance, and route optimization, leading to improved operational planning and resource allocation.	The effectiveness of Industry 4.0 in transportation relies on a robust and reliable infrastructure, including high-speed networks, GPS coverage, and IoT connectivity. Inadequate infrastructure can limit the full potential of Industry 4.0 technologies.	Data analytics and machine learning can be leveraged for predictive maintenance in transportation, allowing for timely maintenance interventions, reducing downtime, and extending the lifespan of vehicles and infrastructure.	
Industry 4.0 facilitates seamless connectivity and integration between different stakeholders in the transportation ecosystem, including shippers, carriers, warehouses, and customers, enabling real-time communication and collaboration.	The implementation of Industry 4.0 technologies in transportation may face regulatory and legal hurdles, such as compliance with privacy regulations, liability concerns, and ethical considerations surrounding autonomous vehicles.	Industry 4.0 technologies enable transportation companies to adopt sustainable practices, such as electric vehicles, energy-efficient routing, and emission monitoring, reducing the environmental impact of transportation operations.	

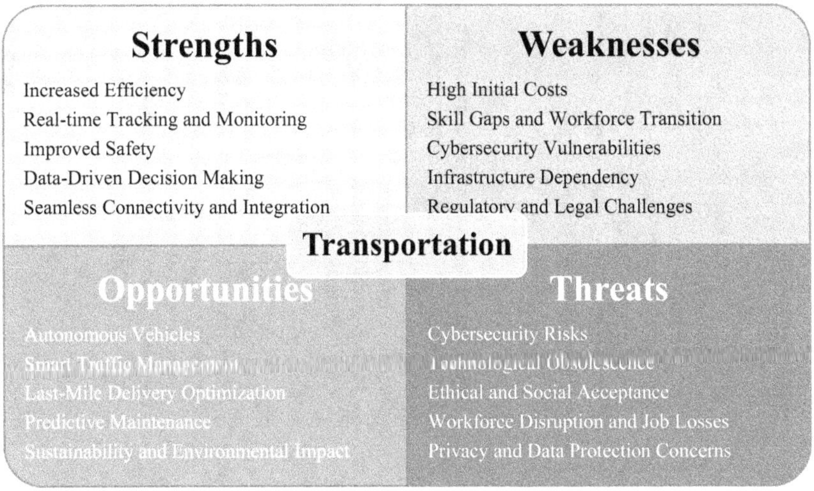

Figure 2.3 Major factors that affect the transportation sector while performing SWOT analysis

operations, enhance the customer experience, and remain competitive in a rapidly evolving industry.

2.3.4 Healthcare Sector

In healthcare, Industry 4.0 presents strengths and weaknesses. The strengths include personalized and proactive healthcare, improved treatment outcomes, and reduced healthcare costs. Industry 4.0 technologies enable remote monitoring, virtual consultations, and self-management tools. Healthcare providers can optimize care delivery, streamline administrative processes, and leverage data-driven insights. However, challenges related to data privacy, security, interoperability, and regulatory compliance exist [28–29]. Protecting patient data, ensuring secure communication channels, and addressing legal and ethical concerns are critical for successful implementation. The detailed SWOT analysis of the healthcare sector is presented in Table 2.4 and the main factors influencing the analysis are provided in Figure 2.4.

Overall, the SWOT analysis of healthcare based on Industry 4.0 provides valuable insights to healthcare organizations, guiding their strategic planning, operational improvements, and risk management. It enables them to harness the benefits of Industry 4.0 technologies, optimize their operations, enhance patient outcomes, and remain competitive in a rapidly evolving healthcare landscape.

In the next section, the benefits of SWOT analysis in diverse fields are explored in detail.

Table 2.4 SWOT Analysis of Industry 4.0 Implementation in the Healthcare Sector

Healthcare			
Strengths	*Weaknesses*	*Opportunities*	*Threats*
Industry 4.0 technologies enable personalized and data-driven healthcare, leading to improved patient care, diagnosis, and treatment outcomes.	The adoption of Industry 4.0 technologies in healthcare raises concerns about data privacy, patient confidentiality, and the security of medical information, requiring robust cybersecurity measures.	Industry 4.0 enables the integration of genomics, patient data, and AI-driven analytics to deliver personalized treatments, precision medicine, and targeted therapies, improving patient outcomes.	The adoption of Industry 4.0 technologies in healthcare may face resistance from healthcare professionals, patients, and regulatory bodies, hindering the pace of implementation and integration.
Automation and digitalization of healthcare processes streamline administrative tasks, reduce errors, and optimize resource utilization, resulting in increased efficiency and productivity.	Integration and interoperability of various healthcare systems and devices can be complex, hindering seamless data exchange and collaboration between different healthcare providers and stakeholders.	Industry 4.0 technologies offer opportunities for remote care delivery and home-based monitoring, reducing healthcare costs, and hospitalizations, and improving patient comfort and satisfaction.	The ethical implications of AI, machine learning, and data-driven healthcare raise concerns about transparency, bias, accountability, and the impact on the doctor–patient relationship, requiring careful ethical frameworks and guidelines.
Industry 4.0 facilitates remote monitoring of a patient's vital signs, enabling proactive and timely interventions, reducing hospital readmissions, and improving patient comfort.	The successful implementation of Industry 4.0 technologies in healthcare requires training and upskilling healthcare professionals to effectively utilize and interpret data from digital systems and connected devices.	Advanced analytics and predictive modeling support the identification of high-risk individuals, enabling proactive interventions, preventive care strategies, and population health management.	The implementation of Industry 4.0 technologies in healthcare must navigate complex regulatory frameworks, compliance requirements, and data privacy regulations, ensuring patient confidentiality and legal adherence.

(*Continued*)

Table 2.4 (Continued) SWOT Analysis of Industry 4.0 Implementation in the Healthcare Sector

Healthcare			
Strengths	*Weaknesses*	*Opportunities*	*Threats*
Advanced analytics and machine learning algorithms enable data-driven decision-making, predictive modeling, and risk assessment, supporting proactive interventions and personalized treatments.	The full potential of Industry 4.0 in healthcare relies on robust and reliable digital infrastructure, including high-speed internet connectivity and interoperable systems, which may not be uniformly available.	Industry 4.0 provides clinical decision support tools, leveraging AI and machine learning, to aid healthcare professionals in diagnosis, treatment planning, and decision-making processes.	The reliability, accuracy, and integrity of healthcare data collected through Industry 4.0 technologies need to be ensured, as erroneous or incomplete data can impact clinical decisions and patient safety.
Industry 4.0 technologies facilitate remote consultations, telemedicine, and virtual care, improving access to healthcare services, especially for underserved areas and individuals with limited mobility.	The high costs associated with implementing and maintaining Industry 4.0 technologies in healthcare can pose challenges to widespread adoption and accessibility, particularly for resource-constrained healthcare settings.	Industry 4.0 technologies enable supply chain optimization in healthcare, improving inventory management, reducing waste, and ensuring the timely availability of medical supplies and medications.	Relying heavily on Industry 4.0 technologies in healthcare creates dependencies on digital systems and connectivity. System failures, technical glitches, or cyberattacks can disrupt healthcare services, highlighting the need for robust backup plans and contingency measures.

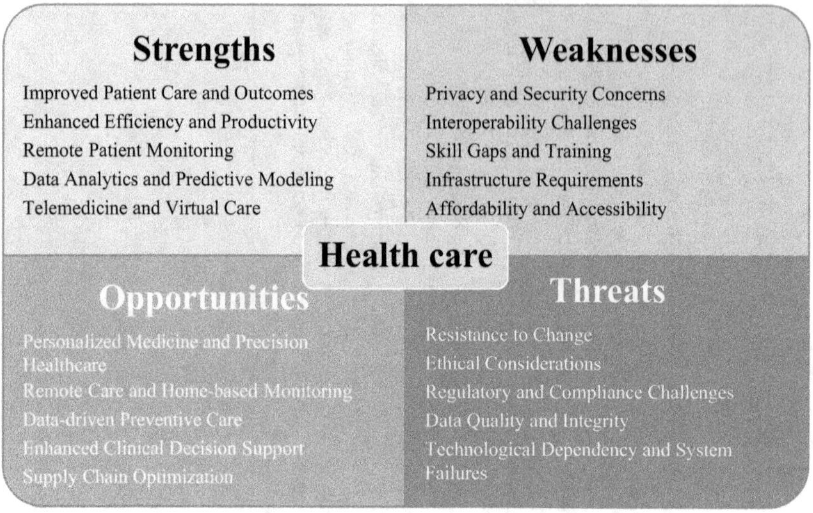

Figure 2.4 Major factors that affect the healthcare sector while performing SWOT analysis

2.4 BENEFITS OF SWOT ANALYSIS

The SWOT analysis of implementing Industry 4.0 in the fields of manufacturing, communication, transportation, and healthcare provides several benefits. Following are some of the key benefits [30–32], which are pictorially shown in Figure 2.5.

2.4.1 Strategic Planning

A SWOT analysis helps organizations in these sectors to assess their internal strengths and weaknesses, as well as external opportunities and threats. By understanding these factors, organizations can develop informed strategies and action plans to leverage their strengths, mitigate weaknesses, capitalize on opportunities, and address potential threats.

2.4.2 Improved Decision-Making

A SWOT analysis provides valuable insights that can aid in decision-making processes. It helps organizations identify areas where they have a competitive advantage and can focus their resources. It also highlights weaknesses and potential threats, allowing organizations to proactively address them and make more informed decisions.

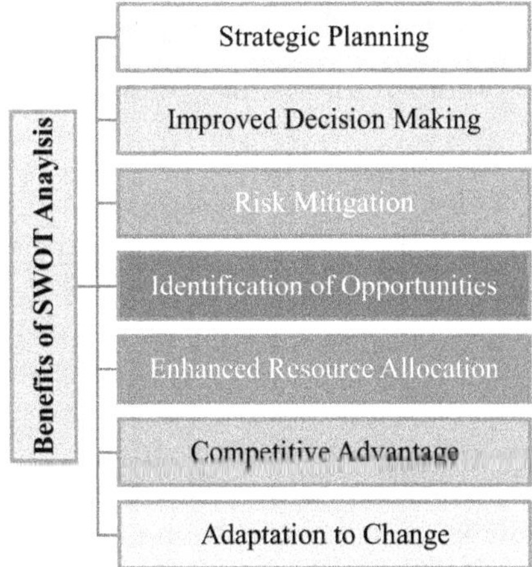

Figure 2.5 Basic parameters to measure the benefits of SWOT analysis

2.4.3 Risk Mitigation

Industry 4.0 implementation involves technological advancements and changes in processes. It helps organizations identify potential risks and challenges associated with the implementation. By understanding these risks, organizations can develop risk mitigation strategies and contingency plans to ensure a smoother transition and minimize disruptions.

2.4.4 Identification of Opportunities

A SWOT analysis helps organizations identify new opportunities that arise from Industry 4.0 implementation. It allows them to spot emerging trends, technologies, and market demands. By leveraging these opportunities, organizations can gain a competitive edge, enter new markets, or develop innovative products and services.

2.4.5 Enhanced Resource Allocation

A SWOT analysis helps organizations understand their resource allocation needs more effectively. It allows them to allocate resources strategically by aligning their strengths with the opportunities available in the market. By optimizing resource allocation, organizations can improve operational efficiency, reduce costs, and maximize return on investment.

2.4.6 Competitive Advantage

By conducting a SWOT analysis, organizations can identify their unique strengths and capabilities. This knowledge helps them develop a competitive advantage in their respective sectors. Industry 4.0 implementation enables organizations to leverage advanced technologies, optimize processes, and deliver innovative solutions, positioning them ahead of their competitors.

2.4.7 Adaptation to Change

Industry 4.0 brings significant changes to various aspects of these sectors. A SWOT analysis facilitates organizations in understanding the potential impacts of these changes and prepares them to adapt and embrace the new paradigm. It helps organizations anticipate and respond to market shifts, technological advancements, and changing customer expectations.

Conducting a SWOT analysis of implementing Industry 4.0 in the manufacturing, communication, transportation, and healthcare sectors provides organizations with valuable insights and benefits. It enables strategic planning, improved decision-making, risk mitigation, identification of opportunities, enhanced resource allocation, competitive advantage, and adaptability to change. These benefits empower organizations to navigate the complexities of Industry 4.0 and thrive in the rapidly evolving business landscape. The comprehensive view of the benefits of Industry 4.0 implementation in diverse fields is presented in Table 2.5.

2.5 CONCLUSION

A SWOT analysis is beneficial in the fields of manufacturing, communication, transportation, and healthcare for several reasons. It provides a structured framework for assessing the internal strengths and weaknesses of an organization and analyzing the external opportunities and threats it faces. It is beneficial in these sectors because it provides a comprehensive overview of the internal and external factors that influence organizational performance. It enables organizations to make informed decisions, capitalize on opportunities, mitigate risks, and develop strategies to stay competitive and sustainable in their respective industries. The analysis can be conducted at various levels, from individual departments to the entire organization, allowing for tailored strategies and action plans.

Overall, the future aspects of SWOT analysis in manufacturing, communication, transportation, and healthcare will be shaped by ongoing technological advancements, changing consumer demands, and emerging trends. The integration of advanced analytics, connectivity, sustainability practices, and personalized approaches will play a significant role in evaluating the strengths, weaknesses, opportunities, and threats in these sectors. The SWOT analysis will continue to evolve as a valuable strategic tool, enabling organizations to adapt and thrive in a rapidly changing business landscape.

Table 2.5 Comprehensive Overview of Benefits of SWOT Analysis for Manufacturing, Communication, Transportation, and Healthcare Sectors

Benefit of SWOT Analysis	*Manufacturing*	*Communication*	*Transportation*	*Healthcare*
Enhanced strategic planning	It provides a structured framework for assessing the internal and external factors influencing manufacturing operations in the context of Industry 4.0. It helps manufacturers identify their strengths and weaknesses, as well as the opportunities and threats present in the industry. This analysis enables more informed strategic planning by aligning manufacturing capabilities with the potential benefits and challenges associated with Industry 4.0.	It helps organizations make informed decisions regarding the adoption and utilization of communication technologies, enabling them to align their communication strategies with the opportunities and challenges presented by Industry 4.0.	It helps transportation companies make informed decisions regarding the adoption and implementation of Industry 4.0 technologies, enabling them to align their strategies with the opportunities and challenges presented by the Fourth Industrial Revolution.	It helps healthcare organizations make informed decisions regarding the adoption and implementation of Industry 4.0 technologies, enabling them to align their strategies with the opportunities and challenges presented by the Fourth Industrial Revolution.

(Continued)

Table 2.5 (Continued) Comprehensive Overview of Benefits of SWOT Analysis for Manufacturing, Communication, Transportation, and Healthcare Sectors

Benefit of SWOT Analysis	*Manufacturing*	*Communication*	*Transportation*	*Healthcare*
Increased competitiveness	By conducting a SWOT analysis, manufacturers can gain insights into their competitive advantages and areas for improvement. It helps them identify opportunities to leverage Industry 4.0 technologies and practices to improve productivity, efficiency, and quality. By addressing weaknesses and capitalizing on strengths, manufacturers can enhance their competitiveness in the market.	By conducting a SWOT analysis, organizations can gain insights into their communication strengths and weaknesses. This analysis helps in identifying areas where communication processes and technologies can be enhanced to improve efficiency, collaboration, and customer engagement. It aids in developing robust communication plans tailored to the requirements of Industry 4.0.	By conducting a SWOT analysis, transportation companies can identify their strengths and weaknesses concerning Industry 4.0 technologies. This analysis allows them to leverage their strengths to optimize operational efficiency and address weaknesses through targeted improvements and investments. It facilitates the adoption of technologies such as IoT, data analytics, and automation to streamline processes, reduce costs, and enhance productivity.	Industry 4.0 technologies in healthcare enable personalized and data-driven approaches to diagnosis, treatment, and patient care. By conducting a SWOT analysis, healthcare organizations can identify their strengths and opportunities to leverage these technologies, leading to improved patient outcomes, enhanced quality of care, and better disease management.

(Continued)

Table 2.5 (Continued) Comprehensive Overview of Benefits of SWOT Analysis for Manufacturing, Communication, Transportation, and Healthcare Sectors

Benefit of SWOT Analysis	*Manufacturing*	*Communication*	*Transportation*	*Healthcare*
Optimal resource allocation	It assists manufacturers in identifying areas where resources, such as investments, technology adoption, and talent development, need to be allocated. It helps prioritize initiatives and investments based on the potential impact on manufacturing operations in the Industry 4.0 landscape. This ensures efficient resource utilization and avoids wastage.	It assists organizations in determining the allocation of resources, such as investments, training, and infrastructure, for communication initiatives in the context of Industry 4.0. It helps prioritize resource allocation based on identified strengths and opportunities while addressing weaknesses and mitigating potential threats. This ensures optimal utilization of resources and maximizes the return on investment in communication technologies.	Industry 4.0 technologies provide opportunities to improve the customer experience in transportation. It helps identify the strengths and opportunities to leverage technologies like real-time tracking, personalized services, and efficient logistics management. By understanding customer needs and aligning them with Industry 4.0 capabilities, transportation companies can enhance customer satisfaction, loyalty, and retention.	It helps healthcare organizations identify resource gaps and allocate resources effectively. By understanding strengths and weaknesses concerning Industry 4.0 technologies, organizations can prioritize investments in infrastructure, training, and technology adoption. This ensures optimal utilization of resources and maximizes the potential benefits of Industry 4.0 in healthcare.

(*Continued*)

Table 2.5 (Continued) Comprehensive Overview of Benefits of SWOT Analysis for Manufacturing, Communication, Transportation, and Healthcare Sectors

Benefit of SWOT Analysis	*Manufacturing*	*Communication*	*Transportation*	*Healthcare*
Risk management	It highlights potential threats and challenges that manufacturers may face when implementing Industry 4.0 initiatives. By identifying these risks, manufacturers can develop risk management strategies to mitigate or minimize their impact. This includes cybersecurity measures, workforce training programs, and contingency plans to address potential disruptions.	It highlights potential threats and challenges related to communication in the Industry 4.0 landscape. By identifying these risks, organizations can develop strategies to mitigate or minimize their impact. This includes implementing cybersecurity measures, ensuring data privacy, and addressing compatibility issues to safeguard communication processes and technologies.	It highlights potential threats and challenges related to transportation in the Industry 4.0 landscape. By identifying these risks, transportation companies can develop strategies to mitigate or minimize their impact. This includes addressing cybersecurity vulnerabilities, ensuring regulatory compliance, and planning for disruptive technologies. It enables transportation companies to proactively manage risks and ensure the smooth operation of their services.	It highlights potential threats and challenges related to the adoption of Industry 4.0 technologies in healthcare, such as data privacy, cybersecurity, and regulatory compliance. By identifying these risks, healthcare organizations can develop strategies to mitigate them, implement appropriate security measures, and ensure compliance with regulations, safeguarding patient data and maintaining trust.

(*Continued*)

Table 2.5 (Continued) Comprehensive Overview of Benefits of SWOT Analysis for Manufacturing, Communication, Transportation, and Healthcare Sectors

Benefit of SWOT Analysis	*Manufacturing*	*Communication*	*Transportation*	*Healthcare*
Adaptation to technological changes	It enables manufacturers to stay abreast of these changes by regularly assessing their strengths and weaknesses concerning emerging technologies. It helps manufacturers proactively adapt and embrace new technologies to stay competitive and remain at the forefront of Industry 4.0 developments.	It helps organizations stay informed about emerging technologies and trends, enabling them to adapt and innovate in their communication strategies. It encourages organizations to embrace new communication tools, platforms, and approaches to leverage the benefits offered by Industry 4.0.	It helps transportation companies stay informed about emerging trends and technologies. It encourages organizations to embrace innovation and adapt their strategies and operations to leverage the benefits of Industry 4.0. By integrating the findings of the analysis into their decision-making processes, transportation companies can drive innovation, explore new business models, and gain a competitive edge in the evolving transportation landscape.	Industry 4.0 technologies provide healthcare organizations with opportunities for advanced research, data analytics, and AI-driven insights. It helps identify research strengths and opportunities to leverage these technologies, leading to accelerated research, the discovery of new treatments, and innovation in healthcare.
Patient-centric care	—	—	—	It enables healthcare organizations to identify opportunities to leverage Industry 4.0 technologies for patient-centric care. For example, telemedicine, remote monitoring, and wearable devices allow for convenient and personalized healthcare services. By embracing these opportunities, healthcare organizations can enhance patient engagement, satisfaction, and access to care.

(*Continued*)

Table 2.5 (Continued) Comprehensive Overview of Benefits of SWOT Analysis for Manufacturing, Communication, Transportation, and Healthcare Sectors

Benefit of SWOT Analysis	*Manufacturing*	*Communication*	*Transportation*	*Healthcare*
Enhanced operational efficiency	—	—	—	It helps identify weaknesses and areas of improvement within healthcare organizations. By leveraging Industry 4.0 technologies, such as electronic health records, automation, and IoT devices, healthcare organizations can streamline administrative tasks, optimize resource utilization, and improve operational efficiency. This leads to cost savings, reduced errors, and enhanced productivity.
Improved patient outcomes	—	—	—	Industry 4.0 technologies in healthcare enable personalized and data-driven approaches to diagnosis, treatment, and patient care. By conducting a SWOT analysis, healthcare organizations can identify their strengths and opportunities to leverage these technologies, leading to improved patient outcomes, enhanced quality of care, and better disease management.

Sources: From [33–39].

REFERENCES

1. Bala, I., Mijwil, M.M., Ali, G. and Sadıkoğlu, E., 2023. Analysing the connection between AI and industry 4.0 from a cybersecurity perspective: Defending the smart revolution. *Mesopotamian Journal of Big Data, 2023*, pp. 63–69.
2. Castagnoli, R., Büchi, G., Coeurderoy, R. and Cugno, M., 2022. Evolution of Industry 4.0 and international business: A systematic literature review and a research agenda. *European Management Journal*, *40*(4), pp. 572–589.
3. Butt, J., 2020. A strategic roadmap for the manufacturing industry to implement Industry 4.0. *Designs*, *4*(2), p. 11.
4. Miśkiewicz, R. and Wolniak, R., 2020. Practical application of the Industry 4.0 concept in a steel company. *Sustainability*, *12*(14), p. 5776.
5. Bala, I., Bhamrah, M.S. and Singh, G., 2017. Capacity in fading environment based on soft sensing information under spectrum sharing constraints. *Wireless Networks*, *23*(2), pp. 519–531.
6. Butt, J., 2020. A conceptual framework to support digital transformation in manufacturing using an integrated business process management approach. *Designs*, *4*(3), p. 17.
7. Bala, I., Bhamrah, M.S. and Singh, G., 2017. Rate and power optimization under received-power constraints for opportunistic spectrum-sharing communication. *Wireless Personal Communications*, *96*(4), pp. 5667–5685.
8. Bala, I., Bhamrah, M.S. and Singh, G., 2019. Investigation on outage capacity of spectrum sharing system using CSI and SSI under received power constraints. *Wireless Networks*, *25*(3), pp. 1047–1056.
9. Dieste, M., Orzes, G., Culot, G., Sartor, M. and Nassimbeni, G., 2023. The "dark side" of Industry 4.0: How can technology be made more sustainable? *International Journal of Operations and Production Management*, 12, pp. 200–213.
10. Gupta, S., Wang, Y. and Czinkota, M., 2023. Reshoring: A road to Industry 4.0 transformation. *British Journal of Management*, *87*, pp. 340–352.
11. Bogoviz, A.V., 2019. Industry 4.0 as a new vector of growth and development of knowledge economy. In *Industry 4.0: Industrial Revolution of the 21st Century*, pp. 85–91. Springer.
12. Bogoviz, A.V., Osipov, V.S., Chistyakova, M.K. and Borisov, M.Y., 2019. Comparative analysis of formation of Industry 4.0 in developed and developing countries. In *Industry 4.0: Industrial Revolution of the 21st Century*, pp. 155–164. Springer.
13. Pedreira, V., Barros, D. and Pinto, P., 2021. A review of attacks, vulnerabilities, and defenses in Industry 4.0 with new challenges on data sovereignty ahead. *Sensors*, *21*(15), p. 5189.
14. Feshina, S.S., Konovalova, O.V. and Sinyavsky, N.G., 2019. Industry 4.0—Transition to new economic reality. In *Industry 4.0: Industrial Revolution of the 21st Century*, pp. 111–120. Springer.
15. Popkova, E.G., Ragulina, Y.V. and Bogoviz, A.V., 2019. Fundamental differences of transition to Industry 4.0 from previous industrial revolutions. In *Industry 4.0: Industrial Revolution of the 21st Century*, pp. 21–29. Springer.

16. Ragulina, Y.V., Alekseev, A.N., Strizhkina, I.V. and Tumanov, A.I., 2019. Methodology of criterial evaluation of consequences of the Industrial Revolution of the 21st century. In *Industry 4.0: Industrial Revolution of the 21st Century*, pp. 235–244. Springer.
17. Bala, I. and Ahuja, K., 2021. Energy-efficient framework for throughput enhancement of cognitive radio network. *International Journal of Communication Systems*, *34*(13), p. e4918.
18. Raj, A., Dwivedi, G., Sharma, A., de Sousa Jabbour, A.B.L. and Rajak, S., 2020. Barriers to the adoption of Industry 4.0 technologies in the manufacturing sector: An inter-country comparative perspective. *International Journal of Production Economics*, *224*, p. 107546.
19. Kumar, V., Vrat, P. and Shankar, R., 2022. Factors influencing the implementation of Industry 4.0 for sustainability in manufacturing. *Global Journal of Flexible Systems Management*, *23*(4), pp. 453–478.
20. Konstantinidis, F.K., Myrillas, N., Mouroutsos, S.G., Koulouriotis, D. and Gasteratos, A., 2022. Assessment of Industry 4.0 for modern manufacturing ecosystem: A systematic survey of surveys. *Machines*, *10*(9), p. 746.
21. Bai, C., Dallasega, P., Orzes, G. and Sarkis, J., 2020. Industry 4.0 technologies assessment: A sustainability perspective. *International Journal of Production Economics*, *229*, p. 107776.
22. Pongboonchai-Empl, T., Antony, J., Garza-Reyes, J.A., Komkowski, T. and Tortorella, G.L., 2023. Integration of Industry 4.0 technologies into lean six sigma DMAIC: A systematic review. *Production Planning and Control*, pp. 1–26.
23. Marinagi, C., Reklitis, P., Trivellas, P. and Sakas, D., 2023. The impact of Industry 4.0 technologies on key performance indicators for a resilient supply chain 4.0. *Sustainability*, *15*(6), p. 5185.
24. Le, V.L.T., Nguyen, T.H. and Pham, K.D., 2023. What drives Industry 4.0 technologies adoption? Evidence from a SEM-neural network approach in the context of Vietnamese firms. *Sustainability*, *15*(7), p. 5969.
25. Müller, J.M., Kiel, D. and Voigt, K.I., 2018. What drives the implementation of Industry 4.0? The role of opportunities and challenges in the context of sustainability. *Sustainability*, *10*(1), p. 247.
26. Ghobakhloo, M., 2020. Industry 4.0, digitization, and opportunities for sustainability. *Journal of Cleaner Production*, *252*, p. 119869.
27. Birkel, H. and Müller, J.M., 2021. Potentials of Industry 4.0 for supply chain management within the triple bottom line of sustainability–A systematic literature review. *Journal of Cleaner Production*, *289*, p. 125612.
28. Bala, I. and Ahuja, K., 2023. Energy-efficient framework for throughput enhancement of cognitive radio network by exploiting transmission mode diversity. *Journal of Ambient Intelligence and Humanized Computing*, *14*(3), pp. 2167–2184.
29. Dalal, S., 2023, April. The smart analysis of Poisson distribution pattern based industrial automation in Industry 4.0. In *2023 International Conference on Distributed Computing and Electrical Circuits and Electronics (ICDCECE)* (pp. 1–6). IEEE.

30. Mijwil, M., Unogwu, O.J., Filali, Y., Bala, I. and Al-Shahwani, H., 2023. Exploring the top five evolving threats in cybersecurity: An in-depth overview. *Mesopotamian Journal of Cybersecurity, 2023*, pp. 57–63.
31. Benzaghta, M.A., Elwalda, A., Mousa, M.M., Erkan, I. and Rahman, M., 2021. SWOT analysis applications: An integrative literature review. *Journal of Global Business Insights*, *6*(1), pp. 55–73.
32. Szum, K. and Nazarko, J., 2020. Exploring the determinants of Industry 4.0 development using an extended SWOT analysis: A regional study. *Energies*, *13*(22), p. 5972.
33. Bala, I., Sharma, A., Tselykh, A. and Kim, B.G., 2022. Throughput optimization of interference limited cognitive radio-based Internet of Things (CR-IoT) network. *Journal of King Saud University – Computer and Information Sciences*, *34*(7), pp. 4233–4243.
34. Bakhtari, A.R., Waris, M.M., Mannan, B., Sanin, C. and Szczerbicki, E., 2020. Assessing Industry 4.0 features using SWOT analysis. In *Intelligent Information and Database Systems: 12th Asian Conference, ACIIDS 2020, Phuket, Thailand, March 23–26, 2020, Proceedings 12* (pp. 216–225). Springer.
35. Szum, K. and Nazarko, J., 2020. Exploring the determinants of Industry 4.0 development using an extended SWOT analysis: A regional study. *Energies*, *13*(22), p. 5972.
36. Sony, M. and Naik, S., 2020. Key ingredients for evaluating Industry 4.0 readiness for organizations: A literature review. *Benchmarking: An International Journal*, *27*(7), pp. 2213–2232.
37. Naciri, L., Gallab, M., Soulhi, A., Merzouk, S. and Di Nardo, M., 2023. Digital technologies' risks and opportunities: Case study of an RFID system. *Applied System Innovation*, *6*(3), p. 54.
38. Kumar, K., Chaudhury, K. and Tripathi, S.L., 2023. Future of machine learning (ML) and deep learning (DL) in healthcare monitoring system. In *Machine Learning Algorithms for Signal and Image Processing*. IEEE, pp. 293–313. doi: 10.1002/9781119861850.ch17.
39. Thillaiarasu, N., Lata Tripathi, S. and Dhinakaran, V. (Eds.), 2022. *Artificial Intelligence for Internet of Things: Design Principle, Modernization, and Techniques* (1st ed.). CRC Press, Boca Raton. doi: 10.1201/9781003335801.

Chapter 3

Role and Impact of Blockchain–IoT-Enabled Supply Chain Management Model for Medical Supply

Inderpal Singh, Balraj Singh, and Arun Kumar Rana

3.1 INTRODUCTION

Supply chain visibility is crucial since each stage must be approved, stamped, and documented, from design, manufacture, and sales to distribution and tracking repairs. The distributed and digital ledger, known as the blockchain, has significantly affected supply chains. Data integrity and immutability are guaranteed without the requirement of a third-party trusted agent. Today's supply networks include many participants and are highly sophisticated. Supply chain companies use the Internet of Things (IoT) and blockchain technologies to keep track of their assets. It is possible to significantly enhance supply networks by enabling the faster and more cost-effective delivery of items, boosting the traceability of products, enhancing coordination between parties, and facilitating access to funding. The entire supply chain may be automated and monitored with the help of IoT.

Organizations must innovate and keep their information systems up to date due to the ever-changing nature of information technology (IT), including numerous software and infrastructure technologies. The rapidly evolving IT development tempts businesses to focus on the attractive benefits of emerging technologies while ignoring the obstacles to their adoption. Such circumstances arise due to a lack of understanding and clear vision of the nature of developing technology such as cloud computing, blockchain, and IoT. Academia and different industrial organizations and sectors pay close attention to these three new emerging technologies [1].

Cloud computing, a prevalent technology used nowadays, provides on-demand services on a pay-as-you-go basis, offering continuous network access and resource pooling with rapid elasticity [2]. The traditional resource management problem can be solved through cloud computing by significantly lowering costs. However, certain limitations persist, such as those concerning shared infrastructure, virtualization, API security, privacy, and legal issues based on service level agreements. In this regard, researchers attempt to solve these issues using various technologies. Blockchain has recently emerged as one of the most popular technologies for solving these problems [3].

 DOI: 10.1201/9781003466949-3

IoT is behind blockchain in the emerging technologies hype cycle and is currently in the trial stage. IoT is necessary for organizations and governments because it boosts productivity, improves the quality of life, enables process automation, enables context-specific applications, and enables real-time creation of rich data, among other benefits. However, there are significant barriers to achieving those values; these barriers include privacy, security attacks, interoperability due to device heterogeneity, high implementation costs, insufficient infrastructure, technological immaturity in storing and processing massive amounts of data, and inadequate regulatory frameworks [4].

3.2 BLOCKCHAIN

A distributed ledger technology based on peer-to-peer networks, encryption technologies, and distributed systems is the blockchain. A public permissionless blockchain is available to everybody, is decentralized, and guarantees user anonymity. In a permissioned private blockchain, transaction validation is performed decentralized. A central authority manages the private permissioned blockchain that is confined to specified trusted users with verified IDs. As a result, transaction validation is centralized on a private blockchain with permissions.

Despite the perceived value that blockchain offers to businesses, blockchain technology is still in its infancy and is being trialed. A recent industry survey identified organizations' top-perceived impediments to blockchain adoption [5]. The decentralization, automation, and consensus mechanisms inherent in blockchain are the sources of innovation [6]. However, these sources of innovation are also sources of technical and architectural risks [7].

The consensus method is susceptible to DDoS attacks [8] and double-spending attacks (i.e., 51% attacks), both of which are pretty likely to occur in private permissioned blockchains. Due to being open, decentralized, and public, the permissionless blockchain is vulnerable to vulnerabilities such as a lack of control over address creation and faulty key generation attacks. The working of blockchain technology is shown in Figure 3.1.

A transaction is entered in the network. Every computer in the network gets the block. The transaction is checked by authorized nodes, which then add the block to the blockchain. The nodes in public blockchain networks are called "miners," and they are usually paid in cryptocurrency through a process called proof of work, or PoW. The network sends out the update, which finishes the transaction.

3.3 IOT

The Internet of Things enables different devices/objects in our surroundings to be addressable, recognized, and locatable via sensor devices. Additionally,

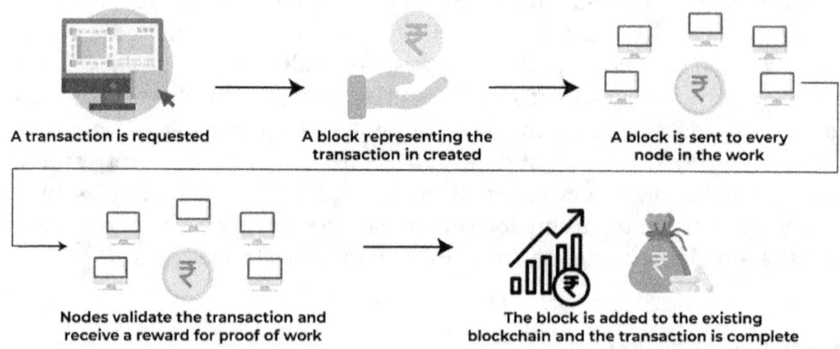

Figure 3.1 Working of blockchain technology

it enables Internet-based control of these devices via wired or wireless communication networks. Everyday items include not just conventional electrical equipment or technological advancements such as cars and phones, but also food, animals, clothing, trees, etc. The primary objective of the IoT system is to enable the connection of diverse things everywhere, at any time, by anyone, ideally via any path/network and any service [9]. The IoT system is capable of interconnecting nearly all physical and virtual items in our surroundings, resulting in the creation of new services and applications, as shown in Figure 3.2. These applications can be implemented in various fields to improve our quality of life.

3.4 ISSUES IN IOT AND THE NEED FOR BLOCKCHAIN

Since the growth of IoT technology, the majority of conventional applications have evolved into smart IoT-based applications. Many efforts have been devoted to the design and protocol of IoT-based applications. The security and privacy concerns must yet be addressed. As described by Singh and Dwivedi [10], IoT technologies face security and privacy problems. Layer-by-layer descriptions of several attack models for IoT-based applications are also provided. The IoT apps are constructed using a framework by Kshetri [11], who identifies eight distinct frameworks and their security and privacy issues for application development. Authentication, data protection, and other security and privacy considerations are the most demanding aspects of developing an Internet of Things application. Lee and Lee [12] discuss how blockchain, fog computing, and machine learning can be utilized to resolve the issue. Tan [13] presents a secure data-collecting framework for the intelligent healthcare system. In a smart healthcare system, important patients are monitored by intelligent technologies. The smart devices are wirelessly or wired connection. In some cases, remote device access is also

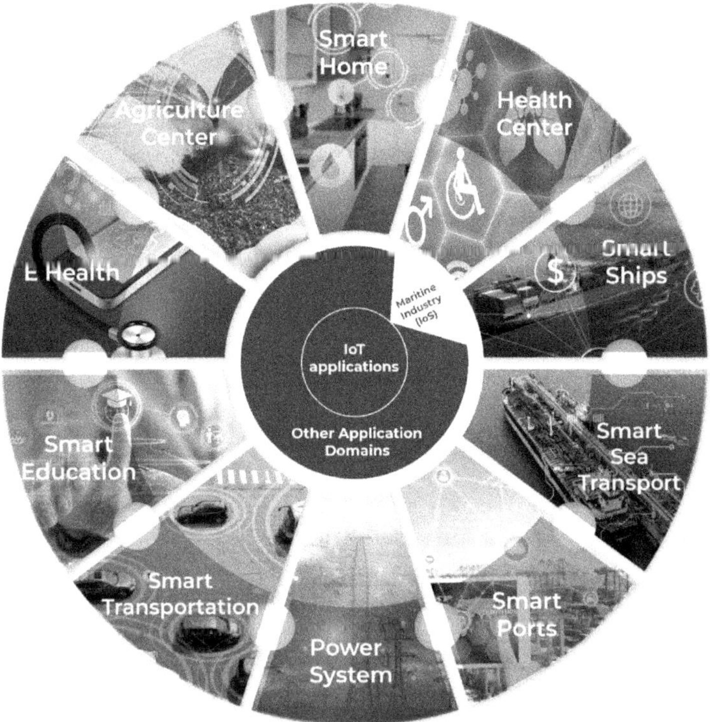

Figure 3.2 IoT application

possible. For connectivity, ZigBee, Bluetooth, and WiFi are utilized. Each of these gadgets is susceptible to various forms of attack. Existing security procedures or algorithms are unsuitable for IoT devices due to their limited resource availability. Lightweight algorithms or protocols are required for IoT devices. In this regard, Zhang [14] proposes the elliptic curve cryptography (ECC)-based technique for IoT applications due to the decreased key size requirements for computation. Three layers comprise the IoT infrastructure: the physical, network, and application layers. There are security concerns in each of these tiers. The following sections discuss of these security and privacy concerns.

3.4.1 Detection Methodology

In IoT, there are two types of attack detection: (1) signature-based detection, which involves gathering specific data from a device, and (2) comparing patterns [15]. These methods, however, cannot detect zero-day attacks. When signatures do not match any predefined rules or practices is also quite challenging to detect attacks [16].

3.4.2 Cryptography Issue

Cryptosystems are designed explicitly for the cipher of integer values that perform simple computations that may influence the results and even help areas where incorrect diagnosis occurs. Obtaining a safe and accurate diagnosis is one of the most difficult challenges in this field. Cryptography is used to protect the privacy of sensors in most cases [17]. Cryptography should keep the encryption keys maintained and secured; it is incapable of dealing with situations where it is necessary to share data with the general public. Variance confidentiality is currently being used for different privacy concerns and works primarily to distribute query results rather than datasets to clients [18].

3.4.3 End User's Privacy

User concerns have recently been raised about breaches to their private information, such as personal data and location, when end users use facilities like cloud computing, IoT, and wireless networks.

Edge computing does not allow data transfer, which is a significant advantage, and is thus regarded as more secure. Edge computing keeps and manages all data on the device that primarily generated it. The data enclosed within the source of truth contained, the creating device remains discrete and secure. Moreover, compared to edge computing, fog computing has a more significant and larger volume to process additional data, which benefits businesses in collecting data from various devices.

Fog computing is best implemented when millions of connected devices are exchanging data. Because fog computing devices are commonly implemented without strict observation and protection, they are vulnerable to many security risks. As a result, increasing trust at the fog level is challenging [19]. This thesis is focused on fog computing due to its weaknesses, such as data security issues and heterogeneity issues. The more blockchain nodes there are, the more difficult it is to manipulate the data [20]. This blockchain-based answer to cloud forensics security and legal challenges comes at a cost. Having blockchain ledgers dispersed widely increases performance costs, resulting in increased latency issues [21].

3.4.4 Heterogeneity Issue

Device mobility and changing application needs are likely to regularly alter the network topology. The environment's fluctuation necessitates dynamic and active system control based on multicriteria resource allotment and the abnormal levels of heterogeneity in IoT devices [22]. Handling dynamic behaviors through improved and enhanced resource allocation includes multicriteria schedulers and resource management systems [23]. The newly developed blockchain refers to any active system management based on multicriteria resource allocation.

3.4.5 Accessibility and Confidentiality Issues

Business and service models are also some of the challenges to be faced. Accessibility challenges arise because a large number of industry stakeholders is present. A hybrid cloud illustration can be deployed using fog, and limited resources can be supplemented with cloud resources. Furthermore, different stakeholders from various IoTs, when combined in a specific order in the cloud, can eventually result in a situation where entirely distinct entities maintain other areas of systems.

When multiple players are involved, it is a challenging task to link IoT facilities with cloud computing and fog services and to observe and manage them. This creates arbitrating roles and permissions issues in IoT [24].

3.5 ROLE OF BLOCKCHAIN AND IOT IN SUPPLY CHAIN MANAGEMENT

In this section, we look at how blockchain, IoT, and supply chain management (SCM) can work together. We assume that if blockchain can improve IoT security, it will also enhance the security of supply chain (SC) systems. Blockchain-based solutions use an IoT system to verify the identities of individuals and assets [25].

Using the blockchain in an SC, it is possible to track the activities of each member of the SC. In addition, some key outcomes and performances may be accurately measured thanks to these features. The role of IoT and its impact on SCM has been examined [26]. IoT for SCM impacts SCM [27], including all the aforementioned activities, plus inventory control, quality assurance, and regular maintenance.

As a result of IoT technologies, SCM can have unparalleled access to all elements of the SC. However, IoT for SCM is still in its infancy. Risks associated with IoT implementation in SCM exist [28]. These risks are categorized into three clusters: environmental, network-related, and organizational. The role of blockchain in medical supply is shown in Figure 3.3.

IoT requires proper security to minimize environmental, network, and organizational threats [29]. IoT can be defined as connecting and monitoring industrial items. Key IoT security issues can be addressed with blockchain-based access management solutions, such as those connected with IP address spoofing [29]. IoT devices must have an identifiable identity. In this

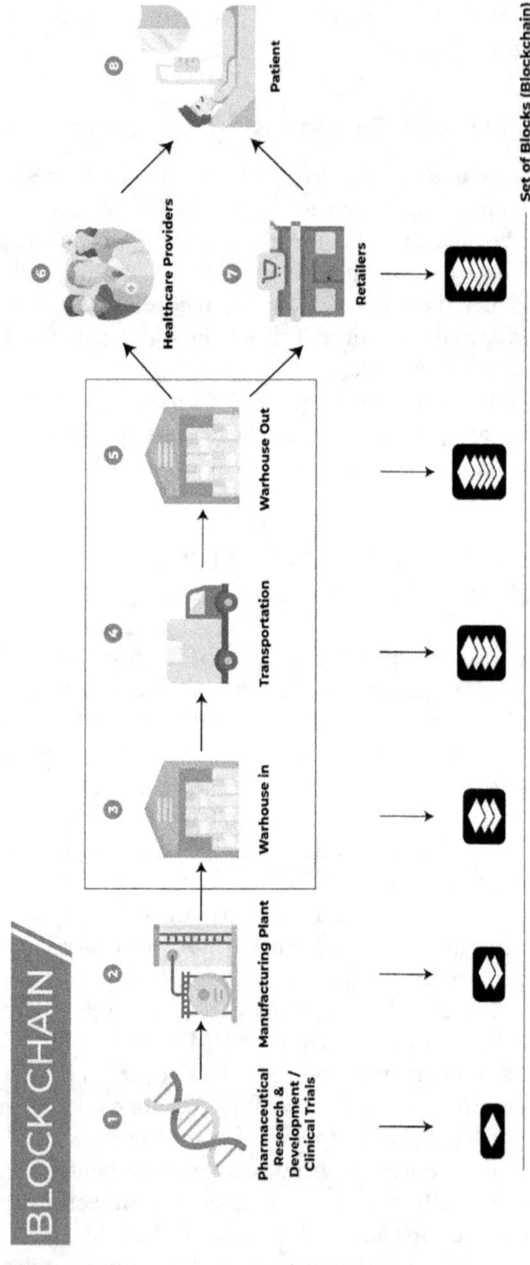

Figure 3.3 Role of blockchain in medical supply

context, the term "blockchain" is the device's origin that can be tracked using decentralized identifiers (DIDs).

The integration of blockchain with IoT is shown in Figure 3.4. The sharing of services and resources is facilitated by using a blockchain and IoT combo. Innovating at the cutting edge of technology opens the door for increased automation and innovation in a safe environment [20].

The blockchain–IoT combo is a formidable one, and it's only going to get stronger. IoT devices can perform autonomous transactions through smart contracts, providing machine-to-machine independent payments, and autonomous communication and decision-making between machines, for example, transforming many sectors [30]. It will also change the way businesses around the world employ IoT equipment. The combination of blockchain, IoT, and SCs may constitute a new opportunity for improvements in data handling for interconnected devices.

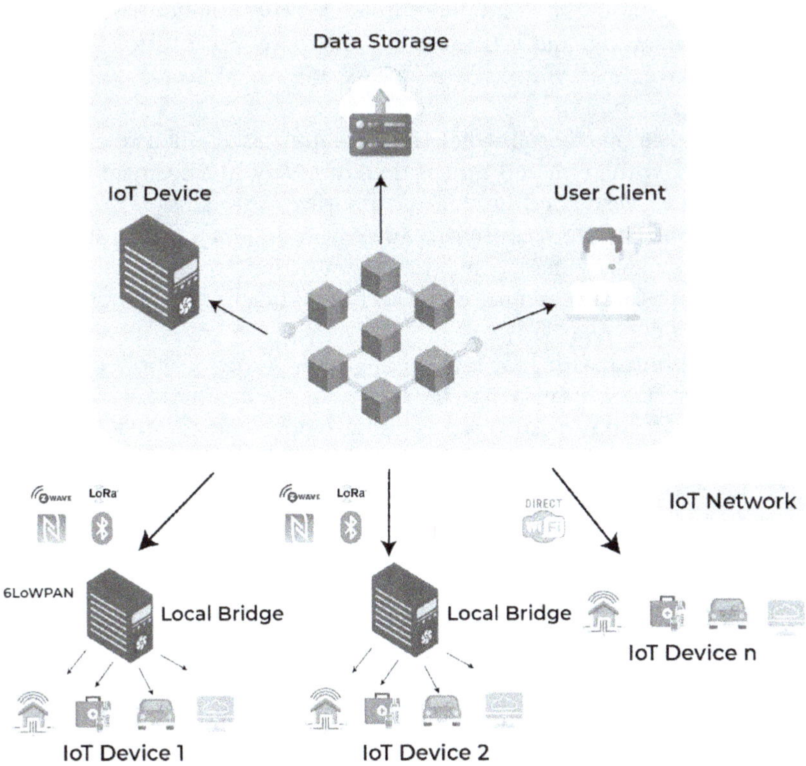

Figure 3.4 Integration of blockchain with IoT

3.6 RELATED STUDIES TO THE ROLES OF IOT AND BLOCKCHAIN IN MEDICAL SUPPLY CHAIN MANAGEMENT

The major downside of cloud computing is that it does not guarantee data protection. The data in the cloud is controlled on a server that may be hacked and attacked. Therefore, anything accessible via the Internet is vulnerable to assault [31]. By utilizing blockchain, attacks can be lessened to some extent. For example, we fathom that it is simpler to take secret data than to take that specific data from the public record. This is where blockchain has an effect [32].

The blockchain can be linked to distributed computing so that its disseminated property of shared organization appears and information can be secured. It is possible to modify data on the framework by hacking a few cloud workers. However, nothing like this will happen if recorded on a public ledger such as blockchain. When we try to answer that precise question, several hubs or miners in the framework will keep track of it, and the hacker will have hundreds of framework hubs, which is nearly inconceivable. Blockchain has a significant advantage [33].

The immaturity of the cloud-computing concept is the source of technical issues, with data loss and leakage being the top concerns. In addition, the top security weaknesses are illegal access, misuse of access controls, and insecure interfaces [34].

The virtual cloud environment can be compromised and its instances can be controlled with escalated rights; therefore, key management and cryptography aren't very good in cloud computing [35]. This problem can be solved using blockchain's consensus and cryptographic mechanisms, which enable secure identity management, authentication, and validation of user authorization to access and use cloud services, and charging for cloud usage via intelligent contracts [36].

When combined with IoT, blockchain could protect supply chains and fight counterfeiters by making the entire supply chain visible and trackable. A tech startup in Australia is using blockchain technology to keep fake goods from getting into the supply chain by making sure they can be tracked, provenanced, and authenticated. Making sure that products can be tracked through the supply chain is a big part of stopping fakes. The growth of global supply chains has made it harder to track goods from the factory floor to the store shelf. At the moment, supply chains are made up of a large number of players, each of which runs its own system. This makes it hard to coordinate and gives brand owners a limited view of how their operations are going. Protecting against fakes usually involves four things: the product itself, its packaging, its label, and the cover that is used to open and close the product.

The World Health Organization (WHO) says that counterfeit drug sales bring in around $200 billion a year and that between 10% and 15% of the global pharmaceutical trade involves fake drugs sold on the black market, on the Internet, or to patients directly through prescriptions. As of April 2018, the group had received about 1,500 reports of fake or poor-quality products since 2013. Also, the US Food and Drug Administration has discussed the problem of unofficial websites and social media platforms being used to sell illegal opioids [37].

Up to 30% of all drugs on the market are fake. This causes up to a million deaths every year, including 450,000 deaths from malaria that could have been prevented. When the WHO looked at more than 48,000 samples from 100 studies conducted from 2007 to 2016, it found that 10.5% of drugs in low- and middle-income countries were fake or not up to par. Since these countries sell nearly $300 billion worth of medicines every year, this means that the trade in fake medicines is a $30 billion business [38].

The Indian pharmaceutical industry is the third largest in the world and makes up 10% of the world's total output. India is the world leader when it comes to making generic drugs and vaccines, which are shipped to more than 200 countries. The bad news is that 35% of fake drugs sold worldwide come from India, according to the WHO. Fake and copied drugs in the supply chain cost the pharmaceutical industry billions of dollars. More worrying is that it puts patients at a higher risk, especially in developing countries where the WHO says that one in ten medical products (like pills, vaccines, and diagnostic kits) is fake or of poor quality. More than a million people worldwide die every year from taking fake medicines. Drug manufacturers are struggling to find a fast, secure, and clear way to find out where these drugs came from or to get the information they need to stop the sale of fake drugs. To keep people trusting the pharmaceuticals India exports, the Indian government is looking for a way to keep track of all the drugs made and shipped out of the country in real time. It also wants to give patients and regulators around the world a way to check if drugs made in India are real [39].

It is important to know how fake drugs get into the supply chain [40]. There are many unchecked and unsafe points of contact:

1. It's harder to figure out where drugs or drug ingredients come from because global supply chains are so complicated.
2. Drugs usually go through several trading companies that don't check their quality before the drugs get to their final destination.
3. One or more of the people in the supply chain could be dishonest. Products can be contaminated, switched out, or mislabeled in the supply chain.
4. The company that made the product might not know that some of the ingredients came from a place that wasn't certified.
5. With the help of fake paperwork, companies that make ingredients or drugs can pass themselves off as real pharmaceutical companies.

It is hard to track the drug supply chain because there are so many points of entry and no strong or secure system is in place [41]. One problem with the current supply chain system is that there isn't a single labeling and identification standard that everyone can use.

1. A supply chain infrastructure can be separated, broken up, and hard to see. There is no clear way to follow a product's path through the supply chain that can show where it came from and where it was handled. There is bad management and monitoring of the cold chain.
2. The drugs are passed between many different people, including the people who package and ship them. This could be a way for fake drugs to get into the system.
3. Different systems are used by different manufacturers. This means that wholesalers and resellers have to keep different types of solutions in their supply chain systems, which can mess up data or delivery and put the consumer at risk.

3.7 CONCLUSION

In both computing and healthcare, blockchain technology is still in its infancy. The qualities and properties of this technology have enormous potential in healthcare subsectors to solve important concerns. Technological advancements may have a profound impact on the entire environment. More research is needed in the early stages of its development, but it must also be conducted in the health insurance and pharmaceutical supply chains. It's important to note that the application of blockchain technology has run into several problems, which will be addressed in future studies. Some of the concerns raised here could lead to better future research.

REFERENCES

1. Y. Zhang and J. Wen, An IoT electric business model based on the protocol of bitcoin. *In Intelligence in Next Generation Networks (ICIN), 2015 18th International Conference on*, 2015, pp. 184–191.
2. S. Schneider and A. Sunyaev, Determinant factors of cloud-sourcing decisions: Reflecting on the IT outsourcing literature in the era of cloud computing. *Journal of Information Technology*, vol. 31, no. 1, pp. 1–31, 2014.
3. J. P. Shim, M. Avital, O. Sheng, C. Sorensen, A. R. Dennis, M. Rossi, and A. M. French, Internet of things: Opportunities and challenges to business, society, and IS research. In *Proceedings of the 38th International Conference on Information Systems*, 2018.
4. L. Atzori, A. Iera, and G. Morabito, Understanding the Internet of things: Definition, potentials, and societal role of a fast-evolving paradigm. *Ad Hoc Networks*, vol. 56, pp. 122–140, 2017.

5. M. Avital, J. L. King, R. Beck, M. Rossi, and R. Teigland, Jumping on the blockchain Bandwagon: Lessons of the past and outlook to the future. In *Proceedings of the 37th International Conference on Information Systems*, 2016.
6. I. Makhdoom, M. Abolhasan, H. Abbas, and W. Ni, Blockchain's adoption in IoT: The challenges, and a way forward. *Journal of Network and Computer Applications*, vol. 125, pp. 251–279, 2019.
7. V. J. Morkunas, J. Paschen, and E. Boon, How blockchain technologies impact your business model. *Business Horizons*, vol. 62, no. 3, pp. 295–306, 2019.
8. S. K. Johansen *A Comprehensive Literature Review on the Blockchain Technology as a Technological Enabler for Innovation*. Department of Information Systems, Mannheim University, 2018.
9. C. Walsh, P. O'Reilly, R. Gleasure, J. Feller, S. Li, and J. Cristoforo, New kid on the block: A strategic archetypes approach to understanding the blockchain. In *Proceedings of the Thirty Seventh International Conference on Information Systems Deloitte (2019)*, 2016.
10. R. Singh and A. Dwivedi, A game theoretic analysis of resource mining in blockchain. *Cluster Computing*, vol. 34, pp. 760–772, 2020.
11. N. Kshetri, Can blockchain strengthen the Internet of things? *IT Professional Magazine*, vol. 19, no 4, 2017.
12. I. Lee and K. Lee, The Internet of Things (IoT): Applications, investments, and challenges for enterprises. *Business Horizons*, vol. 58, no. 4, pp. 431–440, 2015.
13. L. Tan, Blockbench: A framework for analyzing private blockchains. In *Proceedings of the 2017 ACM International Conference on Management of Data, ser. SIGMOD '17*, 2017. New York: ACM, pp. 1085–1100.
14. Y. Zhang, Virtualization for distributed ledger technology (vDLT). *IEEE Access*, vol. 6, pp. 25019–25028.
15. M. Banerjee, J. Lee, and K.-K. R. Choo, A blockchain future for internet-of-things security: A position paper. *Digital Communications and Networks*, vol. 4, no. 3, pp. 149–160, 2018.
16. F. Restuccia and S. D'O r o, and T. Melodia, Securing the internet of things in the age of machine learning and software-defined networking. *IEEE Internet of Things Journal*, vol. 5, no. 6, pp. 4829–4842, 2018.
17. A. Reyna, C. Martín, J. Chen, E. Soler, and M. Díaz, On blockchain and its integration with IoT: Challenges and opportunities. *Future Generation Computer Systems*, vol. 88, pp. 173–190, 2018.
18. Y. Xin, L. Kong, and Z. Liu, et al., Machine learning and deep learning methods for cyber security. *IEEE Access*, vol. 6, pp. 35365–35381, 2018.
19. M. A. Khan and K. Salah, IoT security: Review, blockchain solutions, and open challenges. *Future Generation Computer Systems*, vol. 82, pp. 395–411, 2018.
20. T. Alam and M. Benaida, Blockchain, fog, and IoT integrated framework: Review, architecture, and evaluation. *Technology Reports of Kansai University*, 2020.
21. M. A. Ferrag, L. Shu, X. Yang, A. Derhab, and L. Maglaras, Security and privacy for green IoT-based agriculture: Review, blockchain solutions, and challenges. *IEEE Access*, vol. 8, pp. 32031–32053, 2020.

22. I.-C. Lin and T.-C. Liao, A survey of blockchain security issues and challenges. *International Journal of Network Security*, vol. 19, no. 5, pp. 653–659, 2017.
23. M. Frustaci, P. Pace, G. Aloi, and G. Fortino, Evaluating critical security issues of the IoT world: Present and future challenges. *IEEE Internet of Things Journal*, vol. 5, no. 4, pp. 2483–2495, 2018.
24. G. Lize, W. Jingpei, and S. Bin, Trust management mechanism for the internet of things. *China Communications*, vol. 11, no. 2, pp. 148–156, 2014.
25. Y. Yang, L. Wu, G. Yin, L. Li, and H. Zhao, A survey on security and privacy issues in internet-of-things. *IEEE Internet of Things Journal*, vol. 4, no. 5, pp. 1250–1258, 2017.
26. M. Ammar, G. Russello, and B. Crispo, Internet of things: A survey on the security of IoT frameworks. *Journal of Information Security and Applications*, vol. 38, pp. 8–27, 2018.
27. V. Hassija, V. Chamola, V. Saxena, D. Jain, P. Goyal, and B. Sikdar, A survey on IoT security: Application areas, security threats, solution architectures. *IEEE Access*, vol. 7, pp. 82, 721–782, 743, 2019.
28. K. Jaiswal, S. Sobhanayak, B. K. Mohanta, and D. Jena, IoT-cloud based framework for patient's data collection in smart healthcare system using raspberry-pi. In *2017 International Conference on Electrical and Computing Technologies and Applications (ICECTA)*. IEEE, 2017, pp. 1–4.
29. U. Satapathy, B. K. Mohanta, D. Jena, and S. Sobhanayak, An ECC-based lightweight authentication protocol for mobile phone in smart home. In *2018 IEEE 13th International Conference on Industrial and Information Systems (ICIIS)*. IEEE, 2018, pp. 303–308.
30. S. Biswas, K. Sharif, F. Li, S. Maharjan, S. P. Mohanty, and Y. Wang, PoBT: A lightweight consensus algorithm for scalable IoT business blockchain. *IEEE Internet of Things Journal*, vol. 11, pp. 252–262, 2019.
31. A. Dorri, S. S. Kanhere, R. Jurdak, and P. Gauravaram, Lsb: A lightweight scalable blockchain for IoT security and anonymity. *Journal of Parallel and Distributed Computing*, vol. 134, pp. 180–197, 2019.
32. A. Yu, J. Wright, S. Nepal, L. Zhu, J. Liu, and R. Ranjan, Trustchain: Establishing trust in the IoT-based applications ecosystem using Blockchain. *IEEE Cloud Computing*, vol. 5, no. 4, pp. 12–23, 2018.
33. L. Xie, Y. Ding, H. Yang, and X. Wang, Blockchain-based secure and trustworthy internet of things in SDN-enabled 5G-VANETs. *IEEE Access*, vol. 7, pp. 56, pp. 656–656 666, 2019.
34. L. Zhou, L. Wang, Y. Sun, and P. Lv, Beekeeper: A blockchain-based IoT system with secure storage and homomorphic computation. *IEEE Access*, 2018.
35. M. T. Hammi, B. Hammi, P. Bellot, and A. Serhrouchni, Bubbles of trust: A decentralized Blockchain-based authentication system for IoT. *Computers and Security*, vol. 78, pp. 126–142, 2018.
36. C. Lin, D. He, N. Kumar, X. Huang, P. Vijaykumar, and K.-K. R. Choo, Homechain: A blockchain-based secure mutual authentication system for smart homes. *IEEE Internet of Things Journal*, vol. 11, pp. 300–312, 2019.
37. A. Gauhar, N. Ahmad, Y. Cao, S. Khan, H. Cruickshank, E. A. Qazi, and A. Ali, Blockchain-based cross-domain authentication and authorization framework for internet of things. *IEEE Access*, 2020.

38. M. Shen, X. Tang, L. Zhu, X. Du, and M. Guizani, Privacy-preserving support vector machine training over blockchain-based encrypted IoT data in smart cities. *IEEE Internet of Things Journal*, vol. 6, no. 5, pp. 7702–7712, 2019.
39. P. Lv, L. Wang, H. Zhu, W. Deng, and L. Gu, An Iot-oriented privacy-preserving publish/subscribe model over blockchains. *IEEE Access*, vol. 7, pp. 41, 309–341, 314, 2019.
40. S. Ding, J. Cao, C. Li, K. Fan, and H. Li, A novel attribute-based access control scheme using blockchain for IoT. *IEEE Access*, vol. 7, pp. 38, 431–438, 441, 2019.
41. M. A. Khan, K. Salah, IoT security: Review, blockchain solutions, and open challenges. *Future Generation Computer Systems*, vol. 82, pp. 395–411, 2019.

Chapter 4

The Internet of Things in Healthcare

A Remote Patient Monitoring System

Dev Gupta and Rachit Jain

4.1 INTRODUCTION

The primary applications of wearable technology are discussed in this review of research, including security, personal treatment, health and wellness, therapy efficacy assessment, and early disease detection. Protection, residential treatment, health and wellness, treatment efficacy assessment, and early problem detection are just a few of the applications it covers. This review chapter focuses on current trends in the field of portable sensors and therapeutic devices. It investigates what has to be done to get the sector closer to the clinical application of advanced detectors and devices.

In India, there are more doctors per person than there were five years ago. However, rural areas still lack access to doctors. According to data from India's Ministry of Rural Development, 64.61% of the country's residents live in rural areas. They come from Himachal Pradesh, Bihar, Assam, Odisha, and Meghalaya the most [1]. The World Health Organization (WHO) recommends a doctor–patient ratio of one doctor per thousand people; there are 9.27 lakhs of doctors available for active service in India, according to statistics from the Ministry of Health of India [1]. One method for removing the obstacles to healthcare is a remote patient monitoring system. It offers rural residents specialized healthcare services.

Information and communication technology (ICT) is used. Continuous health and well-being monitoring, in accordance with Patel et al., can support patient therapy [2]. A doctor can remotely check on a patient's health using a remote patient monitoring system at any time or location [3]. Prevention can start when the illness is first detected. The concept in this study supports both the real-time and store-and-forward phases of an Internet of Things (IoT)-based real-time electrocardiogram, or ECG, surveillance system. The security of data is not an issue for the store-and-forward mode, and it doesn't require a strong network. The instant mode is difficult, nevertheless, because dataset integrity may be impacted by transmission latency and packet degradation during instant time distribution, particularly for the transfer of real-time ECG signals. The use of incorrect

DOI: 10.1201/9781003466949-4

health information might lead to a misdiagnosis. In order to advance biomedical engineering, IoT is crucial.

Technologies are referred to as "things" in IoT that are linked together via a network and exchange information for improved outcomes. It can increase advancements in the biomedical area with the aid of the IoT. The configuration of a smartphone's embedded circuit, which is a handheld device, is currently a difficulty. Blood pressure and many other deadly ailments can be monitored by utilizing a smartphone. However, the technology must be affordable for the poor.

Intelligent development provides users with prolonged learning and helps them become experts in their symptoms and treatments. Medical facilities have always ignored important expectations for patient protection, treatment, and financial constraints. There have been several statements that raise severe concerns about the area of acquisition of the involved organizations.

Problems with expensive restoration services and patient safety have been recognized by the National Survey of Health Office, the National Health Prosperity Office, Medicines and Human Administrative Things, the Regulatory Office, the National Wellbeing Organization, Cases Pro, and the Global Wellbeing Affiliation.

A functional cardiac care unit (CCU) is a crucial sign of the health system's capacity to deliver crucial and life-saving operations and therapies. Assam, Jharkhand, Telangana, Uttar Pradesh, Arunachal Pradesh, Manipur, Meghalaya, Sikkim, Tripura, and Andaman and Nicobar were among the states and union territories overall (Figure 4.1).

There are no operational CCUs at district hospitals. By creating at least one CCU for every two districts, Tamil Nadu, Himachal Pradesh, Kerala, West Bengal, Punjab, Maharashtra, Andhra Pradesh, Goa, and union territories have achieved good progress.

Federated learning is suggested as a solution to the privacy and research problem. It is a decentralized machine learning method for large-scale data training [4]. "Making code talk to data, not data talk to code" is the name of this method. Federated learning resolves the data's privacy, ownership, and location concerns by keeping the model parameters rather than the actual data. It is feasible to construct a shared global model while retaining the data in local institutions and by sending local models to end users rather than sending particular data to a centralized server, as discussed in McMahan et al.'s [4] and Konecky et al.'s research [5].

Gboard [6], a virtual touchscreen keyboard for portable devices developed by Google, is the first recommended application, which preserves privacy before uploading local corpus text data from users to the server to enhance word prediction performance. In situations when many institutions desire to enhance the interpretation of their models, federated learning may also

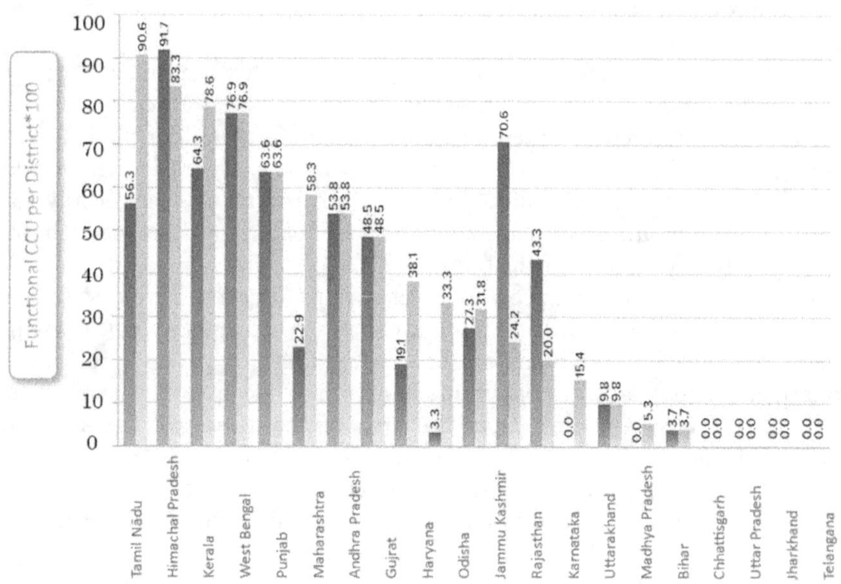

Figure 4.1 Cardiac care units in districts in large Indian states

be employed. It can build a global model out of local ones without breaching privacy laws or disclosing personal medical information. Federated learning also lessens the load on communication networks and improves communication efficiency while building models.

When a machine learning model is developed using either information about a single person (which may be millions of individuals, as in the instance of Gboard) or data from multiple organizations, the data is sent to a central server via traditional routes.

The amount of data being sent puts a strain on the network's infrastructure, and the data may be text corpora, physiological signals, or medical imaging. By creating models locally and sending only instead of sending the entire collection of data, the model parameters are sent to the centralized server, federated learning reduces the strain on communication networks. Wearable sensors have both observational and diagnostic functions. They can now physically and biochemically detect motion. The magnitude of the issues that these innovations may tackle cannot be overstated.

Physiological monitoring may be helpful for both the initial diagnosis and continuous treatment of people with neurological, cardiovascular, and pulmonary conditions such as breathing problems, irregular heartbeats, high blood pressure, and seizures. Home-based tracking of movement might minimize falls while maximizing a person's independence and community participation. Troublesome patient access issues may be resolved by remote monitoring systems.

Only 9% of doctors in the US practice in rural areas, despite the fact that nearly 20% of people live in rural areas [7]. Since millions of unique patients will have access to insurance thanks to the healthcare reform, many organizations predict that access will deteriorate over time [8].

The differences in care that rural populations experience are well discussed in the literature [7]. Rural dwellers see fewer specialists, compared to their metropolitan counterparts, must drive two to three times farther to visit a doctor, and experience worse outcomes for common illnesses like diabetes and coronary artery disease. Wearable sensors and screened surveillance equipment may help reduce poor outcomes by expanding the reach of metropolitan experts into rural communities.

A hypothetical representation of a remote monitoring system is shown in Figure 4.2. Wearables are equipped with sensors to collect movement and physiological data, which allows for the monitoring of patients' conditions, depending on the medical application of interest. For instance, sensors to assess symptoms like heart rate and breathing rate might be utilized while examining people who have a persistent respiratory illness or congestive heart failure.

Patient data transmission to a portable gadget or access point for internet transmission to a remote center depends on wireless communication. Data processing applied throughout the system detects emergency circumstances

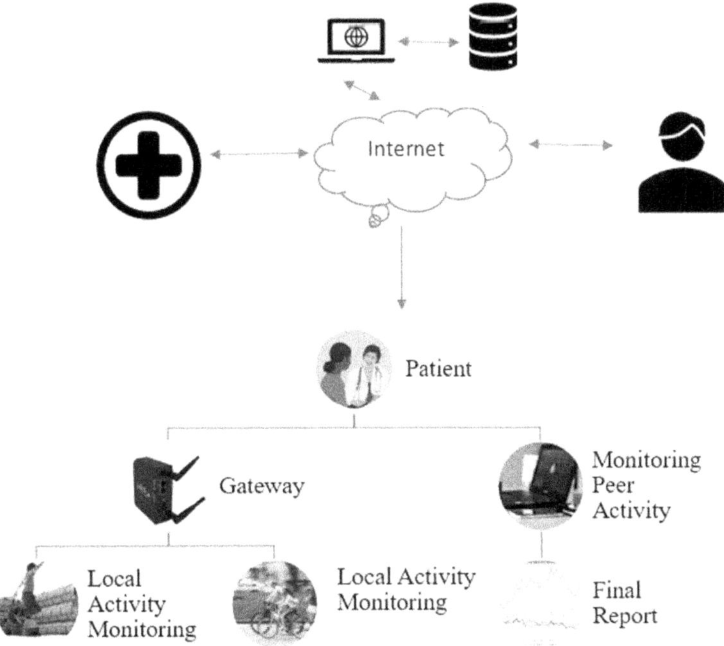

Figure 4.2 An example of a wearable sensor-based remote health tracking system

(such as falls), and in order to provide patients with prompt assistance, a warning message is sent to an urgent care center. In addition to being contacted in cases of emergencies, family members and carers may also be informed when a patient needs help, such as with taking his or her prescriptions. Clinical staff can remotely check on patients and be informed if a healthcare decision has to be made. Clinical practitioners can monitor a patient's status remotely and are informed when a medical choice has to be taken.

Although wearing a sensor-based remote tracking system may have certain advantages such as the ones mentioned earlier, there are still many obstacles to overcome before such a system can be widely used. These difficulties include scientific ones, like the limitations of existing battery technology, and cultural ones, such as the shame attached to using medical equipment for in-home clinical monitoring. The next section goes through the essential technologies that make wearable technology development and screened monitoring technique deployment possible. The following section discusses personal and environmental sensors, which are crucial parts of equipment used to monitor patients at home and in the community. Then, examples of uses for these technologies are given, many of which depended on an examination of European projects with an emphasis on rehabilitation technology that was launched by the National Science Foundation [9]. In the concluding section, we examine our findings and our predictions for the future of wearable technology-based remote patient monitoring.

4.2 KEY ENABLING TECHNOLOGIES

Three key components make up mobile device systems for remote monitoring of individuals [10]: tools for detecting and data collection to obtain information on movement and physiological nature [11]. Using software and hardware that interact, data may be sent to a distant location. Data analysis techniques can be used to glean therapeutically useful information from mental and signal data. Thanks to recent developments in technology for sensors, electronic components, communication, and data analysis techniques, wearable devices for monitoring patients have been created and put into use.

Researchers have relied on developments in the aforementioned domains to solve limitations in ambulatory technology (such as Holter monitors) that previously made it impossible to monitor patients' conditions over time in the residence and community.

In accordance with the healthcare purpose of interest, wearables are fitted with sensors to collect physiological and mobility data, enabling the surveillance of patients' ailments. Sensors, for example, that measure indicators like pulse and breathing might be utilized while examining persons with congestive heart failure or people with chronic respiratory disorders.

Recent advancements in the domain of microelectronics have made it possible for researchers to create tiny circuits with radio transmission, front-end amplification, and microcontroller functionality. An illustration of such technology is the flexible circuit in Figure 4.3, which enables the collecting of physiological data and wirelessly transmitting it to a data recorder. Microelectromechanical system (MEMS) manufacturing technology advancement is particularly relevant to uses in the field of therapy. MEMS technology has made it feasible to create tiny inertial sensors for use in motor activity as well as health rate monitoring systems. The use of batch manufacturing techniques has considerably lowered the size and charge of sensors. System-on-chip implementations are the result of the use of microelectronics to merge several components, such as wireless communications circuits and microprocessors, into one integrated circuit [13].

E-textile–based systems have been made possible by developments in materials science. These technologies enable the incorporation of sensor functionality into clothing. An illustration of how sensors might be woven into fabric to gather electrocardiographic and electromyographic data is shown in Figure 4.3, as well as conductive elastomer-based components that can be printed on fabric to collect movement data by sensing changes in resistance caused by the fabric stretching as a result of movements of the subject. Rapid developments in this area indicate that soon it may be possible to print whole circuit boards on cloth.

Most wearable systems used for health monitoring employ sensors that are paired into a kind of sensor net that is either wholly made up of body-worn sensors or mixes human-worn detectors with ambient sensors. Wearable sensors were originally inserted into body-worn in the early stages of the technology. Sensor networks were created by inserting "wires" through pockets constructed specifically for this purpose (sometimes referred to as the "human body's sensor networks"). The MIThril system is an illustration of this technology [14]. Such techniques were intentionally inconsistent with long-term health monitoring.

Modern wearable systems connect individual sensors to the sensor network using cutting-edge wireless communication technology. We have seen great advancement in this area over the past ten years, including the emergence of a wide range of low-power wireless communication standards.

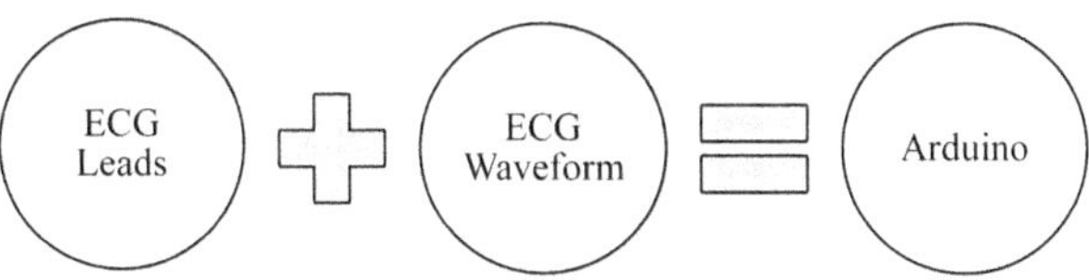

Figure 4.3 Flexible wireless ECG sensor by IMEC with a working microprocessor

Three primary requirements have been taken into consideration when developing these standards: cheap power consumption, tiny transmitters and receivers, and cheap cost are the first three factors.

Due to the adoption of Bluetooth connectivity and IEEE 802.15.4/ZigBee, connected devices are no longer in use [15]. The recently developed IEEE 802.15.4a standard based on applications for low-power, low-cost, yet extremely fast sensor networks is made possible by ultra-wideband (UWB) impulse radio [16]. It has the ability to provide exceptionally precise location predictions.

Most monitoring applications need the sensor network data to be transferred to a distant location, such as a healthcare server, in order to do clinical analysis. Data from the network of sensors can be delivered to a computer or other information gateway, such as a mobile device, to do this. Almost all industrialized countries currently have broadband connectivity.

On a device, sensor data might be integrated and transmitted to a distant place over the internet for in-home monitoring. Furthermore, extensive continuous healthcare and monitoring even when an individual is away from their residence is now possible because of the availability of mobile communications standards like 4G.

Devices for remote monitoring that use wearable sensors have been greatly influenced by mobile phone technology. Applications for monitoring that rely on mobile devices are becoming widespread. A lot of people have access to smartphones, with approximately 220 million devices sold in 2010. The global market for smartphones is anticipated to grow by 35% annually [17]. Smartphones are chosen over traditional data loggers because they provide a platform that is almost "ready to use" for data gathering and transfer to a remote site. Mobile devices may process information in addition to acting as information gateways. The possibility to imagine widespread monitoring of health and intervention applications is made possible by the availability of considerable computational power [18] in portable devices. The GPS tracking technology that is embedded into the majority of portable electronics also makes it easy to locate patients in critical situations.

Health monitoring systems may also become affordable, platform-independent, quickly deployable, and widely accessible as storage and computing move into the cloud [19, 20]. Monitoring devices might become cheaper and easier to operate as computing moves to the cloud. Users are now able to purchase off-the-shelf equipment and utilize cloud services to get specialized monitoring applications [21]. Cloud-based solutions can be particularly helpful for expanding access to healthcare in remote places [22]. Additionally, cloud-based monitoring programs may be quickly updated without having the individual install any software on their specific monitoring equipment, which makes system maintenance simple and convenient.

Finally, to give information that might be therapeutically valuable, it is important to manage and analyze the huge amount of data that may be gathered using wearable technology to monitor a patient's condition. Solutions for monitoring from afar that wouldn't have been practical without the use of artificial intelligence have been made possible by the analysis of data, transmission changes, recognition of patterns, mining of data, and other techniques.

Even though an overview of the different methods used for handling and analyzing adaptable detector data is not covered in this chapter, it is impossible to overstate how crucial data processing and evaluation methods are to the development and design of remote surveillance systems based on wearable devices.

4.3 SENSING TECHNOLOGY

The detectors used in remote surveillance systems are covered in detail in this section. The technologies discussed enable ubiquitous data collection utilizing body-worn (i.e., wearable) sensors. As noted earlier, when monitoring subjects in the home environment, wearable sensors and environmental sensors are commonly coupled, as schematically depicted in Figure 4.4. Multiple uses in the field of portable and ambient sensors in rehabilitation are of great interest.

One could be curious about using wearable sensors to monitor elderly people while adopting treatments to improve balance control and reduce falls. A particular design for data analysis would analyze vital signs and activity data to spot falls. The use of ambient sensors in this scenario may be combined with sensors that are worn to enhance the precision of fall detection and, more critically, make it practical to detect falls even in persons without sensors.

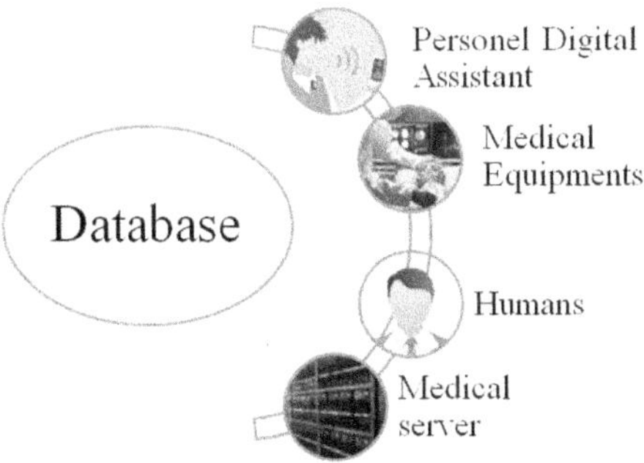

Figure 4.4 Individuals in their own homes can be discreetly observed using ambient sensors

4.4 RELATED WORK

Krishnan et al. [23] report on an end-to-end flow remote monitoring of health systems based on WLAN (wireless local area network). Using medical sensors, the system gathers vital indicators of the patient, including body temperature, oxygen saturation, arterial pressure, and heartbeat. This study did not use real-time ECG data for analysis. The primary CPU and data controller is an Arduino Yun. Following that, the data is transmitted to the internet through WLAN and a programming interface for applications (API).

The internet server can be used by doctors to speak with the patient and to access their medical information. The information will be temporarily kept on the memory card if the gadget loses its WIFI connection.

Once the link has been restored, the system will synchronize the information with the server. A smartphone-based method for remotely monitoring patients was suggested by Lee et al. [24]. This method makes use of an app for smartphones. To discuss the treatment plan through video chat, the patient can use a smartphone. Along with the Advanced Encryption Standard (AES)-style encryption used by Skype, this technique secures the patient's video data. Real-time mode is not supported by this system. The patient must manually input the vital signs onto the server. Roy et al. [25] demonstrated a system for RF-based remote patient monitoring that allows users to get medical information through online and portable software platforms.

The system is composed of the coordination node, web server, databases server, nodes for sensors, and graphical user interface (GUI) elements. Information is gathered by the sensor node. The acquired data is sent to the main server. Users may see the data and assess the results thanks to the GUI. Real-time mode cannot be supported by this system because of transmission latency and a sluggish server response.

Mustapha et al. [26] presented a Web Real-Time Communications (WebRTC) and Edge Cloud–based patient surveillance system, as seen in Figure 4.5. Edge Cloud is a platform for interaction between individuals as well as remote medical monitoring devices in addition to storage. The mechanism has two operating modes: push and pull. If suspicious health data is found when using push mode remote surveillance, the system notifies the user; with pull mode remote surveillance, the user may go back and evaluate the data that has already been acquired.

Raspberry Pi was utilized by Pap et al. to develop the data and video gathered to be examined by the system's analytical engine in an IoT-based e-health system with a major focus on video data processing and communication rather than health data [7]. One specific chart's data was kept in a Node.js server-side application, which also provided a web interface for users to see the chart.

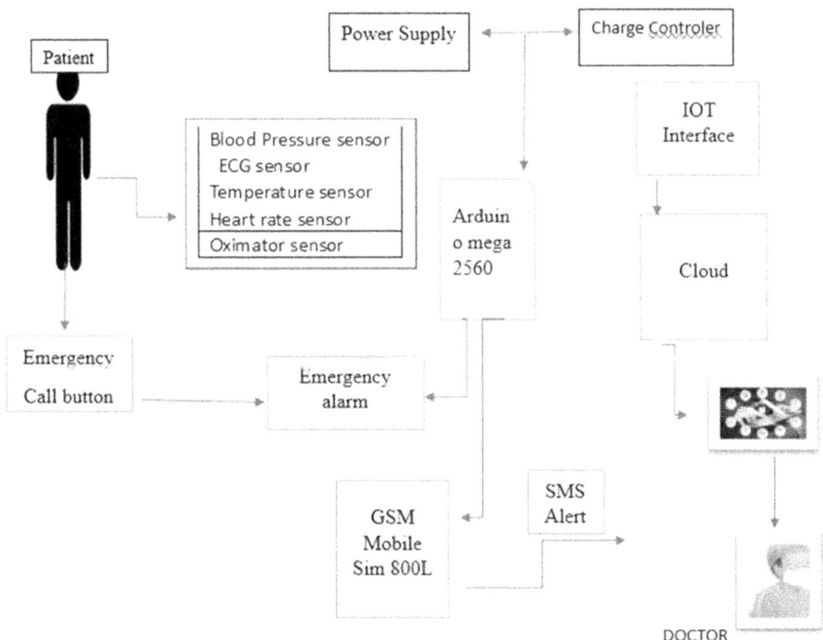

Figure 4.5 Related work for ECG

The e-health system has sensors for blood pressure, temperature, galvanic skin reaction, airflow, and pulse oximetry. With this method, a user can choose to gather data immediately or later. The information won't be saved forever in the real-time mode.

For the duration of the recording session, the data will be retained. An approach to problem identification is considered, and it is recommended.

For longer-term health monitoring using a stream, a WLAN-based system has been used. The device collects inconspicuous vital indicators including body temperature using therapeutic sensors [8].

An ECG flag was not required at the time the work was being done. Arduino Yun is the ideal controller for data handling and analysis. At that point, the data is transferred into the cloud through WLAN and the API. Specialists can access the Online Health Checking Server to receive clinical data and ask devoted server users questions. The information is temporarily kept in the memory flash in the unlikely event that the device loses its WLAN connection.

Once the link to the server has been restored, the structure will organize the data that is sent from it.

Sensor hubs, coordination nodes, customers, web browsers, and database servers with GUIs are all components of the framework [27]. The sensor hub is used to collect the data. The information is delivered to a big server. The GUI may be used by customers to make notes and assess the outcomes.

The network is unable to support real-time approaches because of broadcast disruptions and slow server answers. WebRTC was recommended by Mustapha et al. to create an unknowable monitoring system. Its secondary function is to act as a channel for interaction between patients as well as a more complex silent checking system. Push and pull are the two main working modes of the framework. When employing the push mode when connected to the internet, if aberrant health information is found, the framework alerts the client by sounding an alarm.

The pull mode aims to motivate the customer to assess the knowledge that has already been obtained. Many of the methods through which the cloud server interacts with a variety of frameworks enable WebRTC. The system's interpretative motor assesses the video and the gathered information.

A smartphone-based, inaccessible method of patient monitoring was suggested by Lee et al. [24]. An app for smartphones is run in this context. To discuss the diagnosis.

The patient's video data is protected by this architecture and Skype's AES intelligence encryption. This system does not handle real-time operations. To manually upload the acquired crucial symbol to the server, silence is necessary, a platform for IoT-based remote patient condition monitoring. It is built utilizing a hub-and-spoke design, with the sensor nodes serving as the spokes [9]. Almutairi et al. created an Android-based m-health monitoring system in which device information is gathered online [28]. This procedure uses a gadget to perform medical diagnoses. Gupta et al. developed a system that examines ECG data and delivers alarm signals to the appropriate individual depending on irregularity [29]. Acharya et al. presented an IoT-based smart healthcare monitoring kit that can track vital signs including heartbeat, ECG, body temperature, and breathing [30]. Its ability to provide a flexible connection with IoT data and multipurpose sensor networks that can assist emergency medical services is this system's key benefit. A wearable device based on a nonintrusive sensor that gathers data automatically was introduced by Z. Yang et al. [31]. An Arduino-based mobile device was presented by Trivedi et al. that might be used to continuously monitor vital bodily functions including temperature and heart rate with the right sensors [32].

Here, the sensor's analogue data is transformed into digital data using an internal A/D converter. This digital information is sent through a Wi-Fi module to the monitoring devices. A microprocessor manages all of the sensors, and an LCD displays the Micro control unit's (MCU) findings. But this device couldn't have more than one sensor. The Real-Time Wireless Pharmacological Monitoring System (RTWPMS) should be improved, according to Lin et al.

This system comes with a GPS module, a second-generation cordless phone, and a module for detecting heart rate, blood pressure, and body temperature. An IoT gadget created by Azariadi et al. monitors heart activity and offers medical services for ECG signals [34]. Khalid Abuelas et al. suggested a portable ECG monitoring device that can track the patient's temperature, respiration, and ECG [35].

4.5 EXPERIMENTAL SETUP

To evaluate the efficiency of the recommended solution in various scenarios, two tests have been set up in genuine networking installations. A local area network (LAN), sometimes referred to as a private network, is where the initial experiment is put up. As shown in Figure 4.5, the suggested architecture, data system, and PCs are all connected to the same access point. Assume the proposed system is provided to the hospital patients.

The obtained ECG data are kept on the internal server. Doctors can see ECG data from their offices in real time or as needed. The public wide area network (WAN) setup for the second trial is shown in Figure 4.6. The suggested system is linked to the house's WIFI [12,33]. The immediate time ECG information is sent to the cloud server through the internet. With their own mobile cellular network, doctors can view the patient's real-time ECG by connecting to a cloud server. The number of packet losses and the average jitter delay are used to gauge how well the proposed system performs. The website and Arduino Serial Monitor both displayed the real-time ECG signal. The ECG signal displayed on the Arduino Digital Monitor is the actual time ECG signal obtained by the AD8232 sensor. This ECG signal will be sent by the MQTT broker for storage in the database and display on the website's server.

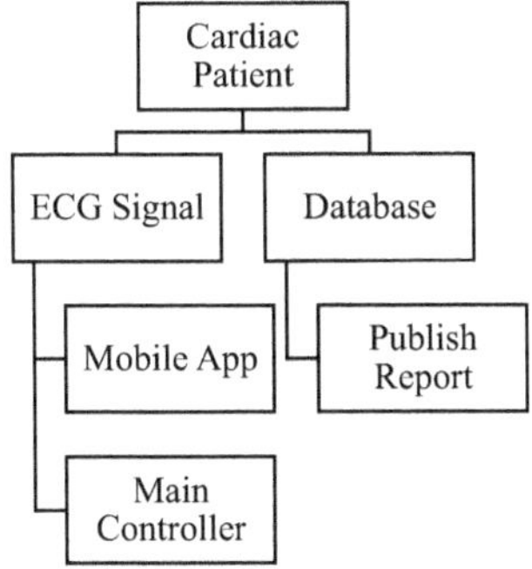

Figure 4.6 Experimental structure of ECG

4.5.1 Health and Wellness Monitoring

Numerous countries are promoting health insurance as the global population ages and healthcare costs grow. "Aging in place" programs enable senior citizens and others with chronic diseases to stay in their homes. They are being remotely watched for safety and to make it easier to implement clinical interventions.

It has been deemed of utmost importance to monitor the actions taken by older persons and those with chronic diseases who are taking part in aging in place programs. The ability of wearable sensors to categorize activities of daily living (ADL) has been the subject of much investigation. Accelerometers may be used to track the ADL performed by older persons being observed in their homes, as demonstrated by Mathie et al. in their study [36].

A set of in-shoe pressure and acceleration sensors was created by Sazonov et al. [37] to identify activities such as sitting, standing, and walking while also being able to determine whether participants were concurrently executing arm-extending motions. Gian Santi et al. [38] developed an accelerometer-based device for Parkinson's disease sufferers to track their steps.

Aziz et al. [39] used wearable sensors to monitor patients' recovery following abdominal surgery. Activity monitoring for wellness applications has been shown in several studies to significantly boost exercise adherence in at-risk groups.

For instance, smartwatches have been used to track physical activity in obese people and to make rehabilitative interventions easier to apply in order to promote a healthy and active lifestyle [40–43]. With commercially available technology, it is possible to gain continuous monitoring of heart rate, blood pressure, oxygen saturation, respiration rate, body temperature, and skin galvanic response. Clinical investigations are now assessing and validating wearable sensor systems' capacity to constantly monitor physiologic data and enhance patient treatment care, such as those with congestive cardiac failure [44, 45].

The clinical evaluation of wearable technology created as part of important research programs is the subject of several active studies. For instance, similar uses are being investigated for Live Net, a system created by the MIT Media Laboratory. Live Net records epileptic episodes and evaluates 3D accelerated motions, ECG, EMG, and electrical skin conductance [46].

A special data recorder called Lifeguard was developed to monitor people's health in dangerous environments (both in space and on Earth) [47]. Tests on the system have been done successfully under difficult circumstances. AMON, a project supported by the FP5 program and funded by the European Commission, employs a wrist-worn gadget that can measure arterial pressure, temperature of the skin, blood oxygen saturation, and ECG [48]. Other noteworthy initiatives that have been carried out as a part of various European Commission programs include My Heart [49],

WEALTHY [50, 51], and Magic [52, 53]. These initiatives resulted in the creation of wearable sensors that can monitor people's overall health when they are at home and in community settings, and are helpful in upcoming 6G [54] technology.

4.6 FINDINGS AND DISCUSSION

According to Figure 4.7, the experiment's findings demonstrate that neither private nor public networks experience packet loss or mistakes. This is due to the checksum mechanism of the MQTT protocol. If subscribers don't receive the packet, it will be resent. The next packet will eventually be sent, although there will be a wait.

On comparing the whole amount of ECG data from the chosen range of 5,000 packets between the sender (main controller) and subscriber to further ensure, there were no packet errors (database system or website). The findings demonstrate that the sender's and subscriber's combined ECG readings are comparable.

Public networks perform around ten times better than private networks in terms of oscillation latency. This is required for the public connection to send data farther than the private network. Since there is a limitation of up to 1 s, the general population's network's delay of 50.08 ms is sufficient [55]. The ECG signal [56] is available on the website and the Arduino Serial Display in both private and public networks.

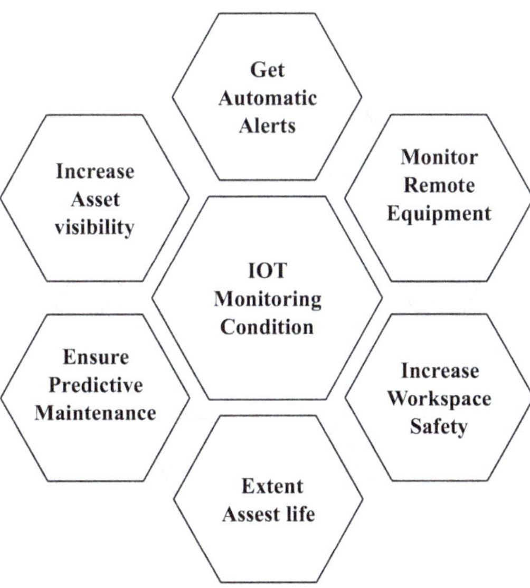

Figure 4.7 IoT asset condition monitoring

4.7 CONCLUSION

Recent studies have shifted focus from smartwatches to monitoring health and well-being, emphasizing the importance of wearable sensors and systems in rehabilitation. This review of research provides an overview of core technologies developed over the past decade, with a primary focus on rehabilitation. The study also emphasizes the use of mobile sensors and systems in clinical applications. House robots will soon be integrated into home surveillance systems, and revenue streams for remote monitoring of older people and those receiving medical treatment will be required. A system for remote monitoring of patients has been tested on public and private networks, demonstrating successful online display and storage of real-time ECG signals on a cloud server. This system can reduce travel time and expenses for patients from remote or suburban locations, allowing clinicians to remotely monitor ECG readings. This approach may improve healthcare delivery across the country. Additional work may include incorporating an ECG self-engine, upgrading the system with additional e-health sensors, and reducing jitter delay and noise signal. Combining IoT with cloud computing can improve the monitoring of elderly patients in retirement communities and other high-quality care facilities. A data gathering and tracking system for temperature, heart rate, blood pressure, and ECG is described, which automatically uploads information to health workers' shared cloud server, ThingSpeak. This system may save medical costs by reducing regular doctor visits and hospital checkups.

REFERENCES

1. Ministry of Health India, Health indicators. Visit http://social.niti.gov.in/ to download this report.
2. Patel S, Park H, Bonato P, Chan L, Rodgers M A review of wearable sensors and systems with application in rehabilitation. *J Neuron Rehab* 2012, 9(1):21.
3. Yew HT, Aditya Y, Satria H, Supriya E, Hua YW Telecardiology system for fourth generation heterogeneous wireless networks. *ARPN J Eng Appl Sci*, 2015, 10(2): 20–31.
4. McMahan HB, Moore E, Ramage D, Hampson S, Arcas BA Communication efficient learning of deep networks from decentralized data. *Proceedings of the 20th International Conference on Artificial Intelligence and Statistics (Proceedings of Machine Learning Research)* (Vol. 54, pp. 1273–1282). PMLR, Fort Lauderdale, FL, 2017.
5. Konecky J, McMahan HB, Felix XY, Tarik PR, Suresh AT, Bacon D Federated learning: Strategies for improving communication efficiency. arrive preprint arXiv:1610.05492 (2016), 2016.
6. Hard A, Rao K, Mathews R, Ramaswamy S, Beaufays F, Augustin S, Eichner H, Kiddon C, Ramage D Federated learning for mobile keyboard prediction. arXiv preprint arXiv:1811.03604 (2018), 2018.

7. Pap IA, Oniga S, Orha I, Alexan A IoT-based eHealth data acquisition system. *2018 IEEE International Conference on Automation, Quality and Testing, Robotics. AQTR 2018 - THETA 21st Ed. Proceedings* (pp. 1–5), 2018.
8. Boopala Krishnan N, Siva Sankara Sai S, Mohanthy SB Real time internet application with distributed flow environment for medical IoT. *2015 International Conference on Green Computing and Internet of Things (ICGCIoT)*, (pp. 832–837). October 2015. https://doi.org/10.1109/ICGCIoT.2015.7380578.
9. Garbhapu VV, Gopalan S IoT based low-cost single sensor node remote health monitoring system. *Procedia Comp. Sci.*, 2017, 113: 408–415.
10. Muennig PA, Glied SA What changes in survival rates tell us about US health care. *Health Affair* 2010, 29:2105–2113.
11. Gulley S, Rasch E, Chan L If we build it, who will come? Working-age adults with chronic health care needs and the medical home. *Medical Care* 2011, 49:149–155.
12. Gulley SP, Rasch EK, Chan L Ongoing coverage for ongoing care: Access, utilization, and out-of-pocket spending among uninsured working-aged adults with chronic health care needs. *Am J Public Health* 2011, 101:368–375.
13. Brand O Microsensor integration into systems-on-chip. *Proceedings of the IEEE* 2006, 94:1160–1176.
14. DeVaul R, Sung M, Gips J, Pentland A MIThril 2003: Applications and architecture. *Seventh IEEE International Symposium on Wearable Computers* (pp. 4–11), 2003.
15. ZigBee Alliance. http://www.zigbee.org.
16. Zhang J, Orlik PV, Sahinoglu Z, Molisch AF, Kinney P UWB systems for wireless sensor networks. *Proceedings of the IEEE* 2009, 97:313–331.
17. Want R iPhone: Smarter than the average phone. *Pervasive Computing IEEE* 2010, 9:6–9.
18. Want R When cell phones become computers. *IEEE Pervasive Computing* 2009, 8:2–5.
19. Botts N, Thoms B, Noamani A, Horan TA Cloud computing architectures for the underserved: Public health cyberinfrastructures through a network of health ATMs. *System Sciences (HICSS), 2010 43rd Hawaii International Conference* (pp. 1–10). 5–8 January 2010.
20. Chang HH, Chou PB, Ramakrishnan S An ecosystem approach for healthcare services cloud. *e-Business Engineering. 2009 ICEBE '09 IEEE International Conference* (pp. 608–612). 21–23 October 2009.
21. Hoang DB, Chen L Mobile cloud for assistive healthcare (MO Cash). *Services Computing Conference (APSCC), 2010 IEEE Asia-Pacific* (pp. 325–332). 6–10 December 2010.
22. Rao GSVRK, Sundararaman K, Parthasarathi J Dhatri - A pervasive cloud initiative for primary healthcare services. *Intelligence in Next Generation Networks (ICIN), 2010 14th International Conference* (pp. 1–6). 11–14 October 2010.
23. Krishnan NB, Sai SSS, Mohanthy SB Real time internet application with distributed flow environment for medical IoT. *Proceedings 2015 International Conference on Green Computing, Internet Things, ICGCIoT 2015* (pp. 832–837), 2016.

24. Lee EK, Wang Y, Davis RA, Egan BM Designing a low-cost adaptable and personalized remote patient monitoring system. In *2017 IEEE International Conference on Bioinformatics and Biomedicine (BIBM)* (pp. 1040–1046), IEEE, 2017.
25. Roy S, Rahman A, Helal M, Kaiser MS, Chowdhury ZI Low-cost RF based online patient monitoring using web and mobile applications, *2016 5th International Conference on Informatics, Electronics Vision, ICIEV 2016* (pp. 869–874), 2016.
26. Moustafa H, Schooler EM, Shen G, Kamath S Remote monitoring and medical devices control in eHealth. *2016 IEEE 12th International Conference on Wireless and Mobile Computing, Networking and Communications (WiMob)* (pp. 1–8), 2016.
27. Iqbal MW, Ahmad N, Shahzad SK, Naqvi MR, Feroz I Usability aspects of adaptive mobile interfaces for colour-blind and vision deficient users. *Int J Comput Netw Inf Secur* 2018, 18(10):179–189.
28. Almotiri SH, Khan MA, Alghamdi MA Mobile health (m-health) system in the context of IoT. *2016 IEEE 4th International Conference on Future Internet of Things and Cloud Workshops (FiCloudW)* (pp. 39–42). IEEE, 2016, August.
29. Gupta P, Agrawal D, Chhabra J, Dhir PK IoT based smart healthcare kit. *2016 International Conference on Computational Techniques in Information and Communication Technologies (ICCTICT)* (pp. 237–242). IEEE, 2016, March.
30. Alsahi QN, Marhoon AF, Hamad AH Remote patient healthcare surveillance system based real-time vital signs. *Al-Khwarizmi Eng J* 2020, 16(4):41–51.
31. Yang Z, Zhou Q, Lei L, Zheng K, Xiang W An IoT-cloud based wearable ECG monitoring system for smart healthcare. *J Med Syst* 2016, 40(12):1–11.
32. Trivedi S, Cheeran AN Android based health parameter monitoring. *2017 International Conference on Intelligent Computing and Control Systems (ICICCS)* (pp. 1145–1149). IEEE, 2017, June.
33. Lin BS, Chou NK, Chong FC, Chen SJ RTWPMS: A real-time wireless physiological monitoring system. *IEEE Transactions on Information Technology in Biomedicine* 2006, 10(4):647–656.
34. Azariadi D, Tsoutsouras V, Xydis S, Soudris D ECG signal analysis and arrhythmia detection on IoT wearable medical devices. *2016 5th International Conference on Modern Circuits and Systems Technologies (MOCAST)* (pp. 1–4). IEEE, 2016, May.
35. Abualsaud K, Chowdhury ME, Gehani A, Yaacoub E, Khattab T, Hammad J A new wearable ECG monitor evaluation and experimental analysis: Proof of concept. *2020 International Wireless Communications and Mobile Computing (IWCMC)* (pp. 1885–1890). IEEE, 2020, June.
36. Mathie MJ, Coster AC, Lovell NH, Celler BG, Lord SR, Tiedemann A A pilot study of long-term monitoring of human movements in the home using accelerometry. *J Telemed Telecare* 2004, 10:144–151.
37. Sazonov ES, Fulk G, Sazonova N, Schuckers S Automatic recognition of postures and activities in stroke patients. *Conference of the IEEE Engineering in Medicine and Biology Society* (pp. 2200–2203), 2009.

38. Giansanti D, Maccioni G, Morelli S An experience of health technology assessment in new models of care for subjects with Parkinson's disease by means of a new wearable device. *Telemed J E Health* 2008, 14:467–472.
39. Aziz O, Atallah L, Lo B, Elhelw M, Wang L, Yang GZ, Darzi A A pervasive body sensor network for measuring postoperative recovery at home. *Surg Innov* 2007, 14:83–90.
40. Amft O, Troster G Recognition of dietary activity events using on-body sensors. *Artif Intell Med* 2008, 42:121–136.
41. Amft O, Kusserow M, Troster G Bite weight prediction from acoustic recognition of chewing. *IEEE Trans Biomed Eng* 2009, 56:1663–1672.
42. Benedetti MG, Di Gioia A, Conti L, Berti L, Esposti LD, Tarrini G, Melchionda N, Giannini S Physical activity monitoring in obese people in the real life environment. *J Neuroeng Rehabil* 2009, 6:17.
43. Sazonov ES, Schuckers SA, Lopez-Meyer P, Makeyev O, Melanson EL, Neuman MR, Hill JO Toward objective monitoring of ingestive behavior in free-living population. *Obesity (Silver Spring)* 2009, 17:1971–1975.
44. Merilahti J, Parkka J, Antila K, Paavilainen P, Mattila E, Malm EJ, Saarinen A, Korhonen I Compliance and technical feasibility of long-term health monitoring with wearable and ambient technologies. *J Telemed Telecare* 2009, 15:302–309.
45. Sciacqua A, Valentini M, Gualtieri A, Perticone F, Faini A, Zacharioudakis G, Karatzanis I, Chiarugi F, Assimakopoulou C, Meriggi P, et al. Validation of a flexible and innovative platform for the home monitoring of heart failure patients: Preliminary results. *Comput Cardiol* 2009, 36:97–100.
46. Sung M, Marci C, Pentland A Wearable feedback systems for rehabilitation. *J Neuroeng Rehabil* 2005, 2:17.
47. Mundt CW, Montgomery KN, Udoh UE, Barker VN, Thonier GC, Tellier AM, Ricks RD, Darling RB, Cagle YD, Cabrol NA, et al. A multiparameter wearable physiologic monitoring system for space and terrestrial applications. *IEEE Trans Inf Technol Biomed* 2005, 9:382–391.
48. Anliker U, Ward JA, Lukowicz P, Troster G, Dolveck F, Baer M, Keita F, Schenker EB, Catarsi F, Coluccini L, et al. AMON: A wearable multiparameter medical monitoring and alert system. *IEEE Trans Inf Technol Biomed* 2004, 8:415–427.
49. Habetha J The MyHeart project–fighting cardiovascular diseases by prevention and early diagnosis. *Conference of the IEEE Engineering in Medicine and Biology Society* (pp. 6746–6749), 2006.
50. Paradiso R, Loriga G, Taccini N Wearable system for vital signs monitoring. *Stud Health Technol Inform* 2004, 108:253–259.
51. Paradiso R, Alonso A, Cianflone D, Milsis A, Vavouras T, Malliopoulos C Remote health monitoring with wearable non-invasive mobile system: The healthwear project. *Conference of the IEEE Engineering in Medicine and Biology Society* (pp. 1699–1702), 2008.
52. Di Rienzo M, Rizzo F, Parati G, Brambilla G, Ferratini M, Castiglioni P MagIC system: A new textile-based wearable device for biological signal monitoring. applicability in daily life and clinical setting. *Conference of the IEEE Engineering in Medicine and Biology Society* (pp. 7167–7169), 2005.

53. Di Rienzo M, Rizzo F, Meriggi P, Bordoni B, Brambilla G, Ferratini M, Castiglioni P Applications of a textile-based wearable system for vital signs monitoring. *Conference of the IEEE Engineering in Medicine and Biology Society* (pp. 2223–2226), 2006.
54. Jain R, Aole K, Mittal S, Ranjan P An analysis on wireless communication in 6G THz network and their challenges. In *Terahertz Devices, Circuits and Systems: Materials, Methods and Applications* (pp. 167–181). Singapore: Springer Nature Singapore, 2022.
55. Yew HT, Supriyanto E, Satria MH, Hau YW Adaptive network selection mechanism for telecardiology system in developing countries. *3rd IEEE EMBS International Conference on Biomedical and Health Informatics, BHI 2016*, 2016.
56. Wijayanto I, Humairani A, Hadiyoso S, Rizal A, Prasanna DL, Tripathi SL Epileptic seizure detection on a compressed EEG signal using energy measurement. *Biomed Signal Process Control*, 2023, 85:104872. https://doi.org/10.1016/j.bspc.2023.104872.

Chapter 5

Revolutionizing Industry 4.0 with Blockchain Technology

Opportunities and Challenges

Ravi Prakash, Shobha Tyagi, and Ratnesh Litoriya

5.1 INTRODUCTION TO INDUSTRY 4.0

Necessity is the mother of all inventions. It goes perfectly well with the various eras of industrial revolution that revolutionized the world as new requirements upgraded technology or revamped lifestyles or changed the operational status of workers [1–5]. Each industrial revolution era produced some remarkable repercussions and accordingly propelled the next generation with greater impetus to think outside the box to produce once-inconceivable innovations. The first generation of the industrial revolution (1760 to 1840) harnessed steam power, which increased and remarkedly changed the efficiency of human labor and transportation. The second generation of the industrial revolution (1863–1947) is primarily acknowledged for the discovery of electricity and enhanced factory production following the assembly line production process, leading to the mass production of products and automobile manufacturing leading to more affordable prices for consumers [6–14]. The third generation of the industrial revolution (1969–2010) paved the path of partial automation with the advent of microprogrammed controls embedded into computers, like robots that could sufficiently handle production lines with less human intervention. The fourth generation of the industrial revolution (2010–present) supports the mantra of staying connected whenever and wherever people go with the amalgamation of advancements in computational intelligence, algorithmic research refinements, and networking technologies. All these developments have considerably accelerated automation and seeded autonomy everywhere whether it is paying bills comfortably from home, entering into smart business contracts securely, planning overseas vacations including booking the flight and hotel and arranging a local taxi for sightseeing, remotely controlling home appliances, or completely automating production lines [15–23].

The industrial revolution characterizes the best traits of information technologies, thus making the world smaller, smarter, and more accessible. The Internet of Things (IoT), self-organizing manufacturing environment, augmented reality, moving from the classic binary bits to the qubits of quantum

DOI: 10.1201/9781003466949-5

computing, ubiquitous computing, mobility of content, and blockchain are some of the applications of the fourth industrial revolution (shown in Figure 5.1). This chapter details how blockchain technology is acting as a transformational ladder to a secure pathway to Industry 4.0 [24–31].

Before discussing how blockchain technology is going to embrace the principles of Industry 4.0, let's dive into the deep ocean of blockchain technology and its entangled principles of architecture, supported by cryptographic techniques.

The chapter is organized into six sections. The first section introduces the basic concepts of industrialization and its growth over time, i.e., the remarkable journey from Industry 1.0 to Industry 4.0 to satisfy our ever-evolving demands. Section 5.2 discusses the background of blockchain technology and the necessity of this secured technology to deal with the voluminous and individualized data in alignment with the revolutionary Industry 4.0. Section 5.3 delineates the blockchain architecture and chronologically provides appropriate examples. Section 5.4 reinforces the contemporary applications underpinned by blockchain technology. Section 5.5 elucidates the societal implications of blockchain technology. The last section is the conclusive discussion of adapting blockchain as a pathway toward Industry 4.0.

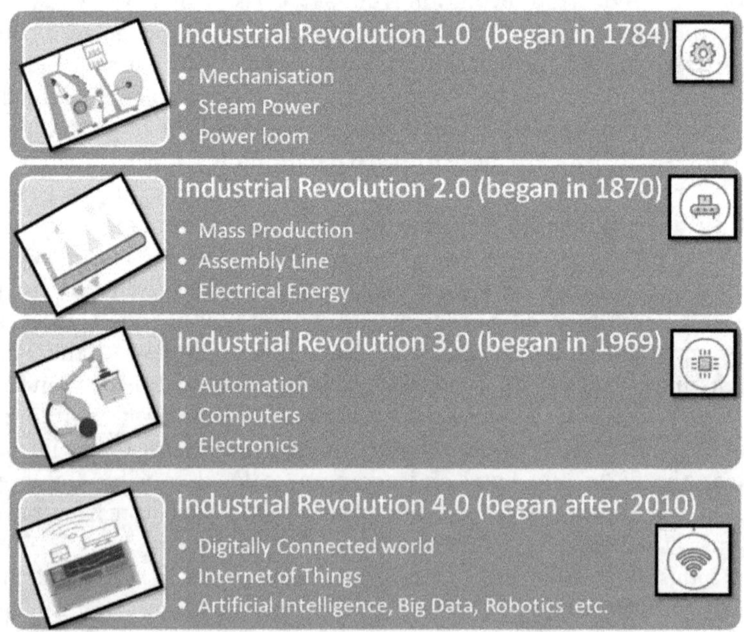

Figure 5.1 Timeline of the industrial revolution from 1.0 to 4.0

5.2 BACKGROUND OF BLOCKCHAIN TECHNOLOGY

Blockchain can be defined as "a collaborated, digitally timestamped integrated environment to bring together all the stakeholders for a particular application on a distributed platform where each piece of information regarding terms and conditions and the transactions are created and verified by all the peer groups and then stored securely in digital ledgers, which cannot be altered by any one stakeholder. The moment blocks are tampered with, the whole transaction gets invalidated" [2]. It is based on the CIA properties and lays the foundation behind making the transactions secure and stored in tamper-proof blocks (shown in Figure 5.2):

C stands for confidentiality, which ensures information remains confined to authorized users.
I represents integrity and ensures that data is accurate and has not been changed by an unauthorized user.
A stands for availability and guarantees that data is accessible only to authorized users.

Blockchain is a contemporary technology that promotes security and transparency in online communications, thereby being able to eliminate counterfeiting and vulnerabilities to a great extent. Blockchain relies on establishing reliable communication networks brimming with secured transactions and their corresponding sealed data records [26].

Blockchain is a technology in which timestamped sequences of immutable blocks are created using cryptographic techniques like asymmetric key cryptography and hash algorithms. These blocks are created in a distributed and cascaded manner (to produce a block at level i + 1 requires

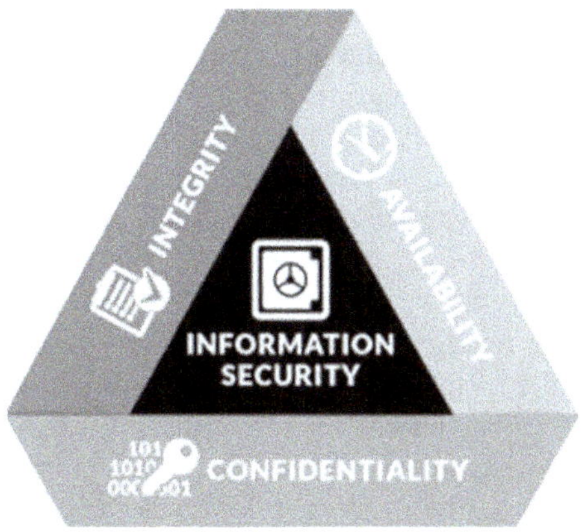

Figure 5.2 The foundation blocks of information security. (Available online at https://images.app.goo.gl/SJoMUrlZqHyXy85P7)

credentials of the block at level i) and are arranged based on timestamps in which they are created and finally weaved into a chain of these produced secured and sealed blocks. Any alteration or tampering in any one block will invalidate the complete series of blockchains for a given transaction. Blockchain technology maintains the transaction database over various computers connected through the internet [32–40].

In blockchain technology contract codes are written that dictate the terms and conditions that all involved parties are legally bound to. This coded or smart contract is encapsulated inside the blockchain, secured through cryptographic algorithms, and cannot be tampered with by any person or authority involved in the transaction [31]. Every involved party can keep track of the data and verify its authenticity. If any stakeholder/attacker tries to tamper with the data stored in the smart contract, then it may invalidate the whole contract and the transaction gets aborted [21]. (A smart contract can also enter the figure of cascaded barcodes in terms of milestones achieved and then some actions are taken or else aborted.) Contracts are executed depending on what rules are satisfied and which actions are being taken [34].

Earlier on there was risk involved because we have to rely on a centralized platform that may or may not be trustworthy. However, blockchain technology solves this issue as the network is decentralized because the computers are physically scattered and the address risk factor is handled by the cryptography techniques to store the data in cipher text so that it is not easily deciphered by the attackers. Availability and a risk-free environment are the two pioneered pillars ensuring security and transparency in all transactions.

Openness and data permanence into blocks, just like data stored in ROM is permanently available and cannot be changed, makes blockchain popular and advantageous to contemporary applications.

An abundance of blockchain technology platforms is available to make transactions secure and distributed, including Hyperledger, Ethereum, Ripple, and Rootstock. These are the platforms on which secure transactions can be implemented with immense transparency among the stakeholders in the business. So in a very simple language, we can see that these blocks contain digitally signed data using the concepts of cryptography which are put inside the ledger once verified by peer groups [18].

Just as data can be stored in a basic variable to hold a single value, sometimes we may require several locations to nurture multiple data like arrays, stacks, heaps, or linked lists. Similarly, implementing blockchain requires a block as a basic data structure where we can capture a lot of transactions depending upon the contract for which the block is created. The size of a block in a blockchain can vary from 1 MB to a maximum of 8 MB [9]. A block can generally contain hundreds of transactions, which may increase or decrease depending on the scope of the application for which the blockchain was created.

5.3 ARCHITECTURE OF BLOCKCHAIN TECHNOLOGY

Bitcoin is a popular terminology used in blockchain and represents the atomic entity that can hold a lot of transactional data (like an agreement signed between X and Y for $10,000 at a particular timestamp, *t* secs, regarding a sale of health equipment). The hash code of this agreement with the hash code of the previous block is calculated using the *SHA-256* hash algorithm to produce a message digest size of 256 bits, which acts as a unique hash code or fingerprint for the document. This produced hash code is entirely dependent upon all the bits of the data, as even a single bit modification in data could entirely change the structure of subsequent hash codes.

Table 5.1 represents a contract signed between two parties X and Y regarding placing an order of 1,000 health equipment and all other details that were a part of the contract, including agreement conditions, location, the amount involved, quality of product, and the date by which the equipment are to be delivered.

Based on contract data (as shown in able 5.1), which has been digitally agreed upon and digitally signed by both the involved parties (X and Y). A hash code of 64 bits (**6d005ae4f4a7508a2265486c2b2ef42f87ad2b30 0930b450f31efaef7c6eb94e**) in hexadecimal (these 64 bits if expanded as 64 × 4 results in 256 bits) is produced (as shown in Figure 5.3).

Whenever a new event or activity is added, a new hash code (**Bbe37 95730dbbd66239536dcfa274e2f9caa9dd9867ff12e3db2a7a0b0d5d0f1**) is produced using the previous hash code and data of the newly added event. Thus a new blockchain is added at the next level as shown in Figure 5.4.

If an attacker tries to tamper the data of any block of blockchain (like the amount involved changed from $10,000 to $1,000,000, as shown in Table 5.2), its hash code changes from **6d005ae4f4a7508a2265486c2b2ef4 2f87ad2b300930b450f31efaef7c6eb94e** to **C80ad064726936340faa51086 408868a5c418f4bf0b8ec43f459bba182e5e589**.

When the hash code of the previous phase changes, it impacts the hash code at the next level (hash code at level 2 changed from **Bbe3795730dbbd6**

Table 5.1 Contract Data between Two Independent Parties X and Y

X: Buyer
Y: Seller
Amount involved: $10000
Time stamp: 10:35pm
Date: 23/06/20
Location: New Jersey
Purpose: Purchased Health Equipment (Equipment Z with precision 10mm and quantity as 100 in no.) from Y
Condition: If Z is not delivered by 26/12/20 then agreement will be ceased and will be irrevocable.

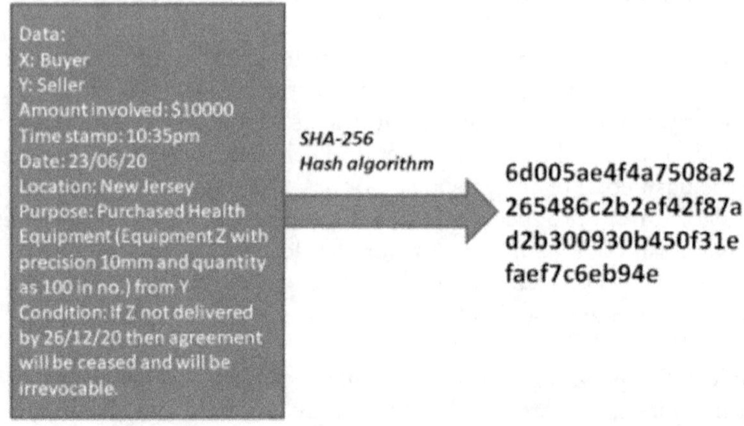

Figure 5.3 The hash code (in hexadecimal code) of the coded contract (shown in shaded block)

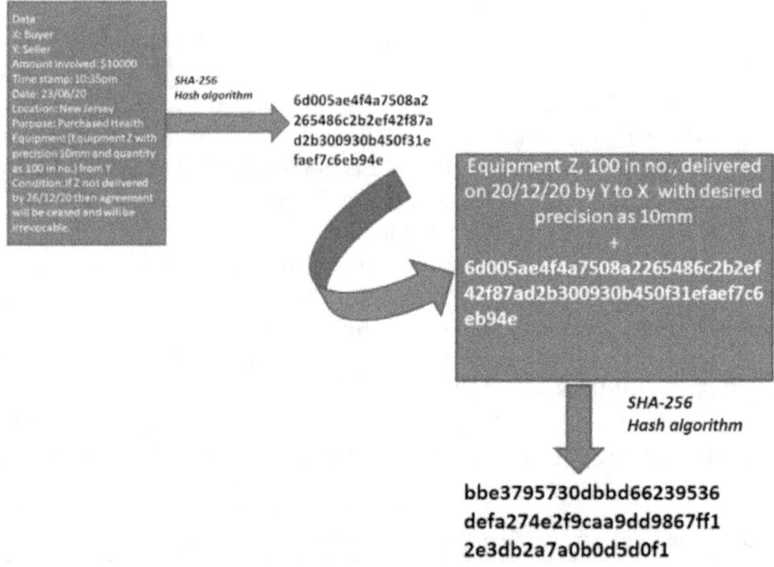

Figure 5.4 The hash code (in hexadecimal code) at the next level when fed with the new contract from the previous level and combined with the credentials at the next level to produce the hash code for the next level (shown in the right-hand shaded block)

Table 5.2 Breaching of Contract Data between Two Independent Parties X and Y by an Attacker

X: Buyer
Y: Seller
Amount involved: $1000000
Time stamp: 10:35pm
Date: 23/06/20
Location: New Jersey
Purpose: Purchased Health Equipment (Equipment Z with precision 10mm and quantity as 100 in no.) from Y
Condition: If Z is not delivered by 26/12/20 then agreement will be ceased and will be irrevocable.

6239536defa274e2f9caa9dd9867ff12e3db2a7a0b0d5d0f1 to 491a280ba57e4976abc0426ce3edb08e6b4ee51b427e25fcd116c245d55a849c).

This change will be sent for verification to all the involved parties, who will verify the data. If they find some discrepancy in block data, the whole blockchain will immediately be invalidated to nullify the undesirable changes done to the block (as shown in Figure 5.5).

The change in the first transaction from $10,000 to $1,000,000 produced a different hash code, and a discrepancy is noticed between the existing hash

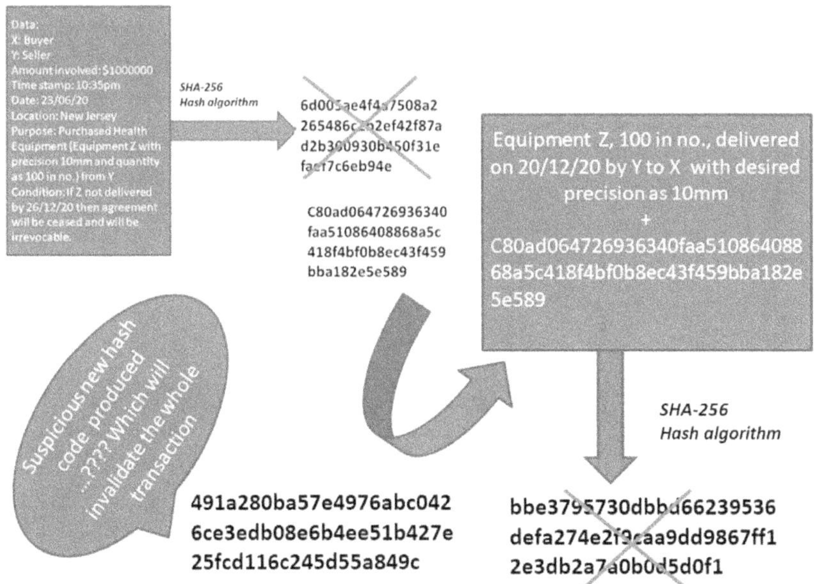

Figure 5.5 Challenging the existing hash code of the block (shown in oval) to a new maliciously fabricated hash code by an attacker gaining illegal access to a block of the blockchain

code and the newly broadcasted hash code (due to the change in amount and timestamp), which is sufficient enough to invalidate the transaction or else the hash code of the subsequent blocks will have to be recomputed, which is computationally very extensive [10]. To further tighten the security, there is another very important concept known as proof of work (PoW), which controls the rate at which the next-level blocks may be created (sets minimum time before which a block at the next level cannot be created). So even if an attacker is able to creep maliciously inside a blockchain, their penetration rate to breach damage to the chain is controlled and before it turns hostile the transaction would be declared as aborted to stop the damage to the integrity of the transaction and it will have to be reinitialized.

A block is a data structure that holds the summary of hashes of all the transactions that are stored in the block [14]. A block maintains the hierarchical structure of all the hashes of all the transactions individually in the form of a tree and then combines two hashes to produce a new hash in the upward direction, as shown in Figure 5.6, forming the Merkle root hash. A single change in the hash value of a transaction or changing its order can discard the entire data of the block.

Each block contains the hash code of the block at the previous level, the hash root of the Merkle tree, and a random number known as the nonce, which is randomly generated for each of the generated blocks.

The nonce effectively helps in adding randomness to the block, thus making the task of an attacker difficult because even if they can get hold of the hash code of a single block, it is almost impossible to randomly generate

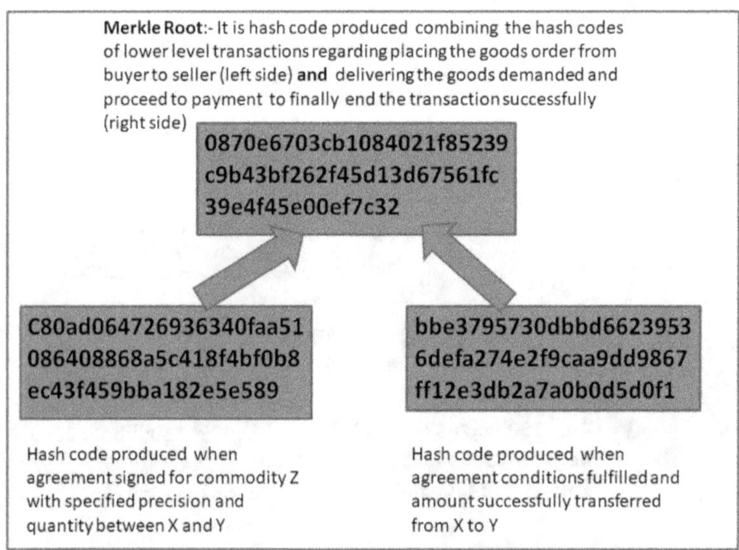

Figure 5.6 A Merkle root hash code is constructed by combining all the descendent hash codes of all the transactions contained in the block in a hierarchical manner

the nonce, which is unique for every data block in the blockchain [19]. The Merkle hash root is the digital footprint of all the digests that are produced for all the transactions that are stored in a block. The route hash for how a Merkle tree is produced is shown diagrammatically in Figure 5.6.

Each block generally has two segments:

Block header. The block header contains information such as the hash code of the previous block, Merkle root tree, and some mining enumeration to compute the hash code of the current block based on the code of the transactions of the block, nonce, date, time, and difficulty level with which the information stored in the block can be hacked (easy or difficult) (see Table 5.3) [28]. All these statistics are essential to building a block and all the transactions that it encapsulates.

A miner verifies the number of transactions and assimilates them into blocks. Each transaction has the attributes listed in Table 5.4.

There are numerous reasons to use this technology, including the creation of blocks that happens in a distributed fashion (eliminates centralized autonomy and a single point of crash), till the time transaction is not complete. Digital blocks are created to store data in an encrypted form, not in plain text, so it cannot be easily attacked.

Every action performed in the transaction is fully transparent to all the entities involved, which prevents the blockchain from being altered.

Table 5.3 Attributes of a Block in Blockchain

Hash: A number that identifies a block uniquely
Confirmations: How many approvals are received for the verification of a block
Timestamp: Timeline at which a block was initiated; both day and time are included
Height: Number of blocks to which the current block is linked
Miner: The one who corroborates the transactions stored in the block
Number of transactions: Cardinality of transactions in the current block
Difficulty: Level with which hash code of this block can be computed
Merkle root: Footprint of the hash code of all the transactions in a hierarchical order, following bottom to top approach
Version: Indicates under which version of blockchain technology the current block belongs to
Bits: A unit of BTC
Weight: Calibrates the size of different transactions in the block with regard to the allotted size of the block technologically
Size: Allocated size of the block as supported by technology
Nonce: Randomly generated value to support proof of work
Transaction volume: Amount of money transactions for the current block in terms of BTC
Block reward: A form of reward calculated frozenly for the person or miner who computed the hash code for the current block after transactions have been verified by the peer groups
Fee reward: A form of the service fee a person or miner charges to calculate the hash code for all the transactions and eventually the hash code of the block (which is governed by all the hash code of descendent transactions)

Table 5.4 Attributes of a Transaction in a Block in Blockchain

Hash: A unique number that identifies a transaction uniquely
Status: Indicates whether transaction has been verified by peer groups or not, accordingly included in a block (confirmed or unconfirmed)
Received time: The date and time at which the transaction was received by the network for verification
Size: Size of the transaction in bytes
Weight: Size of the transaction to that of total size of the block
Included in block: This transaction was committed in which block
Confirmations: Indicates the number of confirmations for a particular transaction from the authorized peer group in the connected network. After being verified, it is added to the block and eventually the blockchain
Total input: How much BTC as input is spent for the given transaction
Total output: How much BTC as output is spent for the given transaction
Fees: Amount spent to get a transaction verified and finally added to the block
Value when transacted: The amount the transaction was initiated in BTC or USD

The blocks created at each level are aligned as a blockchain and remain immutable, even if an attacker or insider tries to breach the integrity of the transaction.

The beauty of the impregnable technology lies in the crux that a change in a single bit of any block record may greatly impact the encrypted form of plain text and propagate this discrepancy into the entire digital ledger, which is enough to invalidate the entire series of transactions. Blockchain technology provides a flexible and open platform to equally and fairly contribute to the ethics of online and secured communications.

Every entity involved in the business network contributes equally to making a transaction secure and transparent, by giving a synchronized set of record transactions, which are accessible to all involved parties. All the events that have happened since the transaction began to the moment it finishes are recorded with a unique timestamp to reveal its transparency and hinder counterfeiting. Each block inherits some of the credentials from its predecessor block and in the same way aids its successor block in assimilating as the transaction process progresses toward completion. For example, all the transactions involved from crop production to its being sold, including quantity, price, location, date, time, transportation, and buyer, are recorded in these digital ledgers, so that no discrepancies can creep in and malign the transaction system at any level. An attacker can easily alter one or two transactions in a conventional security mechanism, without being caught or challenged, but in blockchain, it is almost impossible to alter any single block. If the blockchain is altered, it aborts the transaction and invalidates the whole process.

Blockchain finds its heaviest application in automating supply chain management. For example, in the diamond industry, it can record diamond purity in terms of clarity, weight, cost, color, and certification. Thus it helps customers to get the diamonds worth their price, without any manipulation or interference from its mining to it being sold.

It can be treated as an Economy of Things, which is an ensemble of trust, fairness, and total participation. To exert influence on the origin and purity of diamonds, the Brilliant Earth company used blockchain technology to guide customers about a diamond's authenticity. All diamond certification-related documents are available to the customers with great transparency

In the food industry, blockchain can verify the freshness of food products, whether it be farm products like blueberries and strawberries or seafood like fish or prawns. The concept of food safety and preservation using blockchain technology is shown in Figure 5.7. At every step of food procurement, a barcode is affixed to cartons/boxes in the following sequence:

Farm → Growing crops → Producing crop products → Packing in cartons (information such as name of food item, carton number, type of product [perishable versus nonperishable], number of packets, weight, time, date, starting location, destination, etc. are recorded in the digital ledger) → Transporting of cartons (can be identified using the barcodes and can be tracked anywhere in the world using the distributed digital technology of blockchain) → Delivery to companies that preserve and pack food items in a way that maintains freshness (again credentials added to the block include company name, manufacturing date, expiry date, company location, weight, price, ingredients, barcode) → Retailers → Consumers

Figures 5.8–5.12 represent how a barcode is produced and validated to uniquely identify a particular activity/event using data at every phase of

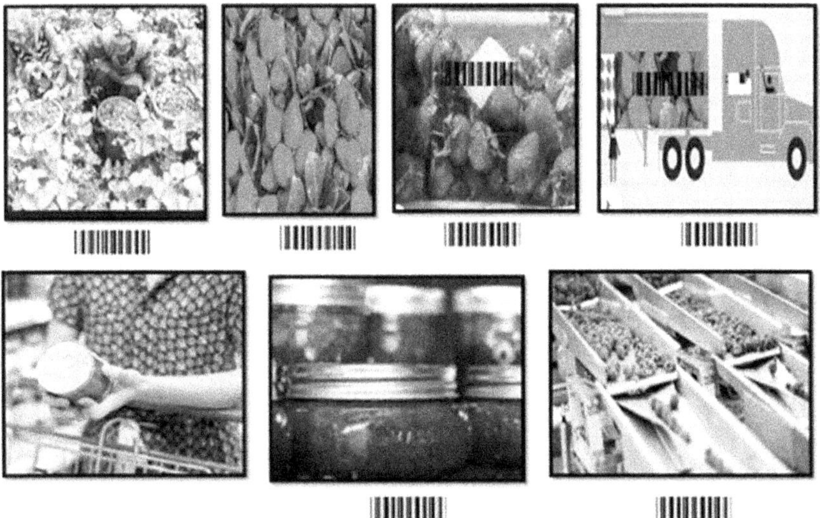

Figure 5.7 Supply chain of food items may be secured and distributed using blockchain technologies, from the stage of procurement of food items from farms to the point of being delivered to customers, maintaining the proof of transparency

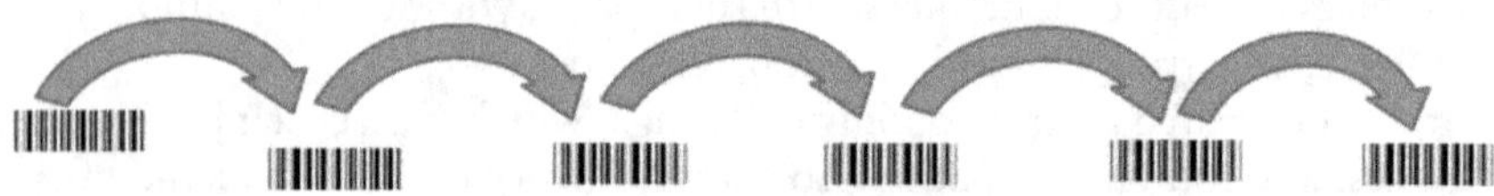

Figure 5.8 Cascading of transactional data contributes to the transparency and uniqueness of the distributed system using blockchain technology

the supply chain through blockchain technology. Figure 5.9 represents the annotations of bar codes produced using blockchain technology, at every stage of supply chain management (taking the example of strawberries produced on a farm until the strawberries are delivered to customers).

Every entity involved in the transactions can keep track of the data stored in the ledger and verify it. These data ledgers are integrated seamlessly to produce a blockchain of complete and consistent data, which is verifiable at any stage to check the authentication of the underlying transactions.

Barcodes	Remarks of produced Barcode at each level of handling product/services
	Farm Barcode (Farm location indicating region, where food is produced)
	Food Barcode (defines the identity of produced food)
	Packed Barcode (Food is packed indicating its freshness and quantity with date and time)
	Transportation Barcode (uniquely defines the transportation date and quantity transported, used generally to track distance covered)
	Food is processed in the food preservative industry (uniquely given a barcode during treating the food using preservatives to elongate its life)
	Food is packed properly in the industry with manufacturing date, expiry date, quantity, ingredients and preservatives used, how to use etc. (Uniquely given barcode during packaging the food item after preservation)

Figure 5.9 Annotations of bar codes produced using blockchain technology

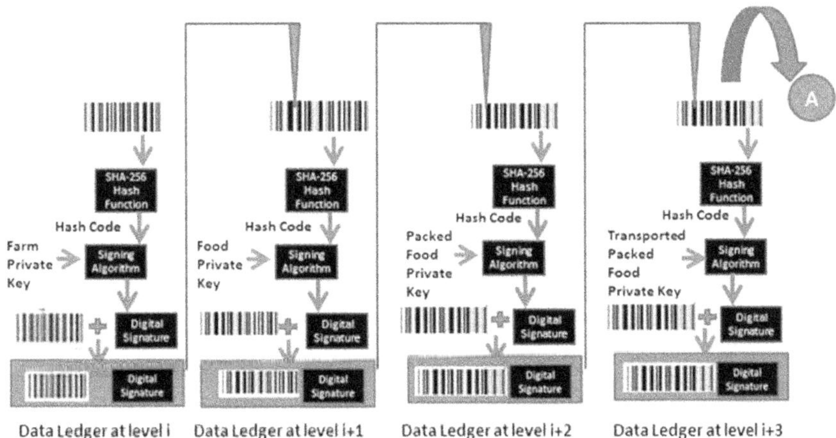

Figure 5.10 Data ledgers are created in a cascaded manner, from procurement to transportation of food items, to preserve transparency and maintain security using the cryptographic techniques in blockchain technology

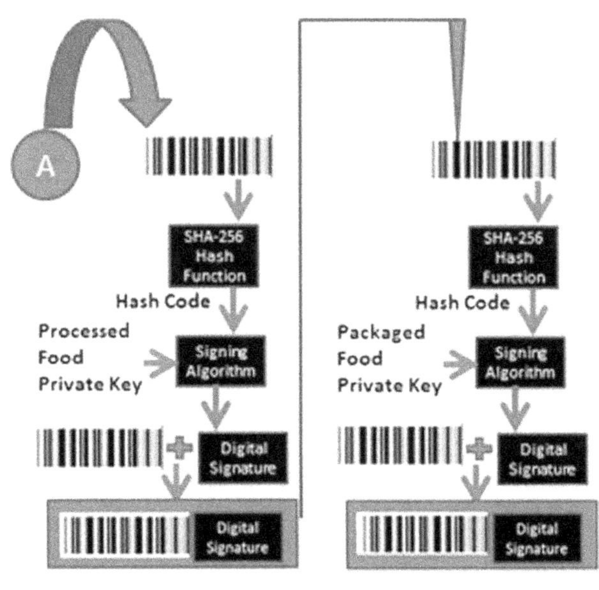

Figure 5.11 Extension of Figure 5.8. Data ledgers in blockchain are further created to accommodate the processing and packaging of the item to be delivered to customers

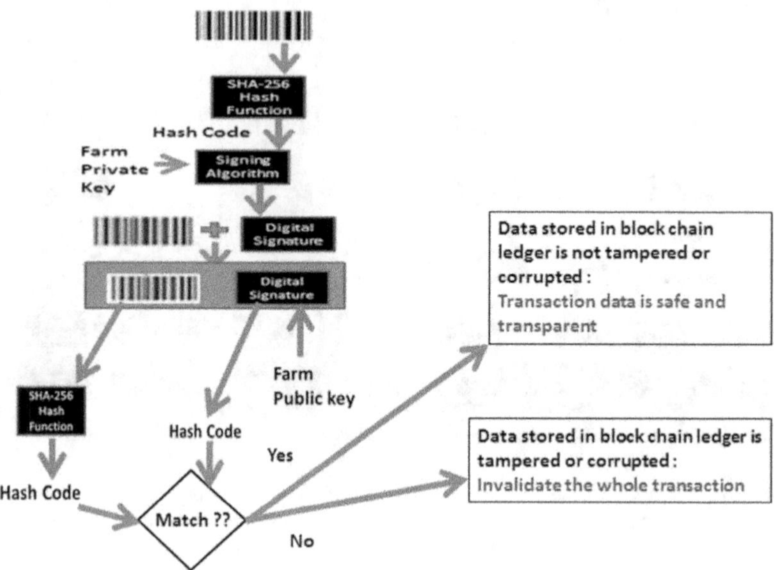

Figure 5.12 Farm data of the transaction can be validated in the blockchain using cryptography. It can be extended to authenticate block data at any level in the sequence

Blockchain technology provides trust among the platform and its intended users. It also helps in maintaining the integrity of supply chain management.

Industry 4.0 applies to automation in all walks of life. For example, as soon as there is any transaction in your bank account regarding a debit or credit, we receive the message, ensuring the safety of our money in the account. Some automatic chatbot systems are deployed by the telecommunication industries. For example, if the customer you are trying to reach is unreachable/switched off/talking to somebody, you can receive an automatic reply ascertaining the status of the person you are trying to reach. Hence, blockchain technology is not only automating the transactions but accomplishing them in a secured manner [41–51].

5.4 APPLICATIONS OF BLOCKCHAIN REINCARNATED BY INDUSTRY 4.0

Early on, developers realized that blockchain technology could be deployed in securities, smart contracts, digital currencies and fraud detection, record-keeping, proof of identity, and healthcare, for example.

Figure 5.13 shows a broader aspect of the application blockchain enveloping every walk of life. The deployment of blockchain technology is

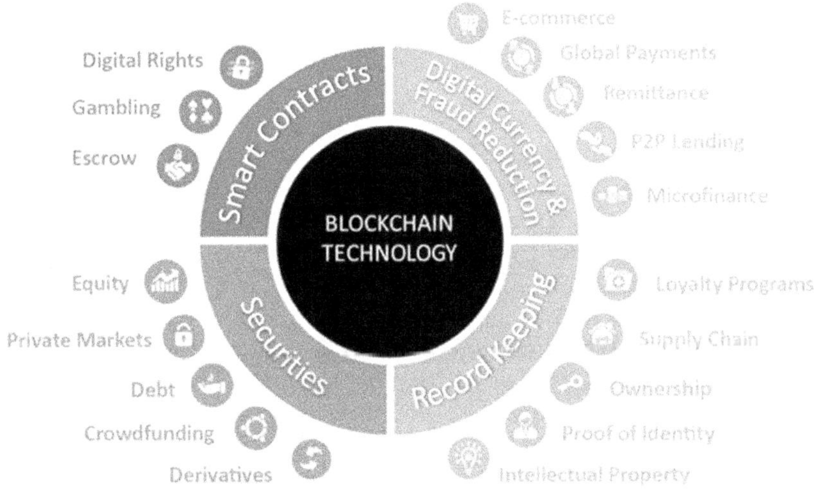

Figure 5.13 Broader spectrum of blockchain applications. (Courtesy of CRI Lab)

prominent in digital currency, fraud detection, and global payment systems. Figure 5.14 depicts the emerging applications of blockchain technology. Each of these contemporary uses is explained next.

5.4.1 Digital Currency and Global Payment System

Digital currency (Bitcoin) came as a surprise to many over conventional currency because it has no dependencies on financial institutions (Satoshi Nakamoto, 2009). In order to establish a digital currency, Bitcoin works on a decentralized blockchain, which does not happen for global currency US dollars. This is the elementary difference between these two. Conventional currency has a centralized system, that is, it works between trusted parties, whereas Bitcoin technology runs on crypto proofs rather than trust and is completely decentralized. Bitcoin does not have a central server. There is a reason behind this and that is it is used for more than profiteering. It has

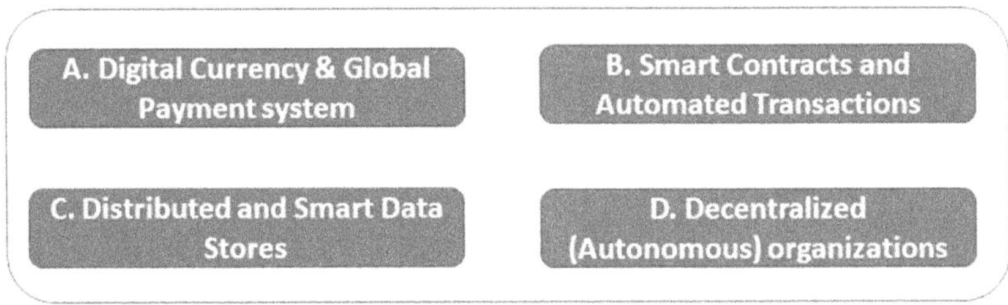

Figure 5.14 Emerging uses of blockchain technology

empowered a new payment system that has the facility for the hassle-free transfer of funds and is applicable globally. Let's compare it to existing payment systems, e.g., Western Union.

A paper-based funds transfer takes days to transfer funds from one account to another globally. Bitcoin has exponentially reduced the funds transfer time to a few minutes, even internationally. The fee for Bitcoin is also quite low compared to other payment systems. One may think that use of the Bitcoin system for funds transfer requires a sophisticated digital infrastructure. However, it just needs a good internet connection and a smart mobile device or a PC. Advocacy of blockchain has surged, and more people are adopting it. The growth is rapid and it can be seen in currency and its imitators. Noted Stanford economist Susan Athey said, "These digital currencies can potentially expand international commerce, support financial inclusion, and transform how we shop, save and do business in ways we probably cannot even yet fully understand." Moreover, it has the potential to deeply penetrate e-commerce functions to the Third World, unleash banking, allow quick and cheaper funds transfer, and broaden the horizon of global remittances.

5.4.2 Smart Contracts and Automated Transactions

Block technology can do more than just power the digital currency. It has appreciably more competence to make our lives simpler and happier. Blockchains are enabling another present-day technology in the name of smart contracts. A smart contract (as shown in Figure 5.15) is a computer code that has three important characteristics: monitoring, execution, and enforcing. A smart contract code can automatically *monitor*, *execute*, and *enforce* a legal agreement. Clauses in the contracts and functional outcomes are mapped as code on the blockchain.

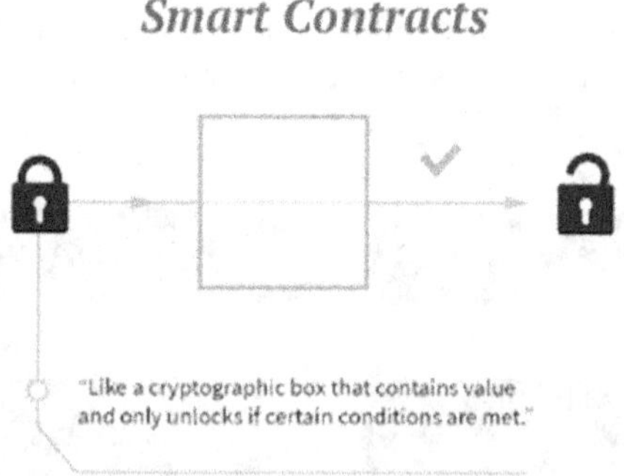

Figure 5.15 How smart contracts are generated. (From the book *Token Economy* by Shermin Voshmgir, 2019; available at https://blockchainhub.net)

If contract execution is automated, then it lowers the dependencies on other parties and the cost of transactions. An important aspect of smart contracts is that they are unmodifiable and final; this is because blockchain impedes retroactive alteration. Automated transactions cannot be reversed or rolled back. As a consequence, it is expected that the contract will be declared void when any action is performed under the respective contract. Blockchain technology enables the verification of the execution of contracts through all the participants in the network. As a result, the execution of the contract is recorded and subsequently monitored by the network for compliance. In smart contracts, all the technical and legal terms are recorded with the coded terms. Nick Szabo (1997) proposed the concept of a smart contract with the help of distributed database systems. This distributed database system is like a blockchain where an occurrence of an event can be confirmed without any intervention of a third party. Szabo says that in a contractual agreement, all the legal provisions are formalized into source codes and this contractual agreement is eventually implemented by smart contracts. It encourages the relationship of contracting parties to be more structured and efficient. Without any intervention, it is likely to be a self-executing process with no ambiguity of words.

> We have a blockchain that is featureless in a sense and it has embedded within it a programming language that allows people to create all sorts of things that run on top of the blockchain architecture. The building block for Ethereum is a smart contract; it is like a virtual machine or autonomous programme that is maintained by everyone in the network.
>
> Vitalik Buterin, founder of Ethereum

There are a few cases wherein new codified relationships have been introduced. The code defines and automatically enforces these relationships. These relationships are, however, nowhere linked to any obligations or underlying contractual rights. As mentioned earlier, to some extent blockchain has the luxury for implementation of self-executing transactions. In this standard contractual agreement, there is no need for any technical input to let parties transact with each other.

Futures, options, derivatives, and swaps are the applications in which smart contracts have been successfully created to execute automatically. This results in the selling of goods over the internet even among random individuals or strangers or unconnected people. It does not require any centralized organization, encouraging the rapid expansion of smart contracts. Counterparty, Ethereum, and Mastercoin are a few open-source projects that have been used to develop programming languages. These programming languages enable the development of sophisticated smart contracts. These smart contracts have been useful for the disbursement of perks to employees on an hourly or daily basis and in real time.

Another application of this technology is administering music royalties instantaneously in real time to both parties, i.e., the composer and performer. Another application is securities. Complicated securities can be represented in smart contracts and this will lead to minimum intervention of technical lead for servicers and trustees. A broad spectrum of activities can be helped with smart contracts and automated transactions.

5.4.3 Distributed and Smart Data Storage

In the cloud structure, there are two storage mechanisms for data: centralized and decentralized. In centralized storage systems, data is stored at a single or a particular location that can be accessed by one or more than one user. In decentralized storage systems, the data is stored on more than one or multiple servers. It means data is not stored at a particular location that can be easily retrieved. In decentralized storage, files are stored and protected with the help of blockchain technology. Here we are talking about the decentralized database and since decentralized databases are encrypted, blockchains have a major impact on how we share and communicate with the data online. The data storage mechanism has an equally dynamic impact on the way the internet has managed to change or upgrade itself over time. This mechanism has also been seen as a facilitator in machine-to-machine communication, particularly when it comes to internet-enabled devices. Blockchain has made a major contribution. It is no longer needed to route files or communication via centralized systems like Dropbox for the exchange of digital files or Yahoo mail for e-mailing (Anjelin and Kumar, 2020).

In blockchain, using decentralized encrypted communication protocols gives users the luxury to retrieve or store data without any risk of intervention. Concerning the exchange of data, from the point of view of security and decentralization, this technology holds true. If required, the information can be encrypted and then published and distributed across many devices. It becomes almost impossible for any entity to sensor access or sensor it. In the early days, people used to access data on their hard drives. The data was stored in a decentralized cloud and blockchain technology was used for security. If we look at it from a user's perspective, then these platforms seem similar to centralized cloud platforms, which are quite popular. Technically they operate differently from one another. A digital currency is provided to users to store the other data. The digital currency can be used to pay for storage of data on someone's computer. In a way, it works as an incentive system wherein people rent out their hard drives to use the services. This way they gain access in the network to collective hard drives. From a design perspective, the decentralized and encrypted behavior of these many platforms makes them reasonably censor-proof. It does not work like this with the centralized organization. On the network, they are not able to view the content of any file. They cannot even stop its transmission.

Do you remember the domain name registry system? It underpins the whole network. Decentralization of data storage is also likely to be considered as a replacement for this. For instance, the Internet Corporation for Assigned Names and Numbers (ICANN) manages domain names like amazon.com or google.com. It is an international organization that maintains the behavior of users who access the internet globally. The advantage is that the blockchain can create a distributed domain name registry system. On distributed databases, this system can store the list of domain names. It is not required to contact any large corporation or government agency to route traffic. New blockchain applications are likely to append this order. If we see the security aspect in this, then we find that a blockchain can extend the existing DNS system. The new DNS system will be more secure and censor-resistant. It costs just a single digital currency transaction.

The ability of blockchain may further make it an efficient foundational tool or base for the utility of IoT. This has become possible because of its ability to manage data from a diversified untrusted source. The composition of an IoT network has billions of internet-enabled devices. Certainly, all the devices cannot be trusted, and a few of them can be malicious. There is a need for a central reference point. This central reference point can facilitate trusted, secure, and private coordination among all the machines.

Blockchain provides one solution, as the devices can be registered with a blockchain. These devices will be identified as smart property and then they will use smart contracts too as explained earlier. With smart contracts, these devices or tangible properties will be controlled over the internet. These devices can be even controlled by other machines. So there are two things to understand. First is the relationship between internet-enabled devices and second is the obligation of the connected devices. These obligations and rights are allocated by smart contracts. The credentials and the relationship can be encoded into the blockchain. There are some cryptographically activated assets (like keys) with regard to which this encoding is made. This ensures that only authorized users have access to the property's features at any given time.

5.4.4 Decentralized (Autonomous) Organizations

When the network system is distributed or decentralized, each device is well facilitated in terms of coordination and interconnectivity. As in the blockchain, in such networks, a variety of smart contracts interact efficiently with one another (Brody and Pureswaran, 2014). Formation of a decentralized or distributed organization (as shown in Figure 5.16 and Figure 5.17) can involve various smart contracts. Now, this distributed organization operates as per the procedures specified by smart contracts and codes. Michael Jensen and William Meckling relate this to their theory. They consider entities as the collection of contracts and relationships into

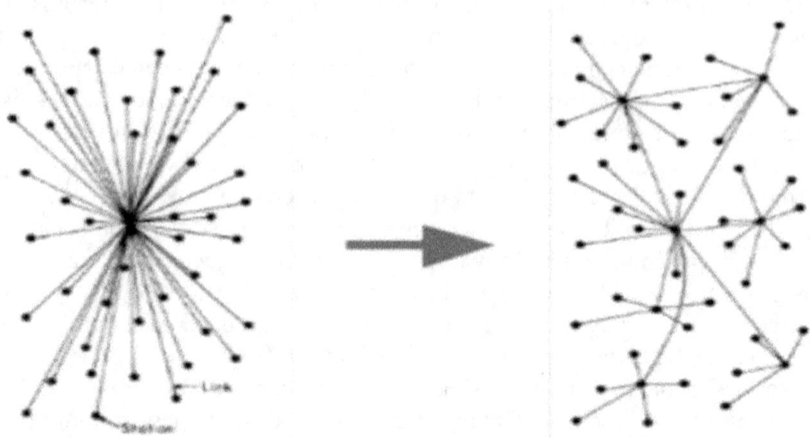

Figure 5.16 The computing paradigm shift from centralization to decentralization

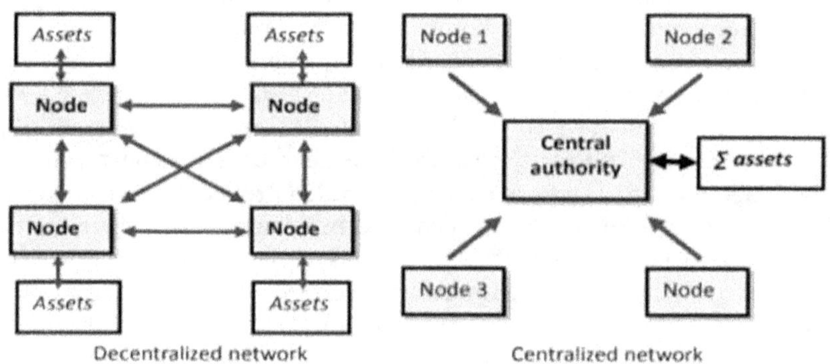

Figure 5.17 Typical representation of a centralized and decentralized network. (From Directorate for Financial and Enterprise Affairs Corporate Governance Committee, Vedat Akgiray, 2018, "Blockchain Technology and Corporate Governance: Technology, Markets, Regulation and Corporate Governance," DAF/CA/CG/RD(2018)1/REV1, Organisation for Economic Co-operation and Development)

reality. How do users coordinate in a blockchain-based decentralized organization? The set of codified smart contracts allows users and machines or both to coordinate.

It is not required to incorporate into conventional business entities. To achieve the governance, it is important to ensure that all the decisions are transparent and auditable. Every transaction is recorded directly to a blockchain, which reduces operational costs. Multiple signature (multi-sig) technology can be used by parties for distributing decision-making. This distributed decision-making power can replicate corporate governance.

This way an action will not be executed until and unless multiple parties agree to a transaction. In conventional organizations, decision-making follows a certain hierarchy.

Decision-making is concentrated at the top, or the executive level. Whereas in a decentralized organization, the decision-making process is encoded directly into the source code. Then how can a shareholder use their decision-making power? Well, in such a distributed system a shareholder adopts decentralized voting. Distributing authority does not require the intervention of any trusted centralized party. So trust and coordination are two important factors facilitated by blockchain. It enables a new form of collaborative action. The whole idea is to understand its potential to overcome existing governance failures. If we see the inherited problems in conventional decision-making, then the opacity can become a major propellent. Distributed systems can potentially solve this in many organizations.

The scenario is different for large organizations. Large hierarchical organizations struggle in terms of perfection and efficiency. The reasons are delegated decision-making, excessive centralization, regulatory capture, and inheritance corruption. However, smart contracts could be a game changer. Smart contracts can predefine the organization and interactions. No need to secure the trust for people to interact with one another or with the machine. Interactions and organizations can be predefined by smart contracts, and people or machines can interact without having to trust the other party. Trust does not rest with the organization, but rather within the security and auditability of the underlying code, whose operations can be scrutinized by millions of eyes. So, with the blockchain, most of the problems in large hierarchical organizations would disappear (De Filippi and Mauro, 2014).

In other sense, decentralized organizations are a kind of open-sourced organizations. Internet-enabled devices are getting more autonomy and hence these devices or machines have started using decentralized organizations. The next step is blockchain. This emerging technology coordinates the interactions of these organizations with the outside world. The emergence of a complex ecosystem of autonomous agents is the result. In this ecosystem, these decentralized organizations (autonomous) are in contractual relationships with the people or users and machines.

As per the hard-wired, set of predetermined or self-enforcing rules these autonomous agents of this ecosystem are interacting with one another. There is a dual advantage of the decentralized autonomous organization. First, it is an autonomous system that does not require a creator or head, and because of this, it has been deployed on the blockchain. Second, it is self-sufficient. It also means that it can have its own capital or digital currency physical assets. The services that are provided by the decentralized systems are paid. This is because the resources used to provide services are not free and hence services are paid. The dark side of this is that if the decentralized autonomous organization is ill-intentioned, then it can be akin to a biological virus.

5.5 SOCIETAL IMPLICATIONS OF BLOCKCHAIN TECHNOLOGY

Blockchain technology has emerged with the potential to minimize the role of the middleman. The middleman has been considered the nation's most important economic and regulatory actor. For instance, in a property transfer, in the conventional process, there would be someone in between to execute the process. The process may not be secure, transparent, or safe. Blockchain allows people to transfer nonsimilar data or ID of digital property to another party in a secure, transparent, or safe manner. It's a very generic example where we see the elimination of the middleman and the end user is the ultimate beneficiary. However, blockchain technology is more than the elimination of human intervention. Broadly, the societal impact of the blockchain has been classified into seven categories as shown in Figure 5.18 (Wright and De Filippi, 2015).

A very elementary understanding of the transition toward decentralization and encryption is end-to-end encryption. One can relate this to current social computing web applications. The deployment of blockchain in digital communications prevents the government from intercepting parties. Since the communication is end-to-end encrypted, it travels between two parties and hence no intervening authority would ever be able to know the contents. In addition, the data is stored in an encrypted format and can be decrypted only by the authorized user.

With automated contractual negotiation, not only have anonymization and decentralization, but smart contracts have significantly impacted our routine lives. The way the internet has reduced the cost of data and information transmission, this technology also minimizes the marginal cost of

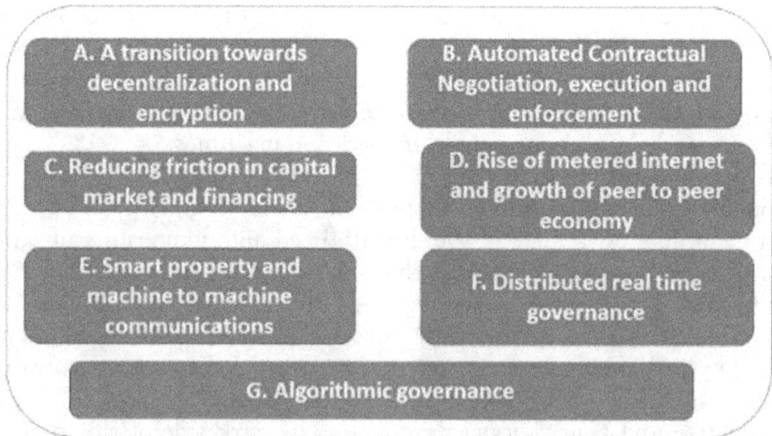

Figure 5.18 Societal implications of blockchain technology

contracting. Interestingly smart contracts have the potential to significantly minimize friction in both society and commerce. It can be achieved by providing speed to transactions and greater clarity.

Capital markets and financing have friction in terms of funding or government policies. Decentralized exchanges and digital assets are very meaningful facilities in the technical framework provided by these technologies. Just imagine the era before blockchain. Without enlisting the support of an attorney, it was difficult to raise funds and allocate equity in any company. But this scenario has been changed in the era of this technology. Think of the services like Koinify or Swarm. With them, a crypto token can be issued by the website to raise funds and reward early adopters. With just a few lines of source code a company can create its own crypto token. This crypto token can represent voting rights or an ownership interest in a company. Friction is almost nil in commerce and finance in this era.

Imagine a situation wherein you got a fine for running a red light. If you are stopped by a police officer, you are supposed to show your license and registration, and later pay the fine in cash or via an online transaction. You might have to complete some paperwork. These papers may also confirm your ownership of the vehicle. But nowadays, using blockchain it is possible to prove ownership without any paper. Blockchain does not allow you to skip the fine, but it will help in the way we transact assets and think of ownership. This is what we call smart property. As depicted in Figure 5.19, there are three characteristics of smart property: secure, interoperable, and intelligent.

Governance, or better yet corporate governance, is all about transparency in the processing through decentralization which allows participating parties to access and verify the data. When citizens and governments share record accessibility, then distrust diminishes. Figure 5.20 depicts three key potential benefits of governance with blockchain. Being a large public data repository, government agencies have been a soft target for hackers. The blockchain data structure has minimized the single point of failure risk. Government agencies need to fulfill their mission while managing scarce resources. Blockchain can be useful in this case. It could reduce redundancy, decrease audit burden, increase security, streamline processes, and ensure data integrity [52].

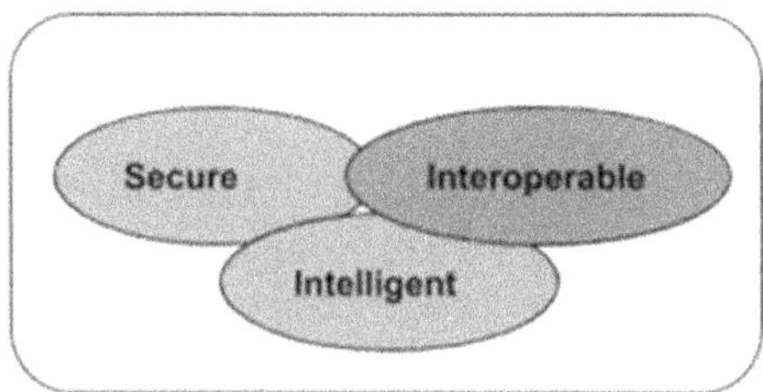

Figure 5.19 Key characteristics of smart property

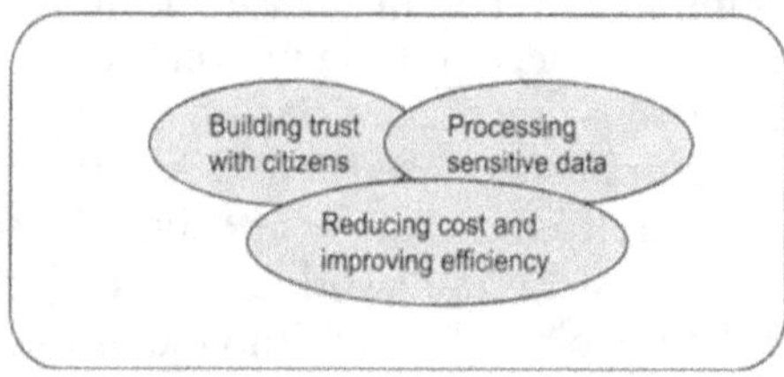

Figure 5.20 Potential benefits of blockchain in governance. (From https://www.boozallen.com/s/insight/blog/3-potential-benefits-of-government-blockchain.html)

5.6 CONCLUSIONS

In this era of Industry 4.0, which is another name for automation and networking, it is possible to be greatly connected to the entire world, where production lines or online transactions are automatic, and everybody can share their experiences and feel connected with a single click. As we move ahead with Industry 4.0, our lives are becoming connected, easier, comfortable, and highly productive because the progress rate has increased many folds, improving resource utilization. Every step in the communication process has been intelligently automated, due to the emergence of Industry 4.0, spanning all walks of life such as healthcare, chatbots, creative arts, drones, finance, agriculture, gaming, space explorations, supply chain management, and social media to name a few. Being connected is one of the prime attributes of Industry 4.0, constantly allowing us to acknowledge our acquaintances regarding their important events like promotions, birthdays, and anniversaries. It also perfectly caters to our needs and demands for knowledge and entertainment, from being producers to consumers, guiding us to popular hang our spots, and to doctors we may frequently visit.

But at the same time, if we look at the unexposed and dark side of this automation, there is a price to pay for this networking and integration, such as exposing our areas of interest and losing privacy, especially when these online platforms continuously monitor our personal and financial data and browsing history, and spoof log-in details of our social media/e-mail accounts. One thing is very much evident: the way we are presented with customized advertisements or recommended content, remote and background daemon algorithms are stalking our actions and capturing our emotions.

Data is the most important asset in today's world of digital technology if used positively and for perpetrating constructive tasks. But it may prove misleading if practiced to influence people's opinions and viewpoints. During online communications, based on patterns of likes, dislikes, and the pages recently visited or browsing history, you may be selectively presented with relevant product advertisements to help you make better choices and accurately predict your behavior. We may be treated as entities who can easily be molded emotionally to be soft targets of online industries/agencies. We are presented with filtered facts to fetch our attention.

Social media platforms like Facebook, WhatsApp, Twitter, and Instagram are acting as a digital fence, where on one side people are more connected, but on the other side, by analyzing the type of connections, followers, and types of posts shared and liked, users are ultimately targeted by certain companies/products/services that want to influence users' opinions and thoughts politically, socially, and economically.

Blockchain is adding another stellar feature to the integrated world of open communications in terms of security. Transactions as a part of operations/tasks/connections are committed only after complete verification, and in a distributed and transparent manner by peer groups, thus ensuring the safety and security of data and the environment at every level. If a security breach is acknowledged at any level, the whole set of transactions rolls back to their original state. Every entity in blockchain equally contributes to honoring the integrity of the transactional data.

After complete verification of all the transactions in a block, it is added to the blockchain. Thus the system is highly transparent and secure. Similarly, the aforementioned lacunae of data breaching during online communications can very well be addressed by incorporating the distributed ledger concept of blockchain, which is not only cost-effective but fast and efficient to implement. Hence to promote Industry 4.0, the security of blockchain is proving very valuable in protecting our much-needed data privacy. As an aware user, one has to be very clear about the choices made while online and remain alert to malicious activities. If something is offered for free, it might have some hidden repercussions.

As a concluding remark about blockchain being a pathway to Industry 4.0, it is a common belief that data captured in the ledger through blockchain technology cannot be tampered with or changed, but this is certainly not completely true and is currently causing a bit of controversy due to certain security breaches instead of being enforced with blockchain security. So the future of Industry 4.0 is yet to evolve, sprawling new dimensions in terms of making blockchain more robust and tougher to breach, giving the propelling force to launch it into a widened orbit of security.

REFERENCES

1. Barnes, D. 2015, "Blockchain Manoeuvres: Applying Bitcoin's Technology to Banking", *The Banker*, May 14.
2. Pilkington, Mark 2016, *Blockchain Technology: Principles and Applications, Research Handbook on Digital Transformations*. Social Science Research Network.

3. Schmidt, E., Cohen, J. 2013, *The New Digital Age: Reshaping the Future of People, Nations and Business*. John Murray, London.
4. Wright, A., De Filippi, P. 2015, "Decentralized Blockchain Technology and the Rise of Lex Cryptographia", March 10. http://ssrn.com/abstract=2580664.
5. Nakomoto, Satoshi 2009, "Bitcoin Open Source Implementation of P2P Currency, P2P FOUNDATION", February 11. http://p2pfoundation.ning.com/forum/topics/bitcoin-opensource.
6. Anjelin, D. Praveena, Kumar, S. Ganesh 2020, "Blockchain Technology for Data Sharing in Decentralized Storage System", Intelligent *Computing* and Applications, pp. 369–382| Part of the Advances in Intelligent Systems and Computing Springer book series (AISC, volume 1172), September 30.
7. Szabo, Nick 1997, "The Idea of Smart Contracts". http://szabo.best.vwh.net/smart_contracts_idea.html (describing the concept of digital "smart" contracts).
8. De Filippi, Primavera, Mauro, Rafaelle 2014, "Ethereum: The Decentralized Platform that Might Displace Today's Institutions", *Internet Policy Review*, August 25. http://policyreview.info/articles/news/ethereum-decentralised-platform-might-displacetodays-institutions/318.
9. Brody, Paul, Pureswaran, Veena 2014, "Device Democracy: Saving the Future of the Internet of Things", *IBM*, September. http://www-01.ibm.com/common/ssi/cgibin/ssialias?subtype=XB&infotype=PM&appname=GBSE_GB_TI_USEN&htmlfid=GBE 03620USEN&attachment=GBE03620USEN.PDF#loaded.
10. Xu, Min, Chen, Xingtong, Kou, Gang 2019, "A Systematic Review of Blockchain", Financial Innovation, Article Number: 27. July 4.
11. Luoa, X., Wang, Z., & Caicd, W. Xiuhua, Lie, Victor CM, Leungaf, 2020, "Application and Evaluation of Payment Channel in Hybrid Decentralized Ethereum Token Exchange", Blockchain: Research and Applications, 1(1–2, December).
12. Bordela, Borja, Alcarriab, Ramón, Roblesa, Tomás 2021, "Denial of Chain: Evaluation and Prediction of a Novel Cyberattack in Blockchain-Supported Systems", *Future Generation Computer Systems*, 116, pp. 426–439, March.
13. Downey, Liang Xi, Bauchot, Frédéric, Röling, Jos 2018, "Blockchain for Business Value: A Contract and Work Flow Management to Reduce Disputes Pilot Project", *IEEE Engineering Management Review*, 46(4), pp. 20–32, December.
14. Ateniese, G., Faonio, A., Magri, B., de Medeiros, B. 2014, "Certified Bitcoins", *Applied Cryptography and Network Security, Lecture Notes in Computer Science*, Vol. 8479. Springer International Publishing, pp. 80–96. doi: 10.1007/978-3-319-07536-5_6.
15. Chen, Wubing, Xu, Zhiying, Shi, Shuyu, Zhao, Yang, Zhao, Jun 2018, "A Survey of Blockchain Applications in Different Domains", *International Conference on Blockchain Technology and Applications (ICBTA) 2018*, China, pp. 17–21, December.
16. Wang, Junyao, Wang, Shenling, Guo, Junqi, Du, Yanchang, Cheng, Shaochi, Li, Xiangyang 2019, "A Summary of Research on Blockchain in the Field of Intellectual Property", Procedia Computer Science, 147, pp. 191–197.

17. Yli-Huumo, Jesse, Ko, Deokyoon, Choi, Sujin, Park, Sooyong, Smolander, Kari 2016, "Where Is Current Research on Blockchain Technology?—A Systematic Review", October 3. doi: 10.1371/journal.pone.0163477.
18. Bitcoinwiki. 2015, Accessed on 24/3/2020 at https://en.bitcoin.it.
19. Antonopoulos AM. 2014, *Mastering Bitcoin: Unlocking Digital Cryptocurrencies.* O'Reilly Media, Inc, USA.
20. Proof-of-Stake. 2016, Accessed: 24/3/2020 at https://en.bitcoin.it/wiki/Proof_of_Stake.
21. Petersen, K., Feldt, R., Mujtaba, S., Mattsson, M. 2008, "Systematic Mapping Studies in Software Engineering", *Proceedings of the 12th International Conference on Evaluation and Assessment in Software Engineering, EASE'08.* Swinton: British Computer Society, pp. 68–77. Available at http://dl.acm.org/citation.cfm?id=2227115.2227123.
22. Dybå, T., Dingsøyr, T. 2008, "Empirical Studies of Agile Software Development: A Systematic Review", *Information and Software Technology,* 50(910), pp. 833–859. doi: 10.1016/j.infsof.2008.01.006.
23. Parra-Moyano, José, Thoroddsen, Tryggvi, Ross, Omri 2019, "Optimised and Dynamic KYC System Based on Blockchain Technology", *International Journal of Blockchains and Cryptocurrencies,* 1(1), pp. 85–106.
24. Anish Dev, J. 2014, "Bitcoin Mining Acceleration and Performance Quantification", *Electrical and Computer Engineering (CCECE), 2014 IEEE 27th Canadian Conference,* pp. 1–6.
25. Cheng, S., Zeng, B., Huang, Y. Z. 2017, "Research on Application Model of Blockchain Technology in Distributed Electricity Market", IOP Conference Series: Earth and Environmental Science, *Conference 1,* 93(1), pp. 300–321.
26. Rana, Q. P., Tyagi, S., Som, Subhranil 2019, "Fuzzy Logic Based Trust Management through Dynamic Multicast Group Formation Provisioning Quality of Service in MANETs", *Journal of Advanced Research in Dynamical and Control Systems,* 10(12), pp. 1243–1271.
27. Paul, G., Sarkar, P., Mukherjee, S. 2014, "Towards a More Democratic Mining in Bitcoins", *Information Systems Security,* Vol. 8880, Lecture Notes in Computer Science. Springer International Publishing, pp. 185–203. doi: 10.1007/978-3-319-13841-1_11.
28. Ghosh, Jaideep 2019, "The Blockchain: Opportunities for Research in Information Systems and Information Technology", *Journal of Global Technology Management,* 22(4), pp. 235–242, 15 October. doi: 10.1080/1097198X.2019.1679954.
29. Litoriya, R., Gulati, A., Yadav, M., Ghosh, R. S., Pandey, P., 2021, "Social, Ethical, and Regulatory Issues of Fog Computing in Healthcare 4.0 Applications", *FOG Computing for Healthcare 4.0 Environments.* Springer, Cham, pp. 593–609. doi: 10.1007/978-3-030-46197-3_23.
30. Sharma, N. et al. 2019, "Designing a Decision Support Framework for Municipal Solid Waste Management", *International Journal on Emerging Technologies,* 10(4), pp. 374–379. doi: 10(4): 374-379(2019).
31. Prateek, P., Ratnesh, L. 2020, "Securing and Authenticating Healthcare Records through Blockchain Technology", *Cryptologia,* 44(4), pp. 341–356. doi: 10.1080/01611194.2019.1706060.

32. Sharma, N. *et al.* 2021, "Modern Approach for the Significance Role of Decision Support System in Solid Waste Management System (SWMS)", in Goyal D., Bălaş V. E., Mukherjee A., Hugo C., de Albuquerque V. G. A. K. (ed.) *Algorithms for Intelligent Systems.* Springer, pp. 619–628. doi: 10.1007/978-981-15-4936-6_67.
33. Bamert, T., Decker, C., Wattenhofer, R., Welten, S. 2014, "BlueWallet: The Secure Bitcoin Wallet", *Security and Trust Management*, Vol. 8743, Lecture Notes in Computer Science. Springer International Publishing, pp. 65–80. doi: 10.1007/978-3-319-11851-2_5.
34. Tyagi, S., Pai, A., Pegado, J., Kamath, A. 2019, "A Proposed Model for Preventing the Spread of Misinformation on Online Social Media Using Machine Learning", *2019 Amity International Conference on Artificial Intelligence (AICAI), IEEE Xplore*, pp. 678–683.
35. Pandey, M., Litoriya, R., Pandey, P. 2019, "Application of Fuzzy DEMATEL Approach in Analyzing Mobile App Issues", *Programming and Computer Software*, 45(5), pp. 268–287. doi: 10.1134/S0361768819050050.
36. Pandey, M., Litoriya, R., Pandey, P. 2019, "Novel Approach for Mobile Based App Development Incorporating MAAF", *Wireless Personal Communications*, 107(4), pp. 1687–1708. doi: 10.1007/s11277-019-06351-9.
37. Prateek, P., Ratnesh, L. 2020, "Promoting Trustless Computation Through Blockchain Technology", *National Academy Science Letters.* doi: 10.1007/s40009-020-00978-0.
38. Prateek, P., Ratnesh, L. 2020, "Fuzzy Cognitive Mapping Analysis to Recommend Machine Learning Based Effort Estimation Technique for Web Applications", *International Journal of Fuzzy Systems*, 22(4), pp. 1212–1223. doi: 10.1007/s40815-020-00815-y.
39. Lone, Auqib Hamid, Mir, Roohie Naaz 2019, "Consensus Protocols as a Model of Trust in Blockchains", *International Journal of Blockchains and Cryptocurrencies*, 1(1), pp. 7–21.
40. Mann, C., Loebenberger, D. 2015, "Two-Factor Authentication for the Bitcoin Protocol", *Security and Trust Management*, Vol. 9331, Lecture Notes in Computer Science. Springer International Publishing, pp. 155–171. doi: 10.1007/978-3-319-24858-5_10.
41. Pandey, P., Litoriya, R. 2019, "Elderly Care through Unusual Behavior Detection: A Disaster Management Approach Using IoT and Intelligence", *IBM Journal of Research and Development*, 64(1), pp. 15:1–15:11. doi: 10.1147/JRD.2019.2947018.
42. Litoriya, R., Ranjan, A., 2010, "Implementation of Relational Algebra Interpreter Using Another Query Language", *2010 International Conference on Data Storage and Data Engineering*, pp. 24–28. doi: 10.1109/DSDE.2010.33.
43. Pandey, M., Litoriya, R., Pandey, P., 2016, "Mobile Applications in Context of Big Data: A Survey", *2016 Symposium on Colossal Data Analysis and Networking (CDAN)*, pp. 1–5. doi: 10.1109/CDAN.2016.7570942.
44. Pandey, P., Litoriya, R. 2020, "Fuzzy AHP Based Identification Model for Efficient Application Development", *Journal of Intelligent and Fuzzy Systems*, 38(3), pp. 3359–3370. doi: 10.3233/JIFS-190508.

45. Singh Bhadauria, S., Sharma, V., Litoriya, R., 2010, "Empirical Analysis of Ethical Issues in the Era of Future Information Technology", *2010 2nd International Conference on Software Technology and Engineering*, pp. V2-31–V2-35. doi: 10.1109/ICSTE.2010.5608757.
46. Sharma, N., Litoriya, R., Sharma, D. 2019, "An Analytical Study on the Importance of Data Mining for Designing a Decision Support System", *Journal of Harmonized Research (JOHR)*, 7(2), pp. 44–48. doi: 10.30876/JOHR.7.2.2019.44-48.
47. Pandey, P., Litoriya, R. 2020, "Ensuring Elderly Well Being during COVID-19 by Using IoT", *Disaster Medicine and Public Health Preparedness*, pp. 1–10. doi: 10.1017/dmp.2020.390.
48. Sharma, N., Bajpai, A., Litoriya, R. 2012, "Comparison the Various Clustering Algorithms of Weka Tools", *International Journal of Emerging Technology and Advanced Engineering*, 2(5), pp. 73–80.
49. Halpin, Harry, Piekarska, Marta 2017, "Introduction to Security and Privacy on the Blockchain", *2017 IEEE European Symposium on Security and Privacy Workshops (EuroS&PW)*, pp. 1–3. doi: 10.1109/EuroSP.2017.26 © 2017, Harry Halpin, Under license to IEEE.
50. Beikverdi, A., Song, J. 2015, "Trend of Centralization in Bitcoin's Distributed Network", *Software Engineering, Artificial Intelligence, Networking and Parallel, Distributed Computing (SNPD), 2015 16th IEEE/ACIS International Conference*, pp. 1–6.
51. Crosby, Michael, Nachiappan, Pradhan Pattanayak, Verma, Sanjeev, Kalyanaraman, Vignesh 2015, *Blockchain Technology Beyond Bitcoin*, Sutardja Center for Entrepreneurship & Technology Technical Report, October 16, pp. 1–35.
52. Prakash, R., Ranjan, R. K., "Role of ICT in Reverse Logistics: An Analytical Approach", pp. 23–27. http://hdl.handle.net/10603/46422.

Chapter 6

Prediction of Breast Cancer Using Machine Learning Techniques for Health Data

Aarti, Saurabh Karling, Pushpendra K Rajput, Surbhi, and Praveen Kumar Malik

6.1 INTRODUCTION

Machine learning (ML) techniques have emerged as powerful tools in various domains, including healthcare. With the availability of large volumes of medical data and advancements in computational resources, ML has the potential to revolutionize healthcare systems. In this section, we provide an introduction to machine learning techniques specifically applied in the context of healthcare.

Machine learning involves the development of algorithms that can learn patterns and make predictions or decisions based on data. In healthcare, these algorithms can analyze complex medical datasets and extract valuable insights for improved diagnosis, treatment, and patient care.

One of the key applications of ML in healthcare is the prediction and early detection of diseases. By training ML models on historical patient data, it is possible to identify patterns and risk factors associated with specific diseases, such as breast cancer. This enables healthcare professionals to intervene at an early stage, potentially saving lives and improving patient outcomes.

ML techniques can leverage various types of healthcare data, including electronic health records (EHRs), medical imaging, genetic information, and wearable sensor data. These diverse data sources provide a comprehensive view of patients' health conditions, allowing ML models to capture intricate relationships and detect subtle patterns that might be missed by human experts.

In the case of breast cancer prediction, ML techniques can utilize features such as age, family history, genetic markers, mammography images, and clinical notes to develop accurate prediction models. By analyzing these features, ML algorithms can identify high-risk individuals who may require further screening or diagnostic tests.

Moreover, ML techniques can assist in personalized treatment decisions. By analyzing patient data, ML models can predict treatment outcomes, recommend optimal therapies, and identify potential adverse reactions to specific medications. This enables healthcare providers to tailor treatment plans to individual patients, maximizing effectiveness and minimizing risks.

DOI: 10.1201/9781003466949-6

Another area where ML techniques have shown promise is in healthcare resource allocation. By analyzing patient data and historical records, ML algorithms can predict hospital readmission rates, emergency department utilization, and patient length of stay. This information can guide resource planning and allocation, leading to more efficient healthcare delivery and improved patient flow.

However, it is essential to address challenges related to privacy, security, and interpretability when implementing ML techniques in healthcare. Patient data must be protected to ensure confidentiality, and ML models should be transparent and interpretable to gain the trust of healthcare professionals and patients.

In conclusion, machine learning techniques have immense potential to transform healthcare by enabling accurate disease prediction, personalized treatment, and efficient resource allocation. By harnessing the power of ML, we can improve patient outcomes, optimize healthcare delivery, and ultimately save lives.

Breast cancer is indeed a serious health issue affecting a significant number of women worldwide. Effective therapy and higher survival rates for breast cancer depend on early diagnosis. One way to detect breast cancer is by making use of tumors. However, accurately identifying malignant tumors is challenging even for specialists. Therefore, there is a need for automatic approaches to detect breast cancer.

Machine learning approaches have been explored in recent studies to diagnose breast cancer and determine its survivability. These algorithms have shown promise in improving the accuracy of breast cancer diagnosis and predicting survival rates. With the help of machine learning, healthcare professionals can make more informed decisions about treatment options for patients with breast cancer.

It is important to note that although machine learning algorithms can assist in breast cancer diagnosis, they should not be used as a substitute for medical advice from a qualified healthcare professional. The results obtained from machine learning algorithms should always be evaluated and interpreted by medical professionals and so with diagnosis and treatment for breast cancer. A doctor's expertise and experience are always crucial for accurate early detection, assessment, and treatment of breast cancer. However, advancements in processing technology have made it easier to gather and analyze large volumes of data, including electronic patient information.

Machine learning approaches have become increasingly popular in recent years for diagnosing breast cancer and identifying patterns in data. Such approaches are used to categorize breast tumors into one of the categories, either malignant or benign. Later, it can help in determining the appropriate treatment options for patients.

In addition to categorizing tumors, machine learning can also be used to model breast cancer and identify hidden patterns and connections in data. This can assist medical practitioners in developing more well-informed patient care decisions and developing hypotheses for further research. Overall, machine learning has shown promise in improving breast cancer diagnosis and treatment. However, one has to remember that these algorithms should only ever be used in combination with medical knowledge and should never be used as a substitute for professional medical advice. The use of artificial intelligence (AI) in clinical areas is growing rapidly, particularly in the clinical analysis of breast cancer. Early identification of breast cancer is essential for better treatment and higher survival rates, as it is the leading cause of death for women globally [16–17].

AI has shown promise in predicting and categorizing breast cancer. The impact of this can help healthcare practitioners by making them more informed about patient care. By analyzing data from various sources, such as electronic medical records and medical imaging, AI algorithms can identify patterns and connections that may be difficult for human experts to detect. In countries like India, where the number of breast cancer cases is low but the number of fatalities is high, early detection through AI could have a significant impact on reducing mortality rates. Overall, AI has proven itself as a potential tool to diagnose breast cancer and offer better opportunities to medical professionals for treatment outcomes. However, it is important to continue researching and refining these algorithms to ensure they are reliable and accurate. Additionally, AI should always be used in conjunction with medical expertise to ensure patients receive the best possible care [13–15].

In Bangladesh, particularly among women, breast cancer is a significant public health problem. With 69% of all disease transmissions, it is the main cause of death for women. The prevalence rate of breast cancer is also significantly higher among Bangladeshi women aged 15 to 44, compared to other types of cancer. Several factors contribute to the high incidence and mortality rates of breast cancer in Bangladesh. These include a lack of awareness about the disease, inadequate screening tests, low trust in clinical care, and inappropriate management of the disease. Furthermore, the stigma associated with cancer and the fear of treatment can prevent patients from seeking medical attention. To address this pressing issue, it is important to raise public awareness about breast cancer and promote early detection through regular screening. Government and healthcare authorities should also prioritize the development of effective screening programs and improve access to affordable cancer treatment options for patients. Finally, efforts to combat the social stigma surrounding cancer and to promote education about the disease should be a priority in Bangladesh.

The study aims to use multiple AI methods to differentiate between malignant and benign breast cancers using publicly available datasets. The main target of the research is to assess the performance of various multi-classifiers to determine the best one for breast cancer classification. Overall, the study demonstrates how AI may enhance the precision and effectiveness of breast cancer detection and therapy [6–12].

Support vector machine (SVM) and artificial neural network (ANN) are two very popular learning algorithms. In reference [1], the authors developed a method for detecting breast cancer using these two approaches. They used the Wisconsin Diagnostic dataset, which contains measurements from fine needle aspirates, to train their SVM model to distinguish between benign and malignant breast tumors. The authors compared their ML approach with traditional statistical methods and found that the ML techniques had the highest reliability, likely due to the advancements in AI and the increasing complexity of data.

In another study, SVM was utilized with naïve Bayes, and J48 was used with a voting classifier approach to improve the accuracy of predicting different types of product classes. The proposed combined approach achieved 97.13 precision. The result shows it was higher than any of the individual classifiers used alone [2].

The F1 scores for each of these models were also quite high, with logistic regression achieving the highest score at 98%. These findings suggest that these models are more reliable than those used in previous studies and that the study's approach can be derived from the review research.

In developing a machine learning model to predict breast cancer progression, it's important to use high-quality data and carefully address concerns about overfitting and underfitting [3, 4]. This can be done through techniques such as cross-validation and regularization. It's also important to involve medical professionals in the development and evaluation of the model to ensure that it aligns with current clinical practice and can be effectively integrated into patient care [18–25]. Overall, machine learning has great potential to improve the early detection and treatment of breast cancer, but it's essential to approach its development and use with care and attention to detail.

We have divided the remainder of the work into distinct sections. In Section 6.2, a discussion of the method is provided along with the experimental approach. It provides more details on how the study was conducted. Section 6.3 analyzes the results of the study, delving deeper into the findings and their implications. Finally, Section 6.4 presents the conclusions of the study, summarizing the key takeaways and potential future directions for research.

6.2 METHOD AND EXPERIMENT METHODOLOGY

The study performed its analysis on a popular dataset, Wisconsin Breast Cancer Diagnostic (WBCD). The dataset is a collection of 569 samples, each of which is associated with 32 features. The features include fine needle aspiration (FNA) data acquired from patient breasts that have been exposed and reflect numerous atomic properties. The dataset is found in a very popular repository, the UCI Machine Learning Repository, which is used for recognized machine learning research.

In FNA, a small needle is put into a bodily fluid or tissue that seems abnormal in order to diagnose or forecast the possibility of cancer. The WBCD dataset contains information on whether each sample was diagnosed as malignant or benign. The class distribution of the dataset is classified as 357 benign and 212 malignant.

The dataset does not have any missing attributes. This means that the dataset is complete and can be used for analysis and modeling without the need for imputation or other data cleaning techniques.

The dataset is first preprocessed by removing the ID column and converting the diagnostic trait columns to numeric values. In the next phase, the features causing the prediction are identified, and the target value is established so that the model can make predictions. For validation of the model, the dataset is split into a training set and a testing set. A ratio of 70% and 30% is kept for training and testing, respectively. The feature scaling is done using standardization.

Our experiment aims to find a reliable and accurate algorithm for detecting breast cancer. To achieve this, we applied various machine learning classifiers, including SVM, logistic regression, and random forests, to the WBCD dataset. We then analyzed the results obtained to determine which model had the highest accuracy.

The proposed approach starts with acquiring the relevant data. Once the data is acquired, preprocessing is performed. The preprocessed data is then fed into machine learning models to predict breast cancer. To assess the performance of these models, we use a set of labeled data to test them. We split the labeled data using the train_test_split method. After a successful run and testing of the models, a comparison of results is performed with the algorithm that showed the performance at a higher side. The objective of the study is to pick the most effective algorithm for identifying breast cancer.

6.2.1 Algorithmic Details

Our project involves using machine learning algorithms for predictive analysis. We applied several algorithms: support vector machine, random forest, and logistic regression.

Support vector machine (SVM) is widely used in various domains, including classification and regression tasks. It is known for its ability to handle both linear and nonlinear data separation through the use of a hyperplane.

The fundamental concept behind SVM is to find an optimal hyperplane. SVM operates by transforming the input data into a higher-dimensional feature space, where the classes can be separated more effectively. This transformation is achieved using kernel functions, which allow SVM to implicitly work in this high-dimensional space without explicitly computing the coordinates of the data points.

One of the key advantages of SVM is its ability to handle data that is not linearly separable by mapping it to a higher-dimensional space. This is accomplished by using different kernel functions such as linear, polynomial, radial basis function (RBF), or sigmoid. The choice of the kernel function depends on the specific characteristics of the data and the desired decision boundary.

In addition to binary classification, SVM can be extended to handle multiclass problems through techniques like one-vs-one or one-vs-all classification. In one-vs-one, SVM builds multiple binary classifiers for each pair of classes, and the final prediction is based on voting between these classifiers. In one-vs-all, each class is treated as a separate binary classification problem, and the class with the highest confidence is chosen as the final prediction.

SVM has been successfully applied in various domains, including image classification, text categorization, bioinformatics, and medical diagnosis. Its ability to handle high-dimensional data and its robustness against overfitting make it an attractive choice for many real-world applications.

Random forest is an ensemble approach utilized for problems like regression and classification. The approach involves constructing multiple decision trees during the training phase and outputs the respective class from the available set of classes (classification) or the mean prediction (regression) of the individual constructed trees. As it employs a set of decision trees, random decision forests correct for the tendency of overfitting training sets.

Logistic regression, which is an extension of linear regression, is a highly effective modeling technique. It is employed to determine the possibility of a disease or health issue based on a risk factor and other related variables. Techniques for simple and complex logistic regression may be used to look at how independent variables, known as predictor variables, relate to one another and a dichotomous dependent variable, also known as the outcome or response variable. The approach is best suited for binary dependent variables or multiclass dependent variables.

6.2.2 Dataset Acquisition

The proposed research employs a popular dataset used for breast cancer diagnosis, the Wisconsin Breast Cancer Diagnostic dataset. The dataset has been sourced from the University of Wisconsin Hospitals Madison Breast Cancer Database [5]. This dataset includes characteristics that have been determined using an image of a breast cancer sample taken by FNA that was digitally captured. The characteristics of the cell nuclei found in the image are determined using these features. The WBCD dataset consists of 569 instances, with 357 instances classified as benign and 212 instances classified as malignant. The dataset has two classes, with 62.74% of the instances classified as benign and 37.26% classified as malignant. It also contains 12 integer-valued attributes, namely, Id, Radius, Diagnosis, Area, Texture, Smoothness, Perimeter, Compactness, Concavity, Symmetry,

Concave points, and Fractal dimension. Table 6.1 describes the details of the dataset.

The proposed machine learning algorithm experiments were carried out using Python as the programming language and the scikit-learn library. Sklearn, a Python library, offers various supportive functions that can be employed for the implementation of machine learning models. It is available for free and includes a range of algorithms for classification, regression, and clustering. It's built to work seamlessly with the scientific and numerical Python libraries SciPy and NumPy.

6.3 RESULTS AND DISCUSSION

Several performance criteria were utilized to assess and compare the models and find the best algorithm. The research was performed by applying various machine learning algorithms to the WBCD dataset. The performance metrics included the confusion matrix, precision, accuracy, F1 score, sensitivity, and ROC (receiver operating characteristic). The confusion matrix is a way of evaluating the performance of a classifier that deals with multiple classes. It's a two-dimensional table with "actual" and "predicted" dimensions, with "true positives (TP)," "false positives (FP)," "true negatives (TN)," and "false negatives (FN)" on both dimensions. The most used performance indicator for classification algorithms is accuracy. The percentage of predictions that were accurate relative to all other predictions is known as accuracy. Precision is another parameter that is used in document retrievals. It depends on the correct number of documents returned by the ML model. The ML model's sensitivity is measured by the number of positive results it returns, and the F1 score provides the harmonic mean of precision and sensitivity.

As confusion matrices are a valuable tool for evaluating classifiers, Table 6.2 show rates for each actual class, while its columns display predictions. The performance metrics of classification are shown in Table 6.3. The data represented is extracted based on the results of the confusion matrix, including precision, recall, and F-measure and ROC scores for both malignant and benign cases.

Table 6.1 Detail of WBCD Dataset

		V2			
		Frequency	*Percent*	*Valid Percent*	*Cumulative Percent*
Valid	B	357	62.7	62.7	62.7
	M	212	37.3	37.3	100.0
	Total	569	100.0	100.0	

Table 6.2 Confusion Matrix for Different Models

Random forest		M	B	Naïve Bayes	M	B	Logistic regression	M	B
	M	201	11		190	22		199	13
	B	5	352		18	339		7	350

Table 6.3 Performance Matrix for Different Models

Technique	*Precision*	*Recall*	*F-Measure*	*ROC*
Random forest	0.93	0.93	0.93	0.98
Naïve Bayes	0.93	0.93	0.93	0.98
Logistic regression	0.965	0.965	0.965	0.989

According to the confusion matrix presented in Table 6.2, the logistic regression accurately predicts 549 out of 569 cases, consisting of 199 correctly predicted malignant cases and 350 correctly predicted benign cases. The remaining 20 cases are predicted incorrectly, with 13 malignant cases predicted as benign and 7 benign cases predicted as malignant. As a result, the precision of logistic regression is better than that of other classification techniques. Logistic regression consistently performs better than other classifiers in the WBCD dataset cancer for both malignant and benign cases. The ROC curves and F-measure of each machine learning algorithm are shown in Figure 6.2, with the area under the ROC curve (AUC) being an important metric for classifier performance. A higher ROC score indicates better classifier performance. In this case, logistic regression has the highest ROC score of 0.989%. Table 6.4 describes that logistic regression has a lower root mean squared error (RMSE) and a higher value of kappa statistic.

Logistic regression consistently outperforms other classifiers in predicting two classes— benign and malignant—in the WBCD. The ROC curves, an important metric for evaluating classifier performance, of each machine learning algorithm are presented in Figure 6.3. The performance of the classifier is calculated using the AUC. A higher area under the curve indicates better performance.

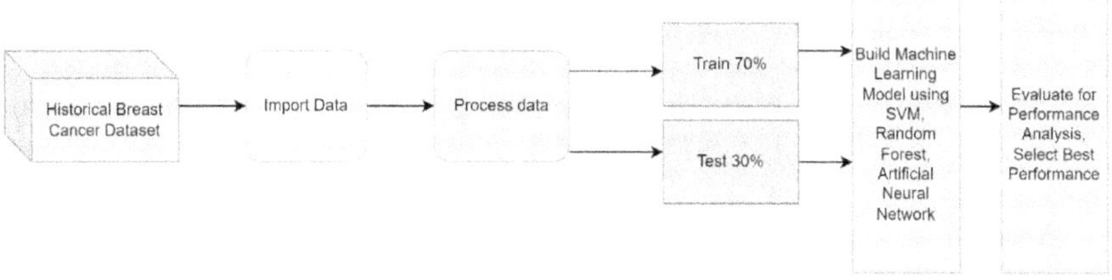

Figure 6.1 Proposed methodology

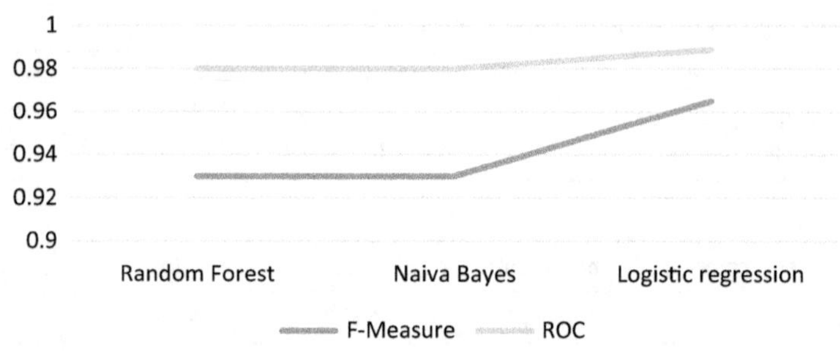

Figure 6.2 ROC curve and F-measure value

Table 6.4 Kappa Statistic, MSE, and RMSE difference

Technique	*Logistic Regression*	*Naïve Bayes*	*Random Forest*
Kappa statistic	0.9395	0.8491	0.9244
MSE	0.0435	0.07	0.0767
RMSE	0.1409	0.2585	0.1743

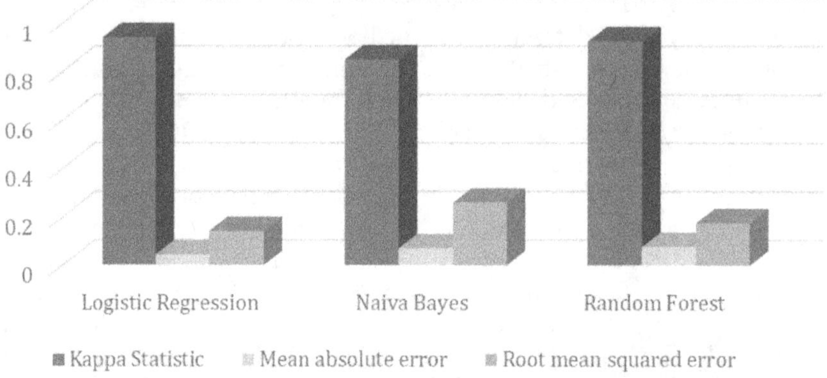

Figure 6.3 Kappa statistic, MSE, and RMSE difference between three classifiers

While ML techniques offer significant promise in the prediction of breast cancer, it is important to acknowledge certain limitations and challenges associated with their application. Understanding these disadvantages is crucial for developing robust and reliable prediction models. Here are some notable drawbacks of using ML for breast cancer prediction:

Data quality and availability. ML models heavily rely on high-quality and diverse datasets for accurate predictions. However, obtaining comprehensive and well-annotated breast cancer data can be challenging. Limited data availability, incomplete records, and inconsistencies in data quality can affect the performance and generalizability of ML models.

Biased or imbalanced datasets. Imbalanced datasets can lead to biased models, with a higher tendency to predict the majority class accurately but struggle with the minority class, which is crucial in breast cancer prediction.

Overfitting and generalizability. Overfitting can occur when the model captures noise or specific patterns unique to the training dataset, leading to poor performance on new samples. Ensuring the generalizability of breast cancer prediction models is essential to avoid inaccurate results.

Ethical considerations. ML models for breast cancer prediction must navigate ethical challenges related to privacy, security, and bias. Ensuring patient data privacy and security is of utmost importance, as sensitive medical information is involved. Additionally, biases in data collection and model training can lead to unfair or discriminatory predictions, exacerbating healthcare disparities.

Clinical integration and validation. Transitioning ML models from research to clinical practice requires thorough validation and integration with existing healthcare systems. Real-world deployment of ML models for breast cancer prediction demands rigorous evaluation, regulatory compliance, and seamless integration with clinical workflows, which can be a complex and resource-intensive process.

Limited domain expertise. Although ML models can analyze vast amounts of data and identify patterns, they may lack the expertise and domain-specific knowledge that healthcare professionals possess. In breast cancer prediction, it is crucial to incorporate the insights and expertise of medical practitioners to ensure accurate and clinically relevant predictions.

Addressing these disadvantages requires a multidisciplinary approach, involving collaboration between data scientists, healthcare professionals, and policymakers. By understanding and mitigating these challenges, ML techniques can be harnessed effectively to enhance breast cancer prediction and improve patient care in a responsible and ethical manner.

6.4 CONCLUSION

In this research, we tested three primary algorithms (random forest, logistic regression, and naïve Bayes). The Wisconsin Breast Cancer Diagnostic (WBCD) dataset was used to find a comparative analysis for breast cancer detection. To find the comparison, the study utilized results obtained based on various metrics such as the confusion matrix, sensitivity, accuracy, precision, and AUC to recognize the most accurate and reliable machine learning algorithm. All algorithms considered for comparison were implemented in Python using the scikit-learn library in the Anaconda environment. After careful analysis, we concluded that logistic regression outperformed all other algorithms. In summary, logistic regression proved to be efficient in predicting and diagnosing breast cancer. However, the study was limited to our findings on the WBCD database. A future scope of the work exists in the form of applying and analyzing algorithms on different datasets. In order to attain more accuracy, we also suggest a future strategy to use additional machine learning algorithms with new parameters on bigger datasets with more disease classes.

REFERENCES

1. Maglogiannis, E., E. Zafiropoulos, and I. Anagnostopoulos (2009), "An intelligent system for automated breast cancer diagnosis and prognosis using SVM based classifiers," *Applied Intelligence*, 30(1), 24–36.
2. Kumar, U. K., M. B. S. Nikhil, and K. Sumangali (2017), "Prediction of breast cancer using voting classifier technique," *Proceedings of the 2017 IEEE International Conference on Smart Technologies and Management for Computing, Communication, Controls, Energy and Materials (ICSTM)*, pp. 108–114, Chennai, August.
3. Zhou, Z.-H., and Y. Jiang (2003), "Medical diagnosis with C4.5 rule preceded by artificial neural network ensemble," *IEEE Transactions on Information Technology in Biomedicine*, 7(1), 37–42.
4. Lundin. (1999), "Artificial neural networks applied to survival prediction in breast cancer," *Oncology*, 57(4), 281–286.
5. "UCI machine learning repository: Breast cancer Wisconsin (diagnostic) data set," *International Journal of Computational Intelligence Studies*, 3(1), 71–89.
6. Swathi, A., Aarti, and S. Kumar (2022), "Review on secure traditional and machine learning algorithms for age prediction using IRIS image, Multimedia Tools and Applications," online link. https://link.springer.com/article/10.1007/s11042-022-13355-4
7. Swathi, A., Aarti, and S. Kumar (2021), A smart application to detect pupil for small dataset with low illumination, *Innovations in Systems and Software Engineering*, 17(1), 29–43.
8. Pal, R., S. Yadav, R. Karnwal, and Aarti (2020), EEWC: Energy-efficient weighted clustering method based on genetic algorithm for HWSNs, *Complex and Intelligent Systems*, 6(2), 391–400.
9. Aarti, G. Sikka, and R. Dhir (2020), "Novel grey relational feature extraction algorithm for software fault-proneness using BBO (B-GRA)," *Arabian Journal for Science and Engineering*, 45(4), 2645–2662.
10. Aarti, G. Sikka, and R. Dhir (2018), "Grey relational classification algorithm for software fault- proneness with SOM clustering," *International Journal of Data Mining, Modelling and Management (IJDMMM), Inderscience*, 12(1), 28–64.
11. Aarti, G. Sikka, and R. Dhir (2016), "An investigation on the effect of cross project data for prediction accuracy," *International Journal of System Assurance Engineering and Management*, 7(1), 1–26.

12. Rajput, P. K., G. Nagpal, and Aarti (2013), "Feature weighted unsupervised classification algorithm and adaptation for software cost estimation," *International Journal of Computational Intelligence Studies*, 3(1), 74–93.
13. Tripathi, M. K., M. Neelakantapp, A. N. Kaulage, K. V. Nabilal, S. N. Patil, and K. D. Bamane (2023), "An enhanced breast cancer diagnosis scheme based on two-step-SVM technique," *International Journal of Advanced Computer Science and Applications*, 8(4), 158–165.
14. Asri, H., H. Mousannif, H. Al Moatassime, and T. Noel (2016), "Using machine learning algorithms for breast cancer risk prediction and diagnosis," *Procedia Computer Science*, 83, 1064–1069.
15. Gayathri, B. M. and C. P. Sumathi (2016), "Comparative study of relevance vector machine with various machine learning techniques used for detecting breast cancer," *2016 IEEE International Conference on Computational Intelligence and Computing Research (ICCIC)*, Chennai, pp. 1–5.
16. Dedeepya, P., A. J. D. Krupa, and S. Dhanalakshmi (2017), "Abnormality detection using weighed particle swarm optimization and smooth support vector machine," *Biomedical Research*, 28(11), 4749–4751.
17. Karim, M. R., G. Wicaksono, I. G. Costa, S. Decker, and O. Beyan (2019), "Prognostically relevant subtypes and survival prediction for breast cancer based on multimodal genomics data," *IEEE Access*, 7, 133850–133864.
18. Akram, Shaik Vaseem, Praveen Kumar Malik, Rajesh Singh, Anita Gehlot, Ashima Juyal, Kayhan Zrar Ghafoor, and Sachin Shrestha (2022), "Implementation of digitalized technologies for fashion Industry 4.0: Opportunities and challenges," *Scientific Programming*. https://doi.org/10.1155/2022/7523246
19. Rokade, Ashay, Manwinder Singh, Praveen Kumar Malik, Rajesh Singh, and Turki Alsuwian (2022), "Intelligent data analytics framework for precision farming using IoT and regressor machine learning algorithms," *Applied Sciences*, 12(19), 9992. https://doi.org/10.3390/app12199992
20. Marwah, Gagan Preet Kour, Anuj Jain, Praveen Kumar Malik, Manwinder Singh, Sudeep Tanwar, Calin Ovidiu Safirescu, Traian Candin Mihaltan, Ravi Sharma, and Ahmed Alkhayyat. "An improved machine learning model with hybrid technique in VANET for robust communication," *Mathematics*, 10(21), 4030. https://doi.org/10.3390/math10214030
21. Kimothi, Sanjeev, Asha Thapliyal, Anita Gehlot, Arwa N. Aledaily, Anish gupta, Naveen Bilandi, Rajesh Singh, Praveen Kumar Malik, and Shaik Vaseem Akram (2023), "Spatio-temporal fluctuations analysis of land surface temperature (LST) using Remote Sensing data (LANDSAT TM5/8) and multifractal technique to characterize the urban heat Islands (UHIs)," *Sustainable Energy Technologies and Assessments*, 55, 102956. https://doi.org/10.1016/j.seta.2022.102956
22. Kumar, Kanak, Kaustav Chaudhury, and Suman Lata Tripathi (2023), "Future of machine learning (ML) and deep learning (DL) in healthcare monitoring system," *Machine Learning Algorithms for Signal and Image Processing*, pp. 293–313. https://doi.org/10.1002/9781119861850.ch17
23. Wijayanto, Inung, Annisa Humairani, Sugondo Hadiyoso, Achmad Rizal, Dasari Lakshmi Prasanna, and Suman Lata Tripathi (2023), "Epileptic seizure detection on a compressed EEG signal using energy measurement," *Biomedical Signal Processing and Control*, 85, 104872. https://doi.org/10.1016/j.bspc.2023.104872

Chapter 7

Design and Development of an IoT-Based Smart Medical Device

Shailesh Khaparkar, Neeta Nathani, and Jagdeesh Kumar Ahirwar

7.1 INTRODUCTION

As wearable technology, telemedicine, and mobile health evolve, remote patient monitoring (RPM) devices are becoming vital tools for healthcare professionals and hold promise for more than just managing chronic health issues. RPM devices use an implantable or external device to gather patient data outside of a conventional healthcare setting before sending the information to medical personnel for analysis. Heart rate, blood pressure, vital signs, temperature, weight, and blood sugar levels are just some of the information they can gather and deliver at any time and any place. Due to the COVID-19 pandemic's limits on in-person visits to avoid the virus' spread, RPM devices were one of the most popular industries in 2020 and 2021. With a compound annual growth rate (CAGR) of 3.3%, the RPM market is predicted to rise from $548.9 million in 2020 to $760 million in 2030.

The COVID-19 epidemic drove the use of virtual care services by medical device companies and patients, which accelerated the creation of mobile care applications, telehealth platforms, and the need for solutions for remote health monitoring. Many patients now place high importance on the comfort and accessibility of at-home care and actively engage in health self-monitoring via fitness trackers, smart watches, smartphones, and mobile applications. According to GlobalData, the wearable technology market will grow to $54.4 billion in value in 2019 from $22.9 billion in 2018, representing a 19% CAGR.

RPM use obstacles like privacy worries and ambiguity about gadget capabilities are vanishing. According to a GlobalData poll of 201 respondents, 66% are more likely to use a remote monitoring device now than they were before the epidemic, despite privacy, effectiveness, or other difficulties. The target market for RPM devices has expanded as a result of this paradigm shift. Continuous remote monitoring continues to be particularly beneficial for patients with chronic diseases like arrhythmias, chronic kidney ailments, and diabetes because any change in their state could necessitate urgent medical intervention. Nevertheless, 37 different companies have released RPM solutions for COVID-19 application cases, according

 DOI: 10.1201/9781003466949-7

to the GlobalData Marketing Solutions database. Other companies have updated the in-use RPM technology to offer at-home solutions for a variety of diagnostic requirements. Medical device businesses are under more pressure to maintain healthcare quality while putting money into data privacy and security for their newest virtual healthcare solutions.

The user-friendliness of at-home devices and improved healthcare access for patients in rural areas and those with restricted mobility will continue to be the main drivers of the RPM industry. For consultations and diagnosis, many specialists can use device data in real time, boosting care for patients who have trouble getting to a testing center. As the world's population ages, effective technology usage will be crucial to preventing the healthcare system from being overloaded.

The structure of the chapter is as follows. The related research on intelligent health monitoring systems is covered in Section 7.2. This is followed by major RPM components that are used to gather health data of patients in Section 7.3. Different IoT cloud platforms that provide options for connectivity are explained in Section 7.4, followed by future RPM devices in Section 7.5. The methodology section (Section 7.6) presents the methodology as well as the workflow for putting the prototype into practice. This section concentrates on the various hardware parts. The system's performance assessment is covered under "Results" together with the collection of patient data. The final section, Section 7.7, contains the summary and prospective research that may be used to improve the efficacy of the IoT-based smart health system.

7.2 RELATED WORK

Numerous academics have focused on health prediction using IoT in smart healthcare. Hamizah Anuar et al. [1] presented the development of a wearable core body temperature (CBT) sensor device based on a single heat-flux idea. According to trials with the sensor on different parts of the body, the forehead has the lowest mean difference between the CBT sensor and clinical thermometer, which is around 0.05°C. Po-Wei Huang et al. demonstrated how to use a neural network regression approach to increase the distance range from 50 to 100 cm. To activate the automated face tracking feature, the human face must be accurately focused while being measured. The information and results are also available via the web and an app [2]. Rahaman et al. focused on the advantages and disadvantages of the technologies used in healthcare systems while discussing the various smart health monitoring system types [3]. Huang and coworkers have developed a wearable temperature measuring system that may be applied to healthcare [4]. The many IoT-based technologies that might be applied to telemedicine and healthcare services for disease prevention were thoroughly analyzed by Albahri et al. [5]. Research was done to monitor student health utilizing a wireless IoT-based gadget that could immediately alert parents or guardians [6]. Along a related research route, many researchers created a remote COVID-19 patient monitoring system with the measurement of important body parameters including photoplethysmography (PPG), electrocardiogram (ECG), and temperature for assessing a patient's health status. Additionally, they discuss the difficulties related to security concerns in IoT-based smart health systems [7].

Bassam et al. used a wearable health monitoring device for COVID-19 patients that included a real-time tracking feature for position tracking using an integrated Global Positioning System (GPS). The complete system is linked to an Android user interface (UI) through an application programming interface (API) to track the patient's recovery and health [8]. Similar frameworks were put out by Paganelli et al. and addressed several architectures that may be utilized to keep track of COVID-19 patients and aid in COVID-19 identification [9]. The application layer, the data distribution layer, and the layer for data collection make up the bulk of the recommended design. The bulk of IoT-based health systems do, however, have a few problems, such as latency and communication delays. All of these problems can be resolved using fog computing and data mining technologies [10]. Patient data security is one of the major problems with IoT-based smart health systems, therefore block encryption-based methods might be utilized to protect data in the cloud [11]. Other parameters, such as gestures, facial expressions, and body language, can be sensed to identify seizure or non-seizure conditions, as well as epilepsy conditions, which can help a doctor decide how to treat a patient through remote monitoring in addition to detecting common diseases by measuring vital body parameters [12]. Bhatia et al.'s work [13] demonstrated the use of an IoT-based home system for identifying infectious illnesses of the urinary tract, such as diabetes, cystines, hepatitis, and liver disease. Another study [14] discussed IoT's possible future engagement in personal health monitoring while focusing on illness management, the patient experience, successful treatment, and the role of 5G in communication.

The issue of using machine learning to analyze and manage cloud data for precise illness prediction was explored in a paper by the Kondaka research team. Deep learning techniques can be used to minimize the flaws and errors in IoT smart health systems [15]. To solve difficulties such as cloud security, storage allocation, communication latency, data retrieval, etc., Li and colleagues carried out an extensive study on the effectiveness of machine learning mixed with big data analytics [16]. Utilizing machine learning techniques, the IoT system might be used to forecast an individual's future conduct by analyzing their actions, gestures, and other health-related indicators [17]. With a focus on important factors like efficiency and security, Onasanya et al. introduced an IoT/wireless sensor network (WSN)-based cloud system for the detection and treatment of cancer patients [18].

Another Internet of Things system was developed for the detection of potential COVID-19 patients with the use of eight different learning algorithms that assisted in differentiating the symptoms of the common cold from those of COVID-19 [19]. One study investigated the use of IoT systems for patient monitoring in smart cities in order for an ambulance and other types of help to reach the patient's location [20].

Wan et al. developed a body-area networked wearable Internet of Things health monitoring system where a variety of sensors continually capture and measure data [21]. All of the IoT technology was installed in a hospital or a house, or was a wearable, therefore in each of these application areas, the system had some issues. Uslu et al. covered some of the elements that must be taken into account while creating and putting into practice an automated IoT health monitoring system, including network traffic, big data analytics, intelligent computing, and IoT layer architecture [22]. A lot of serious issues come up when an IoT-based health monitoring system is built, most notably instances of patient information exploitation, data aggregation, and cybercrime [23]. Using an IoT-based tracking system will enable the government to follow patients and halt the spread of the disease, which is the main objective of tracking COVID-19 occurrences [24]. Real-time monitoring of COVID-19 patients using big data on biological signals may lower the incidence of COVID-19 transmission [25].

7.3 MAJOR RPM COMPONENTS

Similar to how different IoT setup modules can be segmented, an RPM can be segmented. Thus, the following can be said to be the high-level RPM components (as also shown in Figure 7.1):

1) *Personal monitoring devices.* These devices frequently include a Bluetooth module and capture all required patient data. Sensors placed under or over the skin or through wearable technology are used to measure a variety of health variables, including blood pressure and heart rate. For the time being, the US Food and Drug Administration (FDA) will only authorize noninvasive devices that record a basic set of physiological events. Every piece of wearable technology must be able to transmit patient measurements to a healthcare provider. The most popular mechanism for this transmission is the Bluetooth Low Energy (BLE) connection.
2) *Mobile app for patients.* Wearable device data is gathered via a mobile app and given to the physician. To guard against connectivity issues, these apps must be BLE data exchange network compatible and include caching functionality. Fast Healthcare Interoperability Resources (FHIR)-based secure APIs should be used to connect the application to the healthcare provider's system. The program is often made with

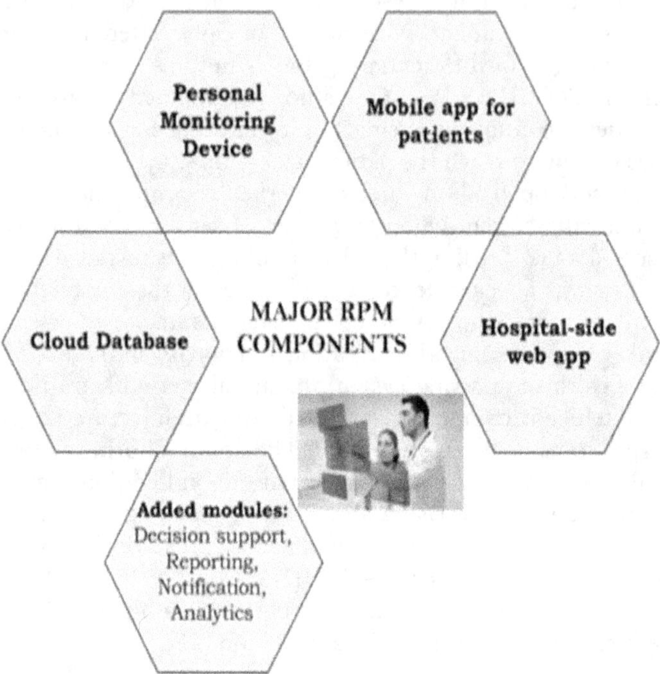

Figure 7.1 RPM components

educational pictures and excellent user experience design to make it fun for patients to use. These applications let users make video calls, access instructional content, and set reminders for taking medications.

3) *Cloud database.* The patient's wearable device may send raw data to the cloud repository. This data is sorted into manageable, labeled clusters using analytics powered by AI. For RPM devices, a number of systems provide direct-to-cloud connectivity, wherein all the recorded data is stored in the cloud.
4) *Hospital-side web app.* The web app used by the hospital, and similar to the patient-side app, satisfies the requirements of the Health Insurance Portability and Accountability Act (HIPAA). It uses Fast Healthcare Interoperability Resources (FHIR)-compatible APIs to interface with the hospital administration's electronic medical records (EMR) system. Furthermore, this software connects directly to the departmental data silos.
5) *Added modules.* Additionally, some or all of the modules listed next are part of the RPM setup:
   i) *Decision support.* Before delivering the patient's vital signs to the doctor, this module copies them from the repository and compares them to the expected values.

ii) *Reporting*. Using all relevant patient metrics and manual inputs, the RPM system provides reports for the medical staff.
iii) *Notification*. If the decision support module notices anomalies in the patient data, a warning message is sent to the relevant physician or consultant.

6) *Analytics*. Real-time conclusions are drawn from the patient data using business intelligence (BI) and AI-enabled data visualization tools. These inferences can be used by doctors to forecast hazards and make informed treatment choices.

7.4 IOT CLOUD PLATFORM

In order to deliver end-to-end service, IoT cloud platforms must combine the capabilities of cloud platforms and IoT devices. An IoT device is connected to the cloud and all of its various sensors through a gateway. The internet is connected to numerous devices, and IoT devices handle enormous amounts of data while interacting with several apps. There are three distinct ways to build an IoT cloud: PaaS (platform as a service), IaaS (infrastructure as a service), and SaaS (software as a service). It is atop other general clouds like Microsoft, Amazon, Google, and others. The duty of extending and analyzing data and processing it through the cloud and devices is handled by IoT cloud platforms.

In the modern era, enormous amounts of data are produced and kept in the cloud. Data minimization with the use of analytics is one of the key promises of the primary purpose, which is to support processing by utilizing the current infrastructure. Instead of a novel storage system, the impetus for this chapter's direction comes from data created from many other sources, including the communication, healthcare industry, mobile sensors, and messaging networks. The three views of descriptive analytics, predictive analytics, and prescriptive analytics are used in data reduction approaches for big data. The cost of storage in a pay-as-you-go cloud environment can be high. The top cloud computing services for IoT development include:

1) *AWS IoT*. In hospitals, houses, cars, and different locations, there are billions of devices. Even when internet access is lost, AWS enables users to gather, store, and analyze device data. Some of the services it provides include AWS IoT Core, IoT device management, and IoT device protection. They can analyze their IoT data using AWS IoT analytics services. Users only have to pay for what they use if they use it on a scale. It provides tools for monitoring and auditing security rules, access control, and encryption as security features. For example, Symantec Network utilizes IoT for the backend, while Anel

Commercial uses IoT for energy management (creating green glass enabling gateways for houses). It is advantageous for linked homes, commercial and industrial undertakings, and industrial purposes.

2) *Microsoft Azure IoT Hub.* Accessing computing services like networking and storage from the service provider Azure via the internet is known as cloud computing. Cloud computing occurs when we keep images online rather than in a phone gallery. Using selected technologies and frameworks, it offers services for delivering applications across a vast worldwide network. It is applied to solving commercial problems. It is a Microsoft product, making it more dependable, more secure, and less expensive to use. When demands vary, the size of the storage resources can be adjusted on Azure. Tools and services for hybrid cloud applications will be managed by it. With all the languages, we can create a framework that can be deployed anywhere. When utilizing Azure, experts offer assistance.
3) *Salesforce IoT.* Constructing an application requires a lot of effort, but with the aid of Salesforce, it becomes simple and takes up less time because it offers the quickest route from considering constructing an app to actually doing it. Tools and infrastructure are not a concern. Anyone with access to the internet and the cloud can utilize it from any location. It can develop with the business, whose applications change according to the seasons. It aids small enterprises and startups. For users and developers, it offers software solutions and platforms. Upgrades and infrastructure are carried out automatically. Services offered to customers include app exchange, sales cloud, service cloud, and exact target market cloud. Businesses can use the services offered by the Salesforce IoT cloud to process and store Internet of Things data. Salesforce manages enormous amounts of data produced by gadgets, websites, sensors, etc., and responds to the information supplied by clients.
4) *Google Cloud IoT.* It is used to gather and analyze data, which is then stored locally and in the cloud. It is a fully managed, scalable cloud service. Users can learn more about the company using the services offered by Google Cloud IoT data. Google BigQuery is used to perform ad hoc analysis. Users learn more about the Google Cloud IoT platform's device performance. Google Maps may be used to track assets in real time and visualize their locations. It offers security while posing less risks. It has intelligent asset monitoring and management.
5) *IBM Watson IoT platform.* IBM Watson is a hosted cloud service that facilitates data storage, communication, management, and quick visualization. Using the intelligent and scalable platform, users can obtain real-time analysis of user and machine data, including speech, text, and video. Users can make wiser business judgments thanks to this. Through ecosystems, it can link IoT devices, networks, and gateways (using HTTPS-based standard-based communication). Both

organized and unstructured data are analyzed by it. We can analyze, alter, and retrieve historical data. IoT applications may be integrated.

6) *Oracle-integrated cloud for IoT.* Oracle IoT is an SaaS product that is based on highly scalable IoT platforms and cloud infrastructure powered by Oracle. It offers built-in expansion capabilities and integrations that allow businesses to expand, including enterprise resource planning. Real-time visibility into the data will be provided, allowing for increased productivity and the extraction of applications' economic benefits. With each device having a distinct identification and authorization of proof-of-origin data, security is extremely available. REST APIs (RESTFul API) are used to link various devices to enterprise applications. It can create clever IoT solutions thanks to its built in intelligence and machine learning capabilities.
7) *ThingSpeak.* These interconnected gadgets of IoT exchange information with people and other objects, and frequently send sensor data to cloud storage and cloud computing resources for processing and analysis to produce significant insights. This trend is made possible by reduced cloud computing costs and improved device connectivity. IoT solutions are designed for a variety of vertical applications, such as home automation, environmental monitoring and control, industrial monitoring and control, health monitoring, and vehicle fleet monitoring. Figure 7.2 can be used to describe several IoT systems at a high level. The advantages of using ThingSpeak include hosting channels for free; simple visualization; and adding new functionality to Ruby, Node.js, and Python. The drawbacks include limited API data uploading and, for new users, the ThingSpeak API can be challenging.

Monitoring, analysis, and control of environments based on information gathered from a network of sensors reflect the perspective of this chapter. With the help of the IoT idea, every object may be recognized and given networking, sensing, and processing capabilities. The items can communicate with other online devices or services as well as with one another. They will be commonplace and aware of their surroundings. This chapter's goal is to illustrate the present state of the development, trends, and research on the Internet of Things as it is used in e-health through examination. The current method uses a heartbeat sensor to determine the heart rate and displays it on the liquid crystal display (LCD) panel. The transmitting circuit uses a microcontroller from the AVR family that is connected to an LCD screen and is powered by a 12V transformer. Similar to the sending circuit, the receiving circuit has a 12V transformer, an AVR family microcontroller, and a radio frequency (RF) receiver. The receiver circuit has a light-emitting diode (LED) light and a buzzer that is used to warn the person monitoring the patient's heartbeat rate. The LED light and buzzer are activated as soon as the patient's heartbeat level deviates from the typical heartbeat level established.

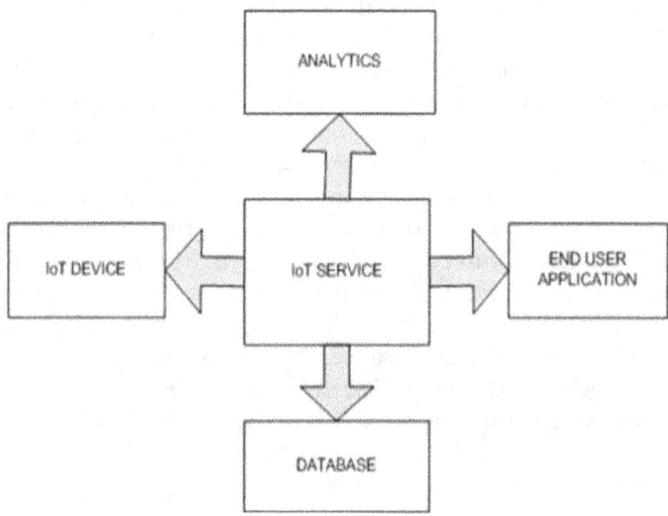

Figure 7.2 ThingSpeak's function

7.5 FUTURE PROTOTYPES AND COMMON RPM DEVICES

According to a 2020 IHS Markit poll, more than five million patients will be monitored remotely globally by the end of 2023. The following are a few of the devices that are dominating the medical device market:

1) *Microsampling devices.* Devices for collecting samples remotely are becoming more common, particularly those that use the volumetric absorptive microsampling (VAMS) method. Blood from the fingertip is sufficient thanks to current analytics tools because it has a volumetric variation of less than 5%. VAMS does away with the requirement for traditional phlebotomy and venous blood collection.
2) *Continuous glucose monitors.* These devices can detect high blood sugar levels using a sensor placed under the skin while monitoring blood sugar levels throughout the day. Parents of children with type I diabetes can monitor their children's readings and act swiftly when readings reach hazardous levels. Clinicians can also use these devices remotely.
3) *Inexpensive surgical automation.* Surgeons can now accurately reach various areas of the human body thanks to these technologies. Despite the high cost of robotic process automation (RPA) for surgical tools, many companies, notably Riverfield and Stryker, are exploring ways to mass-produce these instruments at cost-effective prices. These tools would provide surgeons with advanced technology to securely reach the organs as well as expand projections of the targeted organ.

4) *Intelligent vision.* By the end of 2021, AI will improve computer vision, making it possible to use it to obtain visual features of patient vitals more quickly. The initial use of this technique will be to measure blood loss or hemorrhaging in women during or after delivery. This technique will be especially important in remote and hard-to-reach locations where gynecological intervention is scarce.

RPM systems assist individuals in taking a more active role in their health management, in addition to assisting doctors in treating a significantly bigger volume of patients. When unforeseen accessibility challenges are anticipated to arise in the upcoming years, these technologies will continue to gain in importance. Additionally, doctors would be able to use RPMs' cloud computing and AI-enabled data analytics for better diagnostic and treatment precision.

7.6 USE CASE: METHODOLOGY FOR PROPOSED TELEMEDICINE MONITORING SYSTEM

An extremely effective technique separates IoT-based health monitoring systems from traditional healthcare systems. As a result, using IoT to produce the desired results and performances becomes quite difficult. The embedded world and working with IoT are related because sensors use electronic data signals. Sensors, detectors, monitors, and microcontrollers are initially connected for synchronization. The monitoring system, in summary, is an essential part of the online healthcare service. The performance of health applications depends on the correctness of the data, which may even directly affect patients' lives. In turn, this study encourages data-driven research for future advancements by providing a novel method for continually interacting via commonly used wireless network protocols and monitoring patients' health. The main contributions of this chapter are described in Figure 7.3 and summarized as follows:

- Enable telemedicine and data-driven research by leveraging crucial medical indicators like SpO2, heart rate, and body temperature to generate health recommendations based on trends seen in vast volumes of data that have been accumulated over time [26].
- Low-cost hardware that allows for real-time data observation [27].
- Proactive or preventive approach to cardiovascular diseases (CVDs).

Three sensors are included in the proposed system: sensors 1 and 2 for health monitoring and sensors 3 for imaging the tongue and eyes of the patient and, if necessary, video calling. The SpO2, heart rate, and body temperature of a person have all been measured using these noise- and

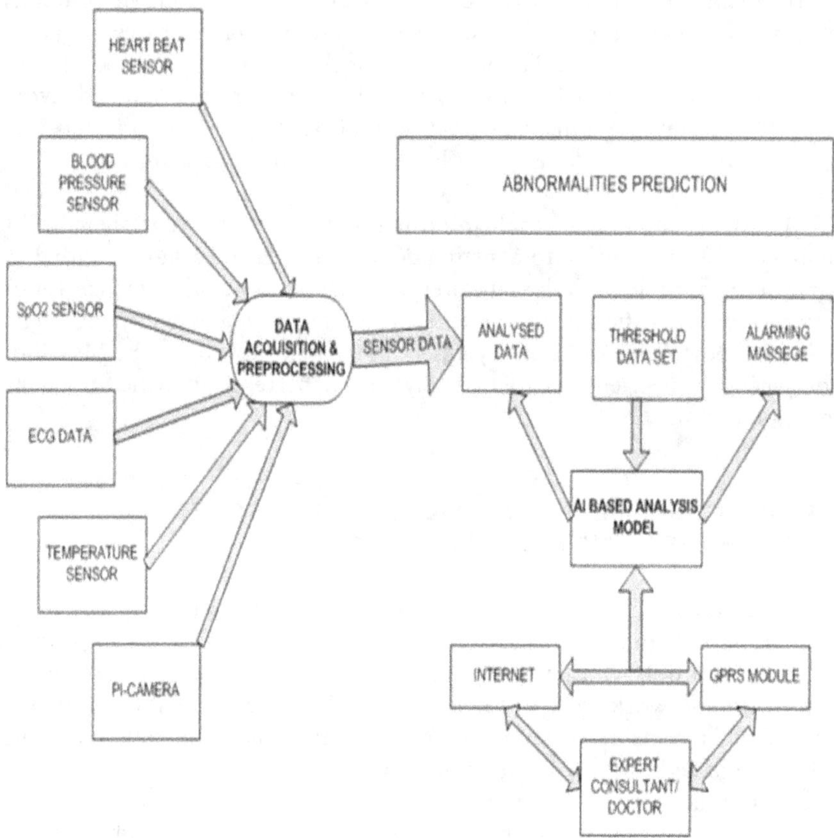

Figure 7.3 Block diagram of proposed remote patient monitoring (RPM)

power-efficient sensors [28]. The signals are recorded and the obtained data is compared to a predefined threshold level on the cloud server, which receives the signals from the ESP-8266 module. A warning message is issued to the patient, hospitals, and patient families if any irregularities are discovered. The devised method also suggests a qualified physician for an online video consultation. Figure 7.4 shows the suggested IoT-based telemedicine monitoring system with different sensors used as follows:

1) *MLX90614 Sensor.* The temperature of a particular item may be ascertained using the MLX90614 Contactless Infrared Digital Temperature Sensor, which has a temperature range of –70°C to 382.2°C. The sensor communicates with the microcontroller via the I2C protocol and uses infrared (IR) rays to monitor temperature without any physical touch. It is used in many commercial, medical, and residential applications because of its high accuracy and precision,

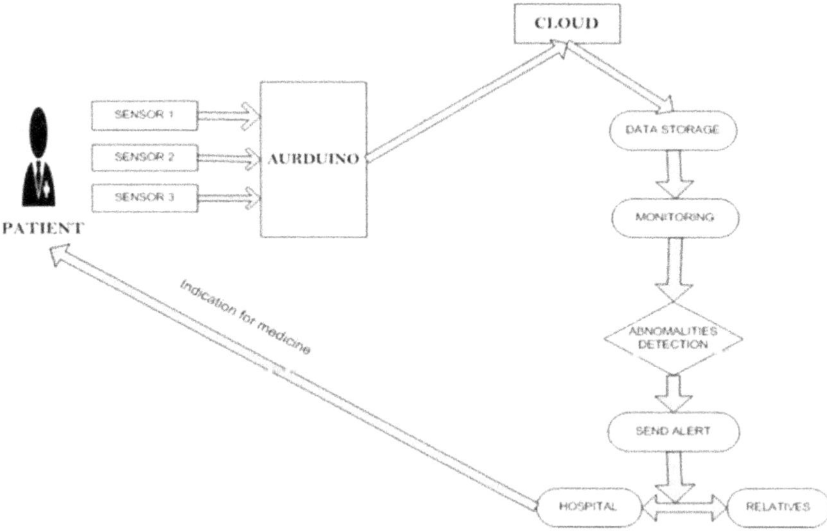

Figure 7.4 Proposed telemedicine monitoring system

including the monitoring of environmental temperature and the measurement of body temperature.

2) *MAX30100 Sensor.* The MAX30100 is a sensor system that measures pulse oximetry and heart rate. It has improved optics, a photodetector, two LEDs, and low-noise analogue data processing. These qualities enable it to detect pulse oximetry and heart rate signals. It needs 1.8V and 3.3V power sources to function.
3) *WeMos D1 R1.* The WeMos D1 Wi-Fi development board is built on the ESP8266 12E. Despite the hardware being a duplicate of the Arduino UNO, NODE-MCU functions more like the Arduino UNO.
4) *IoT cloud.* The IoT cloud is a massive network that supports IoT devices and applications. AWS IoT Platform, Microsoft Azure IoT Suite, ThingSpeak IoT Platform, Google Cloud's IoT Platform, IBM Watson IoT Platform, Kaa IoT Platform, Salesforce IoT Cloud, Oracle IoT Platform, Cisco IoT Cloud Connect, and GE Predix IoT Platform are some of the leading cloud platforms. ThingSpeak is used as the IoT cloud platform in the proposed work. Users may gather and store sensor data in the cloud using the open-source software ThingSpeak. The app can be used with MATLAB to analyze and visualize data. Raspberry Pi, Arduino, or Beaglebone can be used to transmit sensor data. To save data, a different channel can be built. ThingSpeak's features include: collecting data in private channels, event scheduling, app integration, and MATLAB analytics and visualization.
5) *Arduino IDE.* The Arduino Software is another name for the Integrated Development Environment (IDE) for Arduino. It features

menus, a message box, a text terminal, a toolbar with buttons for frequently used operations, and a text editor for writing code. It joins the Arduino hardware for communication and code upload.

6) *Video calling.* The Patient Engagement System now includes a video calling consultation option, allowing patients to access online video consultations with doctors as needed. The created system stores a list of expert doctors along with their contact information and video call link. After checking the vital indicators, it recommends a doctor for online consultation. Face-to-face online consultation services assist doctors in better understanding patients for use in future procedures and accurate diagnosis. The technology is connected with the Google Meet online meeting platform. The sensor data is downloaded to a Google document where it is stored and patient data is recorded for later use.

7.6.1 Hardware Setup

The sensor reading is read by the Node-MCU hardware board before the program is put into action. The cloud Sheets and the IoT platform Blynk get the sensor data after that. A Node-MCU board is simultaneously reading the sensor-1. Python is a computer language that uses an indirect method to send data to the cloud. Python is used to read the data from the serial port before sending it to cloud Sheets using the Google Drive API. The hardware configuration of the suggested system is shown in Figure 7.5 together with its layout in Figure 7.6.

As shown in Figure 7.7, the proposed system begins with reading sensor data. After the sensor reading, data is preprocessed for the minimal threshold check. A minimal threshold examination is done to look for any physiological parameter irregularities in the patient. Following the abnormality check, the report is shown and uploaded to the cloud platform, and a connection is made between the patient and the healthcare provider using a communication device that makes use of the camera module. The health

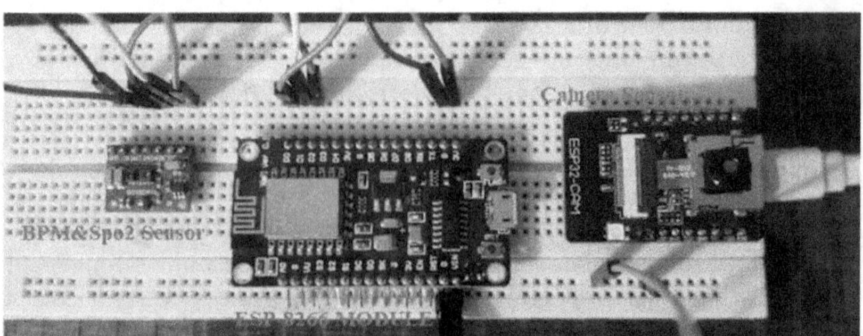

Figure 7.5 Hardware setup of the proposed system

Wemos D1 R1

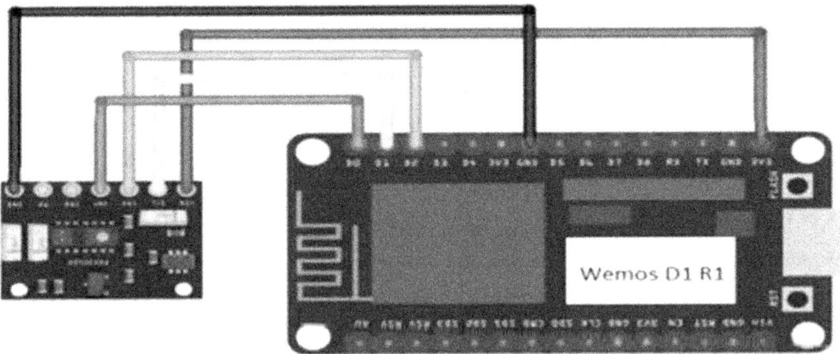

Figure 7.6 Layout of the proposed system

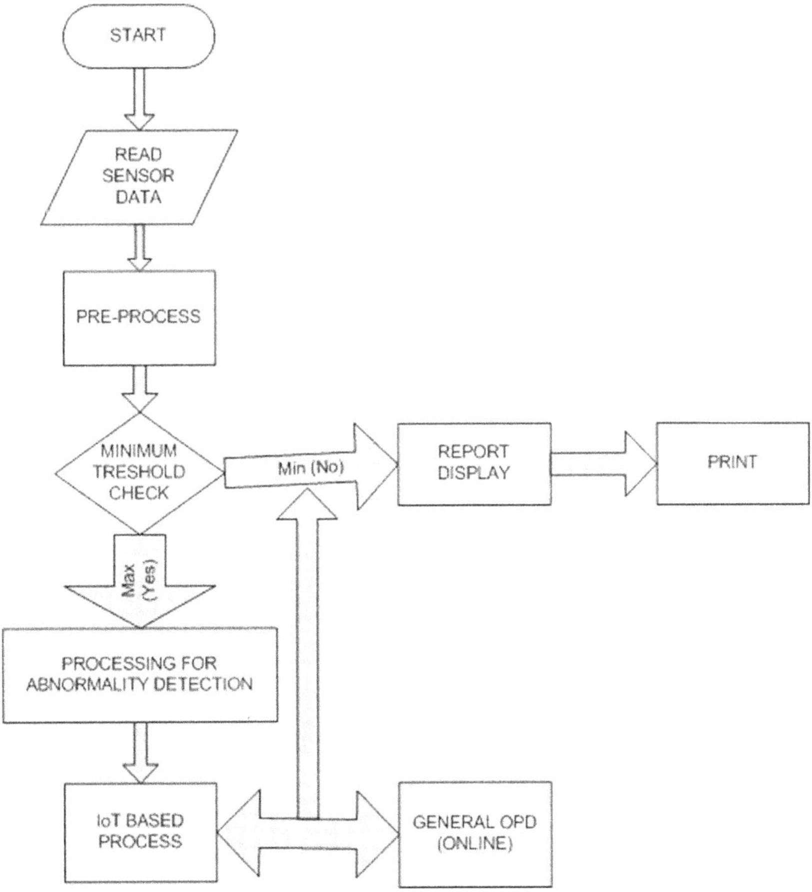

START
READ SENSOR DATA
PRE-PROCESS
MINIMUM TRESHOLD CHECK
Min (No)
REPORT DISPLAY
PRINT
Max (Yes)
PROCESSING FOR ABNORMALITY DETECTION
IoT BASED PROCESS
GENERAL OPD (ONLINE)

Figure 7.7 Flowchart of working of the proposed system

care practitioner is given the various necessary readings and visual feeds of the patient's eyes and tongue with the aid of the camera module and sensor unit to continue evaluating the patient's health status and to assist them in giving the patient the precise solution.

7.6.2 Results

A wide array of extremely sophisticated commercial wireless sensors are used to monitor the characteristics of this system. This system presents a cloud- and IoT-based health monitoring system for telemedicine applications. The method that has been proposed evaluates the many health indicators that may be drawn from sensor data. Thanks to this method, which captures data via the internet and communication devices before linking it to cloud services, people may obtain faster and more reliable medical treatment. The data gathered from the cloud server is updated in real time according to the internet speed of the service provider. The random temperature, SpO2, and heart rate readings from the dashboard are shown in Figure 7.8.

On the operator's mobile phone, the same dashboard will be viewable. The data transferred from the sensor to the cloud also includes real-time date and timestamp changes. By monitoring the physiological traits, the suggested system has also undergone real-time functional testing. Health anomalies are identified using the heart rate and SpO2 level.

7.7 CONCLUSION

The current goal is to enable data-driven research while continually monitoring individual health, aberrant heartbeats, SpO2, body temperature, alerts, and notifications using well-known wireless communication channels. The recommended solution enables patient data-driven research,

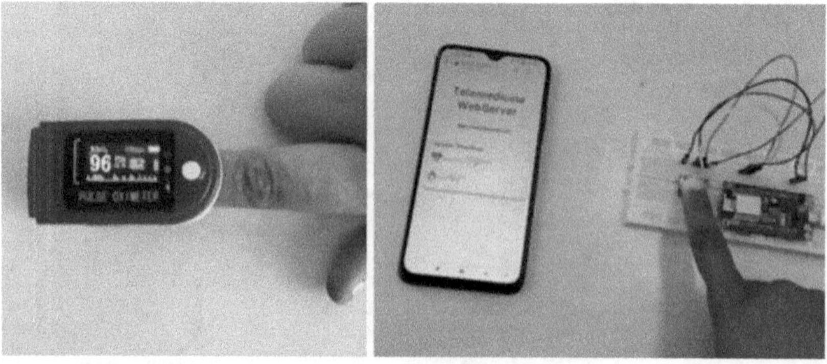

Figure 7.8 Recording of vital parameters using the setup

connectivity over popular wireless network protocols, and ongoing individual health monitoring. Remote diagnosis is made possible by the proposed paradigm, which speeds up treatment intervention. Even though they are far apart, a patient and doctor can consult with one another. This framework also shows patients' heartbeats recorded live data with timestamps over the internet and alert management systems inside the clinics or hospitals to aid in localization and early action for the treatment of cardiovascular patients. Real-time wearable monitoring sensors are accurate enough. A telemedicine system utilizing a cloud interface and the cloud Sheets API has been built based on the MLX 90614 sensor and the MAX30100 with WeMos D1 R1. The filtered data is received by the Android mobile device, which then sends it to a cloud server for storage and ongoing patient monitoring. The system has undergone validation testing on a number of users, and the outcomes are thought to be favorable. Therefore, the deployment of a smart health monitoring system based on the Internet of Things enables contactless tracking and treatment of patients. The key issues with the prototype are protecting patient data and providing the data to the doctor with the least amount of delay within the specified time limit. One strategy for defending data from security lapses is data encryption. By using edge computing technology, which would make on-demand patient data available for research, this would be made possible. Future automatic cardiac diagnosis will utilize a cloud server and an appropriate convolutional neural network.

REFERENCES

1. Anuar, H, Leow, PL. Non-invasive core body temperature sensor for continuous monitoring. *2019 IEEE International Conference on Sensors and Nanotechnology*, 2019. DOI: 10.1109/SENSORSNANO44414.2019.8940040. Published in 2023.
2. Huang, PW, Chang, TH, Lee, MJ, Lin, TM, Chung, ML, Wu, BF. An embedded non-contact body temperature measurement system with automatic face tracking and neural network regression. *2016 International Automatic Control Conference (CACS)*, 2016. DOI: 10.1109/CACS.2016.7973902. Published in 2017.
3. Rahaman, A, Islam, MM, Sadi, MS. Developing IoT based smart health monitoring systems: A review. *Intelligent Information and Engineering Technology Association* 2019; 33(6):435–440. DOI: 10.18280/ria.330605.
4. Huang, T, Tang, C, Kanaya, S. A wearable thermometry for core body temperature measurement and its experimental verification. *IEEE Journal of Biomedical and Health Informatics* 2017;21(3):708–714. DOI: 10.1109/JBHI.2016.2532933.
5. Albahri, AS, Alwan, JK, Taha, ZK., Ismail, SF., Hamid, RA., Zaidan, AA, Alamoodi, AH, Alsalem, MA. IoT-based telemedicine for disease prevention and health promotion: State-of-the-Art. *Journal of Network and Computer Applications* 2021;173:102873. DOI: 10.1016/j.jnca.2020.102873.

6. Tan, Hua, Muthu, Sivaparthipan. Big data and ambient intelligence in IoT-based wireless student health monitoring system. *Aggression and Violent Behavior* 2021. DOI: 10.1016/j.avb.2021.101601.
7. Sharma, N, Mangla, M, Mohanty, SN, Gupta, D, Tiwari, P, Shorfuzzaman, M, Rawashdeh, M. A smart ontology-based IoT framework for remote patient monitoring. *Biomedical Signal Processing and Control* 2021;68:102717. DOI: 10.1016/j.bspc.2021.102717.
8. Bassam, Hussain, Qaraghuli, Khan, Sumesh, Lavanya. IoT based wearable device to monitor the signs of quarantined remote patients of COVID-19. *Informatics in Medicine Unlocked* 2021;24:100588. DOI: 10.1016/j.imu.2021.100588.
9. Paganelli, AI, Velmovitsky, PE, Miranda, P, Branco, A, Alencar, P, Cowan, D, Endler, M, Morita, PP. A conceptual IoT-based early-warning architecture for remote monitoring of COVID-19 patients in wards and at home. *Internet Things* 2021. DOI: 10.1016/j.iot.2021.100399.
10. Moghadas, E, Rezazadeh, J, Farahbakhsh, R. An IoT patient monitoring based on fog computing and data mining: Cardiac arrhythmia usecase. *Internet Things* 2020;11:100251. DOI: 10.1016/j.iot.2020.100251.
11. Akhbarifar, Javadi, Hossein, Jadeh. A secure remote health monitoring model for early disease diagnosis in cloud-based IoT environment. *Personal and Ubiquitous Computing* 2020. DOI: 10.1007/s00779-020-01475-3.
12. Alhussein, Muhammad, Hossain, Amin. Cognitive IoT-cloud integration for smart healthcare: Case study for epileptic seizure detection and monitoring. *Mobile Networks and Applications* 2018;23(6):1624–1635. DOI: 10.1007/s11036-018-1113-0.
13. Bhatia, M, Kaur, S, Sood, SK. IoT-inspired smart home based urine infection prediction. *Journal of Ambient Intelligence and Humanized Computing* 2020. DOI: 10.1007/s12652-020-01952-w.
14. Kadhim, Alsahlany, Wadi, Kadhum. An overview of patient's health status monitoring system based on internet of things (IoT). *Wireless Personal Communications* 2020;114(3):2235–2262. DOI: 10.1007/s11277-020-07474-0.
15. Kondaka, Sudha, Thenmozhi, Kohli. An intensive healthcare monitoring paradigm by using IoT based machine learning strategies. *Multimedia Tools and Applications* 2021. DOI: 10.1007/s11042-021-11111-8.
16. Li, W, Chai, Y, Jan, V, Menon, L. A comprehensive survey on machine learning-based big data analytics for IoT-enabled smart healthcare system. *Mobile Networks and Applications* 2021;26(1):234–252. DOI: 10.1007/s11036-020-01700-6.
17. Manocha, Kumar, Bhatia, Sharma. IoT-inspired machine learning-assisted sedentary behavior analysis in smart healthcare industry. *Journal of Ambient Intelligence and Humanized Computing* 2021. DOI: 10.1007/s12652-021-03371-x.
18. Onasanya, Elshakankiri. Smart integrated IoT healthcare system for cancer care. *Wireless Networks* 2019;27(6):4297–4312. DOI: 10.1007/s11276-018-01932-1.

19. Otoom, M, Otoum, N, Alzubaidi, MA, Etoom, Y, Banihani, R. An IoT-based framework for early identification and monitoring of COVID-19 cases. *Biomedical Signal Processing and Control* 2020;62:102149. DOI: 10.1016/j.bspc.2020.102149.
20. Poongodi, Sharma, Hamdi, Chilamkruti. Smart healthcare in smart cities: Wireless patient monitoring system using IoT. *Journal of Supercomputing* 2021;7(11):12230–12255. DOI: 10.1007/s11227-021-03765-w.
21. Wan, Munassar. Al-awlaqi, Grady, Gu, Wang, Cao. Wearable IoT enabled real-time health monitoring system. *EURASIP Journal on Wireless Communications and Networking* 2018;2018(1):298. DOI: 10.1186/s13638-018-1308-x.
22. Uslu Okay, Dursun. Analysis of factors affecting IoT-based smart hospital design. *Journal of Cloud Computing* 2020;9(1):67. DOI: 10.1186/s13677-020-00215-5.
23. Singh, RP, Javaid, M, Haleem, A, Suman, R. Internet of things (IoT) applications to fight against COVID-19 pandemic. *Diabetology & Metabolic Syndrome* 2020;14(4):521–524. DOI: 10.1016/j.dsx.2020.04.041.
24. Kumar, K, Kumar, N, Shah, R. Role of IoT to avoid spreading of COVID-19. *Intelligent Journal of Intelligent Networks* 2020;1:32–35.
25. Sheares, GJ. Internet of Things-enabled smart devices, biomedical big data, and real-time clinical monitoring in COVID-19 patient health prediction. *American Journal of Medical Research* 2020;7(2):64–70. DOI: 10.22381/AJMR7220209.
26. Khaparkar, Shailesh, Mishra, Agya. A smart tele-healthcare system for real-time health monitoring and remote consultation. *2023 1st International Conference on Innovations in High Speed Communication and Signal Processing (IHCSP)*, 2023.
27. Tripathi, Suman Lata, Mahmud, Mufti *Explainable Machine Learning Models and Architecture*, Wiley & Scrivener Publishing LLC 2023. DOI: 10.1002/9781394186570.
28. Kumar, Kanak, Sharma, Anchal, Tripathi, Suman Lata *"Sensors and Their Application" Electronic Device and Circuits Design Challenges to Implement Biomedical Applications*, Elsevier 2021. ISBN: 978-0-323-85172-5. DOI: 10.1016/B978-0-323-85172-5.00021-6.

Chapter 8

Revolutionary Finance

Impact of Blockchain and Distributed Ledger Technology on the Financial Industry

Pooja Jain and Rachit Jain

8.1 INTRODUCTION

As a result of new technologies, the world is changing. A wide spectrum of people now have simple access to high-speed technology advancements thanks to the availability of an online connection and smartphone-enabled services (Sunyaev, 2020). Significant changes to the economy and society are referred to as "Industry 5.0" and as a whole have resulted from global technological breakthroughs that have altered internal and external application models to enhance digital process interactions. One of the biggest financial industry revolutions is frequently referred to as fintech (Natarajan et al., 2017). It has advanced swiftly, owing in part to the sharing economy, supportive regulations, and technological improvements. The development of new technologies-based fintech is a continuous process that involves finance and technology. Mobile and digital payment methods remain the key fintech vehicle. Fintech companies are rapidly increasing around the world, providing services in a wide range of industries such as credit management, asset management, electronic payment systems, and insurance goods and services. This technology is well-designed to assist organizations in adapting to standards in an effective and resourceful manner (Hughes et al., 2019).

According to McLean and Deane-Johns (2016), several elements of blockchain distributed ledger technology can be used to provide new financial services. Blockchain is beginning to have an impact on the internet's communication networks. Networks are an important component of the digital technologies that are revolutionizing the majority of industries and have the potential to change the way things work. Blockchain technology will profoundly disrupt the banking and finance sectors in the same way that information technology has enabled peer-to-peer (P2P) and media connections. Blockchain enables the general population to send and receive money swiftly, securely, and for a small transfer fee, which decreases or eliminates the danger of hacking enabling rapid transactions, without any need for third-party interference (Ellervee et al., 2017; Deshpande et al., 2017). Due to other elements of the fourth industrial age, such as blockchain networks

 DOI: 10.1201/9781003466949-8

and financial technology businesses' readiness for the digital platform and other services, the digitization of banking and financial services has not yet been fully completed. Digitalized banking services assess old business models and procedures in order to give faster response times and competence in providing secure and simple payment methods.

The remaining sections of the chapter are arranged as follows. A theoretical background and a literature review are presented in Section 8.2. Section 8.3 outlines the chapter's objectives. Section 8.4 presents the hypothesis formulation and conceptual relationships, and Section 8.5 explains the empirical results and data analysis. Section 8.6 presents the findings and discussion, and the final section explains the conclusion.

8.2 THEORETICAL BACKGROUND AND REVIEW OF LITERATURE

8.2.1 Distributed Ledger Technology

Distributed ledger technology (DLT) is a sort of digital ledger that enables data to be securely recorded, exchanged, and updated among various network participants or nodes. In contrast to typical centralized ledgers, which store data in a single location or are managed by a central authority, DLT distributes data among numerous nodes, making it decentralized (Trump et al., 2018). DLT's capacity to produce a transparent and immutable record of transactions is one of its fundamental advantages (Janowicz et al., 2018). DLT transactions are often encrypted, time-stamped, and connected to prior transactions, establishing a chain of blocks known as a blockchain.

Three categories of DLT exist: consortium, private, and public blockchains. Anyone can join a public blockchain network, participate in the consensus process, and access the ledger (Ribitzky et al., 2018). In a private blockchain, access to the network and participation in the consensus process are restricted to a small set of players, often within a single organization. Businesses frequently employ private blockchains for internal purposes such as supply chain management or record-keeping (Hamilton, 2020).

Consortium blockchains are a cross between public and private blockchains in which a group of organizations controls the network and participates in the consensus process. Due to its potential to upend sectors, including finance, logistics, medical care, and residential real estate, DLT has attracted a lot of attention. It provides advantages such as increased security, transparency, efficiency, and transaction traceability, which can lead to cost savings, improved procedures, and new business models (Howell et al., 2019). However, it is vital to highlight that DLT is still a developing technology with numerous problems to overcome, including scalability, interoperability, regulatory compliance, and privacy. Nevertheless, DLT has the potential to revolutionize how data and value are stored, shared, and transferred in various industries, offering new opportunities and possibilities for businesses and individuals alike (Bonnet & Teuteberg, 2023).

8.2.2 Distributed Ledger Technology and Transaction Processing

A type of digital database that is dispersed across numerous network nodes or computers is known as distributed ledger technology. The ledger is maintained by each node in the network, and any updates are verified and recorded by node consensus. DLT's distributed and consensus-based nature offers data stored in the ledger with openness, security, and integrity (Ølnes et al., 2017). In the context of DLT, transaction processing entails the creation, validation, and recording of transactions on the ledger. Financial transactions, digital assets, and contractual agreements are all examples of transactions (Kakavand et al., 2017). The transaction processing process typically consists of multiple steps, which may differ based on the specific DLT implementation but generally follow a similar pattern.

First, the transaction creation is started by a user who creates a transaction request. This could be a digital asset transfer, a financial payment, or any other sort of data that must be recorded on the ledger (Gangwar et al., 2014). Then the transaction request is evaluated to ensure that it complies with the DLT network's stated rules and standards. This could entail checking for appropriate dollars or assets, as well as ensuring that the transaction complies with any applicable smart contracts or business logic. Once the transaction has been validated, it must be authorized by consensus among the DLT network nodes. This usually entails a majority of the nodes agreeing on the transaction's authenticity before it can be entered into the ledger. Different DLT implementations employ different consensus methods to obtain consensus among nodes, such as proof-of-work, proof-of-stake, or delegated proof-of-stake. The transaction is recorded on the ledger as a new block of data. The recorded transaction becomes immutable, which means it cannot be changed or erased, and is stored across all network nodes. This ensures that the transaction is secure, transparent, and tamper-proof. Then the user receives confirmation that the transaction has been successfully processed once it has been entered on the ledger. This confirmation may include a transaction ID, which serves as the transaction's unique identification, and can be used for verification or auditing (Natarajan et al., 2017).

Additional steps may be necessary for some DLT implementations, such as finalizing the transaction by clearing and settling any associated financial obligations or updating applicable smart contracts. These stages ensure that the transaction is fully completed and that the necessary changes are applied to the ledger.

DLT and transaction processing have gained significant attention due to their potential to revolutionize industries such as finance, supply chain management, real estate, and more. By providing a decentralized, transparent, and secure approach to recording and processing transactions, DLT has the potential to streamline business processes, reduce fraud, lower costs, and increase trust among participants in a network (Wallace & Sheetz, 2014). However, it's important to note that DLT is still an emerging technology, and its widespread adoption and implementation are ongoing processes that require careful consideration of various technical, regulatory, and operational factors (Lule et al., 2012).

8.2.3 Role of Distributed Ledger Technology in Banks and Financial Institutions

DLT can have a transformative role in banks and financial institutions in several ways.

DLT provides a decentralized and tamper-proof ledger, which can dramatically improve financial transaction security. Transactions on a DLT are encrypted, time-stamped, and spread across numerous nodes, making unauthorized access, fraud, or data modification difficult. This can assist banks and financial institutions in mitigating risks connected with data breaches, cyberattacks, and fraud, hence improving overall operational security (McLean & Deane-Johns, 2016).

DLT enables transparent and traceable record-keeping since all transactions are recorded on a shared ledger that multiple parties may see and verify. This can assist banks and financial organizations in improving transparency in their operations, such as tracking the transfer of cash, validating asset legitimacy, and maintaining regulatory compliance. Transparency and traceability improvements can also lead to more efficient auditing and regulatory reporting processes (Hughes et al., 2019).

DLT can improve the efficiency of bank and financial institution settlement and clearing operations. Traditional financial industry settlement and clearing processes can be time-consuming, complex, and costly, including several intermediaries and reconciliations (Deshpande et al., 2017). DLT can enable real-time and automated settlement and clearing, eliminating the need for intermediaries, decreasing errors, and speeding the settlement process. Banks and financial institutions may benefit from faster, more efficient, and cost-effective transactions as a result of this (Coppi & Fast, 2019).

For banks and financial organizations, DLT offers the potential to cut costs and increase operational efficiency. DLT can minimize operational costs and reduce the risk of errors by eliminating the need for intermediaries, minimizing human processes, and automating reconciliations (Sunyaev, 2020). Furthermore, DLT can enable speedier transaction processing, minimizing the need for time-consuming and expensive reconciliation operations. For banks and financial organizations, this can result in significant cost savings and enhanced operating efficiency.

Cross-border payments can be complicated and time-consuming because they include various intermediaries, different currencies, and different legal requirements. DLT has the potential to ease cross-border payments by getting all parties involved with a single, transparent, and verifiable ledger. This can minimize the time, cost, and complexity of cross-border payments, hence enhancing the overall efficiency of international transactions for banks and financial institutions (Trump et al., 2018).

DLT can help banks and financial institutions improve the efficiency and security of their digital identity and KYC (know your customer) processes. DLT can streamline the client onboarding process, minimize the risk of identity fraud, and improve compliance with KYC rules by securely storing and sharing identification information on a distributed ledger. This can lead to better customer experiences, lower operating costs, and improved regulatory compliance for banks and financial institutions (Janowicz et al., 2018).

DLT has the potential to enable new financial industry business models. It can, for example, promote peer-to-peer financing, decentralized marketplaces, and asset tokenization, among other things. These innovative business models can allow banks and financial institutions to innovate, establish new revenue streams, and expand their offerings to meet changing client expectations (Treiblmaier & Clohessy, 2020).

Regulatory compliance, connectivity, scalability, and privacy are just a few of the issues and factors that need to be taken into account as DLT adoption in banks and other financial institutions continues to develop. DLT, however, has the potential to have a big impact on the financial sector by fostering innovation, security, and efficiency in a number of banking and financial services domains (Ribitzky et al., 2018).

8.2.4 Impact of Distributed Ledger Technology on Banking and Financial Industry

DLT has the potential to have a significant impact on the financial industry and the broader economy. Following are some key areas where DLT can have an impact.

DLT can streamline and automate complicated financial industry procedures like clearing and settlement, decreasing the need for intermediaries and paperwork. This can contribute to faster transaction processing times, lower costs, and higher operational efficiency, thereby saving financial institutions money and improving client experiences (Hamilton, 2020). DLT's distributed and immutable nature provides transparent and auditable record-keeping, lowering the risk of fraud, manipulation, and errors in financial transactions. This can boost participant trust and confidence, leading to increased security and accountability in the financial industry (Howell et al., 2019).

DLT, which enables transactions between peers without the use of middlemen like banks, has the potential to upend established financial intermediaries. This can reduce transaction costs and restrictions, increasing access to financial services for underprivileged communities, encouraging financial inclusion, and lowering reliance on traditional banking institutions (Jain et al., 2022).

DLT has the potential to enable new business models as well as novel financial goods and services. It can, for example, permit the tokenization of assets such as real estate and securities, releasing liquidity and opening new investment options. Decentralized finance (DeFi) applications, such as decentralized loans and decentralized exchanges, can also be enabled by DLT, providing alternative and creative financial services (Bonnet & Teuteberg, 2023). DLT offers the ability to simplify and expedite cross-border transactions and remittances while lowering costs and enhancing efficiency. Transparent and traceable cross-border transactions can be provided by DLT-based systems, decreasing the need for several intermediaries and increasing the speed and cost-effectiveness of cross-border transfers (Ølnes et al., 2017).

Central bank digital currencies (CBDCs), which are digital representations of fiat currencies issued by central banks, can be issued and managed using DLT. CBDCs may have ramifications for monetary policy, payment systems, and financial stability, and they may transform the way central banks create, circulate, and manage money (Kakavand et al., 2017).

Through features such as transparent and traceable transactions, smart contracts, and data integrity, DLT can improve regulatory compliance and risk management in the financial industry. This can assist financial organizations in meeting regulatory requirements, reducing risks, and improving regulatory reporting and auditing. However, DLT is not without its obstacles and considerations, such as legislative frameworks, privacy and security concerns, interoperability, scalability, and energy usage. Addressing these difficulties would necessitate careful planning, stakeholder participation, and effective technical solutions (Treiblmaier & Clohessy, 2020).

8.3 OBJECTIVES

The management and trading of financial assets are both being transformed by DLT. It has the ability to displace established financial intermediaries and democratize access to investment possibilities. This study will analyze how blockchain and distributed ledger technology influence banking and financial services. Based on the aforementioned research inquiries, the objectives addressed in this study are as follows:

1. To analyze the effect of blockchain and distributed ledger technology on banking and financial services.

2. To empirically assess the relationship among variables in the hypothesized measurement model.
3. To analyze structural relationships between perceived usefulness, perceived ease of use, accessibility, security, transparency, and attitude toward adoption intention of distributed ledger technology.

8.4 HYPOTHESIS FORMULATION AND CONCEPTUAL RELATIONSHIPS

The present analysis identifies and examines the following hypotheses for the perception of bank employees toward distributed ledger technology and its effect on banking and financial services based on literature analysis.

8.4.1 Perceived Usefulness and Attitude Toward Adoption Intention of Distributed Ledger Technology

Published research on the relationship between perceived utility and attitude toward DLT adoption intention offers important insights into the variables affecting people's adoption and acceptance of this technology. The perceived utility has continuously been highlighted in prior studies as a critical factor influencing people's attitudes and intentions toward utilizing technology. Studies have indicated that people are more inclined to acquire favorable views toward the adoption of DLT when they believe it will improve their productivity, efficiency, security, transparency, and ability to cut costs (Tung et al., 2008).

H1: There is a significant relationship between perceived usefulness and attitude toward the adoption intention of distributed ledger technology (DLT).

8.4.2 Perceived Ease of Use and Attitude Toward Adoption Intention of Distributed Ledger Technology

The work examining the connection between DLT perceived ease of use and attitude toward adoption intention sheds light on important aspects affecting people's acceptance and willingness to use this technology. Previous studies consistently highlight the significance of perceived ease of use as a critical determinant of individuals' attitudes and intentions toward adopting DLT. According to research, people are more likely to adopt favorable attitudes toward the adoption of DLT when they believe it to be simple to use, requiring little effort and technical expertise. The reduction of complexity, facilitation of user-friendly interactions, and promotion of user acceptance of technology are all attributed to ease of use. Studies have also revealed that perceived ease of use serves as a mediator between the intention to use a technology and acceptance of the technology, suggesting that the perceived ease of use of DLT encourages positive feelings. To investigate and validate these links, theoretical frameworks like the technology acceptance model (TAM) and the unified theory of acceptance and use of technology (UTAUT) have frequently been used (Wu et al., 2005). The research emphasizes the significance of perceived ease of use and how it affects people's attitudes toward their desire to embrace DLT, offering information that can direct efforts to encourage the effective implementation and wide adoption of DLT in a variety of scenarios (Jain & Agarwal, 2019).

H2: There is a significant relationship between perceived ease of use and attitude toward the adoption intention of distributed ledger technology (DLT).

8.4.3 Accessibility and Attitude Toward Adoption Intention of Distributed Ledger Technology

Previous research consistently emphasizes the importance of accessibility as a significant determinant of individuals' attitudes and intentions toward adopting DLT. Accessibility refers to the ease of access to technological platforms, applications, and services, including factors such as availability, affordability, usability, and infrastructure support (Scherer et al., 2019). Studies have shown that when DLT is readily accessible, individuals are more likely to develop positive attitudes toward its adoption. The availability of user-friendly interfaces, seamless integration with existing systems, and widespread accessibility through various devices and connectivity options contribute to a favorable perception of DLT's adoption potential (Sharma & Jain, 2021).

H3: There is a significant relationship between accessibility and attitude toward the adoption intention of distributed ledger technology (DLT).

8.4.4 Security and Attitude Toward Adoption Intention of Distributed Ledger Technology

The literature exploring the relationship between security and attitude toward the adoption intention of new technology offers valuable insights into the factors influencing individuals' acceptance and willingness to adopt this technology (Koul & Eydgahi, 2018). Previous research consistently emphasizes the critical role of security as a determinant of individuals' attitudes and intentions toward adopting DLT. Security concerns encompass aspects such as data protection, privacy, integrity, and resistance to malicious activities or attacks. Studies indicate that when individuals perceive DLT as secure, with robust cryptographic mechanisms, tamper-resistant data storage, and enhanced privacy features, they are more likely to develop positive attitudes toward its adoption. Security concerns are particularly relevant in the context of DLT, as it promises enhanced trust and immutability of transactions (Lai, 2017). Furthermore, research highlights the mediating role of attitude in the relationship between security and adoption intention, suggesting that positive attitudes act as intermediaries between perceived security and the intention to adopt DLT. The literature underscores the importance of security and its impact on individuals' attitudes toward the adoption intention of technology, providing insights that can inform strategies to enhance security measures and promote the widespread adoption of technology in various domains (Çelik & Yilmaz, 2011).

H4: There is a significant relationship between security and attitude toward the adoption intention of distributed ledger technology (DLT).

8.4.5 Transparency and Attitude Toward Adoption Intention of Distributed Ledger Technology

The literature on transparency and attitude toward the adoption intention of DLT provides valuable insights into the factors influencing individuals' acceptance and willingness to adopt this technology (Al-Khasawneh et al., 2022). Previous research consistently highlights the significance of transparency as a critical determinant of individuals' attitudes and intentions toward adopting DLT. Transparency in DLT refers to the visibility and traceability of transactions and data recorded on the blockchain, providing a decentralized and immutable ledger. ElKheshin and Saleeb (2020) have shown that when individuals perceive DLT as transparent, enabling enhanced accountability, and auditability, and eliminating the need for intermediaries, they are more likely to develop positive attitudes toward its adoption. Transparent systems are often associated with increased trust, reduced fraud, and improved efficiency. Furthermore, research has also highlighted the mediating role of attitude in the relationship between transparency and adoption intention, suggesting that positive attitudes act as intermediaries between perceived transparency and the intention to adopt DLT. Theoretical frameworks, such as TAM and UTAUT, have been applied to investigate and validate these relationships (Marakarkandy et al., 2017). Overall, the literature underscores the importance of transparency and its influence on individuals' attitudes toward the adoption intention of DLT, offering insights that can inform strategies to enhance transparency measures and promote widespread adoption of DLT in various domains.

H5: There is a significant relationship between transparency and attitude toward the adoption intention of distributed ledger technology (DLT).

8.5 RESULTS AND DATA ANALYSIS

The results specify that all five hypotheses are supported as there is a substantial relationship among the analyzed variables (see Table 8.1), as presented

Table 8.1 Descriptive Statistics of Sample

Variable	*Gender*	*N (223)*	*%*	*Mean*	*Standard Deviation*	*Standard Error Mean*
Perceived usefulness (PU)	Male	165	73.9	148.5212	21.38999	1.66521
	Female	58	22.1	142.0345	31.85161	4.18232
Perceived ease of use (PEOU)	Male	165	73.9	58.1212	10.01328	.77953
	Female	58	22.1	49.2759	11.91901	1.56504
Accessibility (Acc)	Male	165	73.9	62.2970	11.18918	.87108
	Female	58	22.1	64.2069	8.68101	1.13987
Security (Sec)	Male	165	73.9	40.5697	7.99865	.62269
	Female	58	22.1	41.9655	6.03489	.79242
Transparency (Tra)	Male	165	73.9	39.5697	7.99865	.62269
	Female	58	22.1	40.9655	6.03489	.79242
Attitude toward adoption intention (ATA)	Male	165	73.9	41.4697	7.99865	.62269
	Female	58	22.1	42.4655	6.03489	.79242

in Table 8.2. Results indicated that all alternative hypotheses supported the analysis. For instance, the hypothesized path between PU and ATT with a CR value of 2.102 was statistically significant (p = .005), while PEOU and ATT with a CR value of 2.774 were statistically significant (p = .005). It was found that ACC and ATT with a CR value of 2.633 were statistically significant (p = .005), and SEC and ATT with a CR value of 3.275 were statistically significant (p = .005). Subsequently, TRA and ATT with a CR value of 8.175 were statistically significant (p = .005). Additionally, ATT and ATA with a CR value of 9.623 were statistically significant (p = .005).

A sample of 223 respondents was used for the SEM analysis in order to evaluate the association between the independent variables. Table 8.3 displays the SEM model's goodness of fit metrics. The obtained value of x2 was 28.899; the df value was 13, and the x2/df value was 2.223. RMSEA was 0.031 in each case. GFI was 0.921 and AGFI was 0.924, indicating an excellent match for the model. NFI = .955, RFI = 0.912, IFI = 0.956, TLI = 0.923, and CFI = 0.922 are the incremental fit measures. PRATIO, PNFI, and PCFI had respective values of 0.673, 0.665, and 0.653. According to the goodness of fit numbers, the model adequately fits the data. There was no need for improvement or adjustment.

8.6 FINDINGS AND DISCUSSION

Based on the data analysis of the measurement model through SEM analysis, this section discusses the findings of the study.

Table 8.2 Hypothesis Testing

No.	*Hypothesis*	*Standard Error*	*Critical Ratio*	*p-Value*	*Path Coefficient β Value*	*t-Value*	*Findings*
H1	PU→ATT	.071	2.102	.005	0.090	0.386	Supported
H2	PEOU→ATT	.034	2.774	.005	0.056	0.097	Supported
H3	ACC→ATT	.012	2.633	.005	0.425	4.218	Supported
H4	SEC→ATT	.057	3.275	.005	0.090	1.289	Supported
H5	TRA→ATT	.191	8.175	.005	0.121	0.924	Supported

The findings indicate that there is a notable and positive relationship between the perceived usefulness of distributed ledger technology and the attitude toward its adoption. This outcome aligns with previous research by AlSoufi and Ali (2014), which demonstrated that technology can foster financial inclusion and facilitate digitalization in developing countries.

Similarly, the findings demonstrate a significant positive association between the perceived ease of use of distributed ledger technology and bank workers' attitudes toward its adoption. This finding is similar to prior research by Kalayou et al. (2020), which found that perceived ease of use had a positive impact on the intention to embrace new technologies. They discovered that when people perceive a technology to be simple to use, they are more likely to have a favorable attitude toward adopting it. This favorable attitude enhances their willingness to adopt the technology (Abd Ghani et al., 2017).

Furthermore, the study reveals that accessibility and security also play vital roles in shaping the attitude toward the adoption of distributed ledger technology among bank employees. These findings align with the previous research by Teeroovengadum et al. (2017), which emphasized the positive influence of accessibility and security on the attitude toward adopting new technology. They found that when individuals perceive a technology as accessible and secure, it positively influences their attitude toward adopting it. The availability and ease of access to the technology, as well as the perceived security measures in place, contribute to building a favorable attitude toward its adoption (Soneka & Phiri, 2019).

Additionally, the study found a strong correlation between transparency and bank workers' attitudes regarding the implementation of distributed ledger technology. This finding is in line with earlier research conducted by Kakavand et al. (2017), which showed the beneficial effects of transparency on attitudes toward embracing new technology.

Additionally, the study finds a substantial correlation between bank workers' general attitudes and their inclination to use distributed ledger

Table 8.3 Goodness of Fit Indices of Final SEM Model

			Absolute Fit Measures					
	χ2 (Chi Square)	*DF (Degree of Freedom)*	*χ2/DF (Chi Square/Degree of Freedom)*	*GFI (Goodness of Fit Index)*	*AGFI (Adjusted Goodness of Fit Index)*	*RMSEA (Root Mean Square Error of Approximation)*		
Criteria			1< X 3	≥0.90	≥0.90	<0.05		
Obtained	28.899	13	2.223	0.921	0.924	0.031		
	Incremental Fit Measures					*Parsimony Fit Indices*		
	NFI (Normed Fit Index)	*RFI (Relative fit Indices)*	*IFI (Incremental Fit Index)*	*TLI (Tucker–Lewis Coefficient)*	*CFI (Comparative Fit Index)*	*PRATIO (Parsimony Ratio)*	*PNFI (Parsimony Adjustment to NFI)*	*PCFI (Parsimony Adjustment to CFI)*
Criteria	≥0.90	≥0.90	≥0.90	≥0.90	≥0.90	≥0.50	≥0.50	≥0.50
Obtained	0.955	0.912	0.956	0.923	0.922	0.673	0.665	0.653

technology. This finding is consistent with earlier research by Ølnes et al. (2017), which showed that adoption intentions are influenced by attitudes regarding the use of distributed ledger technology. People are more likely to declare an intention to adopt and utilize technology in their work or organization when they have a favorable perception of it and good thoughts about its advantages.

8.7 CONCLUSION

In conclusion, the study provides valuable insights into the elements that affect bank workers' attitudes regarding the implementation of distributed ledger technology. The results show that perceived usefulness, perceived ease of use, accessibility, security, transparency, and overall attitude all play a significant role in influencing people's intentions to use DLT.

According to the findings, the perceived usefulness of DLT has a favorable link with attitudes toward its implementation. This demonstrates that those who view DLT as beneficial and significant are more likely to adopt it and have a positive attitude toward it. Similar to how the perceived simplicity of use of DLT boosts attitudes toward adoption, those who find the technology to be simple to use are more likely to have a positive attitude and want to adopt it.

Furthermore, accessibility and security emerged as important factors in shaping the attitude toward DLT adoption. When individuals perceive DLT as accessible and secure, it positively influences their attitude and willingness to adopt the technology. This highlights the significance of ensuring convenient access and robust security measures when introducing DLT in a banking context.

The study emphasizes the association between transparency and a favorable view of DLT adoption. People who believe DLT to be a transparent technology are more likely to be in favor of its implementation. This emphasizes the importance of promoting transparency in DLT systems to foster trust and acceptance among bank employees.

Importantly, the study reveals that the overall attitude toward DLT significantly influences the intention to adopt it. When bank employees hold a positive attitude and favorable beliefs about the benefits and advantages of DLT, they are more likely to express an intention to adopt and implement it in their work or organization. This highlights the value of developing a positive perception of DLT to drive successful adoption and implementation.

In conclusion, DLT has the potential to disrupt and transform the financial industry and the broader economy by improving efficiency, transparency, security, and inclusivity in financial transactions, enabling new business models and innovative financial products, and reshaping the way money is managed and circulated. However, successful implementation of

DLT in the financial industry requires careful consideration of regulatory, technical, and social aspects, and further research, experimentation, and collaboration among stakeholders are needed to fully realize its potential impact.

Overall, the study adds to the corpus of previous research by presenting actual evidence of the factors impacting bank workers' attitudes regarding the adoption of DLT. The results highlight how perceived usefulness, perceived ease of use, accessibility, security, transparency, and overall attitude influence people's intentions to use DLT. These findings can guide policies and initiatives that aim to encourage DLT acceptance and use in the banking industry, eventually advancing digitalization and fostering financial inclusion.

REFERENCES

Abd Ghani, M., Rahi, S., Yasin, N. M., & Alnaser, F. M. (2017). Adoption of internet banking: Extending the role of technology acceptance model (TAM) with e-customer service and customer satisfaction. *World Applied Sciences Journal*, *35*(9), 1918–1929.

Al-Khasawneh, M., Sharabati, A., Al-Haddad, S., Tbakhi, R., & Abusaimeh, H. (2022). The adoption of TikTok application using TAM model. *International Journal of Data and Network Science*, *6*(4), 1389–1402.

AlSoufi, A., & Ali, H. (2014). Customers perception of mbanking adoption in Kingdom of Bahrain: An empirical assessment of an extended tam model. *arXiv Preprint ArXiv:1403.2828*.

Bonnet, S., & Teuteberg, F. (2023). Impact of blockchain and distributed ledger technology for the management of the intellectual property life cycle: A multiple case study analysis. *Computers in Industry*, *144*, 103789.

Çelik, H. E., & Yilmaz, V. (2011). Extending the technology acceptance model for adoption of e-shopping by consumers in Turkey. *Journal of Electronic Commerce Research*, *12*(2), 152.

Coppi, G., & Fast, L. (2019). *Blockchain and Distributed Ledger Technologies in the Humanitarian Sector.* HPG Commissioned Report.

Deshpande, A., Stewart, K., Lepetit, L., & Gunashekar, S. (2017). Distributed Ledger Technologies/Blockchain: Challenges, opportunities and the prospects for standards. *Overview Report the British Standards Institution (BSI)*, *40*, 40.

ElKheshin, S. A., & Saleeb, N. (2020). Assessing the adoption of e-government using TAM model: Case of Egypt. *International Journal of Managing Information Technology (IJMIT)*, *12*(1), 1–14.

Ellervee, A., Matulevicius, R., & Mayer, N. (2017, November). A comprehensive reference model for blockchain-based distributed ledger technology. In: ER Forum/Demos (pp. 306–319).

Gangwar, H., Date, H., & Raoot, A. D. (2014). Review on IT adoption: Insights from recent technologies. *Journal of Enterprise Information Management*, *27*(4), 488–502.

Hamilton, M. (2020). Blockchain distributed ledger technology: An introduction and focus on smart contracts. *Journal of Corporate Accounting and Finance, 31*(2), 7–12.

Howell, B. E., Potgieter, P. H., & Sadowski, B. M. (2019). Governance of blockchain and distributed ledger technology projects. *Available at SSRN 3365519.*

Hughes, A., Park, A., Kietzmann, J., & Archer-Brown, C. (2019). Beyond Bitcoin: What blockchain and distributed ledger technologies mean for firms. *Business Horizons, 62*(3), 273–281.

Jain, P., & Agarwal, G. (2019). Factors affecting mobile banking adoption: An empirical study in Gwalior region. *The International Journal of Digital Accounting Research, 19*(4), 79–101.

Jain, P., Sharma, B. K., Jain, R., Pandey, A. K., & Khare, S. (2022, May). Mobile banking adoption for digital financial inclusion. In: 2022 7th International Conference on Business and Industrial Research (ICBIR) (pp. 254–258). IEEE.

Janowicz, K., Regalia, B., Hitzler, P., Mai, G., Delbecque, S., Fröhlich, M., Martinent, P., & Lazarus, T. (2018). On the prospects of blockchain and distributed ledger technologies for open science and academic publishing. *Semantic Web, 9*(5), 545–555.

Kakavand, H., Kost De Sevres, N., & Chilton, B. (2017). The blockchain revolution: An analysis of regulation and technology related to distributed ledger technologies. Available at SSRN 2849251.

Kalayou, M. H., Endehabtu, B. F., & Tilahun, B. (2020). The applicability of the modified technology acceptance model (TAM) On the sustainable adoption of ehealth systems in resource-limited settings. *Journal of Multidisciplinary Healthcare*, 1827–1837.

Koul, S., & Eydgahi, A. (2018). Utilizing technology acceptance model (TAM) for driverless car technology adoption. *Journal of Technology Management and Innovation, 13*(4), 37–46.

Lai, P. C. (2017). The literature review of technology adoption models and theories for the novelty technology. *JISTEM-Journal of Information Systems and Technology Management, 14*(1), 21–38.

Lule, I., Omwansa, T. K., & Waema, T. M. (2012). Application of technology acceptance model (TAM) in m-banking adoption in Kenya. *International Journal of Computing & ICT Research, 6*(1).

Marakarkandy, B., Yajnik, N., & Dasgupta, C. (2017). Enabling internet banking adoption: An empirical examination with an augmented technology acceptance model (TAM). *Journal of Enterprise Information Management, 30*(2), 263–294.

McLean, S., & Deane-Johns, S. (2016). Demystifying blockchain and distributed ledger technology–hype or hero? *Computer Law Review International, 17*(4), 97–102.

Natarajan, H., Krause, S., & Gradstein, H. (2017). *Distributed Ledger Technology and Blockchain.*

Ølnes, S., Ubacht, J., & Janssen, M. (2017). Blockchain in government: Benefits and implications of distributed ledger technology for information sharing. *Government Information Quarterly, 34*(3), 355–364.

Ribitzky, R., Clair, J. S., Houlding, D. I., McFarlane, C. T., Ahier, B., Gould, M., Flannery, H. L., Pupo, E., & Clauson, K. A. (2018). Pragmatic, interdisciplinary perspectives on blockchain and distributed ledger technology: Paving the future for healthcare. *Blockchain in Healthcare Today.*

Scherer, R., Siddiq, F., & Tondeur, J. (2019). The technology acceptance model (TAM): A meta-analytic structural equation modeling approach to explaining teachers' adoption of digital technology in education. *Computers and Education, 128*, 13–35.

Sharma, B. K., & Jain, P. (2021). Financial inclusion: Impact of accessibility, availability, and usage of financial services-a study on household workers in Madhya Pradesh, India. *International Journal of Public Sector Performance Management*, 7(1), 1–19.

Soneka, P. N., & Phiri, J. (2019). A model for improving e-tax systems adoption in rural Zambia based on the TAM model. *Open Journal of Business and Management*, 7(2), 908–918.

Sunyaev, A. (2020). Distributed ledger technology. *Internet Computing: Principles of Distributed Systems and Emerging Internet-Based Technologies*, 265–299.

Teeroovengadum, V., Heeraman, N., & Jugurnath, B. (2017). Examining the antecedents of ICT adoption in education using an extended technology acceptance model (TAM). *International Journal of Education and Development Using ICT, 13*(3).

Treiblmaier, H., & Clohessy, T. (2020). *Blockchain and Distributed Ledger Technology Use Cases.* Cham, Switzerland: Springer.

Trump, B. D., Florin, M. V., Matthews, H. S., Sicker, D., & Linkov, I. (2018). Governing the use of blockchain and distributed ledger technologies: Not one-size-fits-all. *IEEE Engineering Management Review*, 46(3), 56–62.

Tung, F. C., Chang, S. C., & Chou, C. M. (2008). An extension of trust and TAM model with IDT in the adoption of the electronic logistics information system in HIS in the medical industry. *International Journal of Medical Informatics*, 77(5), 324–335.

Wallace, L. G., & Sheetz, S. D. (2014). The adoption of software measures: A technology acceptance model (TAM) perspective. *Information and Management*, *51*(2), 249–259.

Wu, L., & Chen, J. L. (2005). An extension of trust and TAM model with TPB in the initial adoption of on-line tax: An empirical study. *International Journal of Human-Computer Studies*, 62(6), 784–808.

Chapter 9

Barriers and Benefits of Blockchain Adoption in the Healthcare System

Kuldeep Pal and Mukesh Kumar

9.1 INTRODUCTION

"Blockchain" is one of the most popular buzzwords used in the medical technology industry. This is valid justification. Simply put, blockchain has the power to completely transform the healthcare industry. Patients will be at the center of all operations with the full implementation of blockchain, which will also completely redesign operations with greater security, privacy, and accessibility. But how precisely does blockchain make this possible? How is the health sector making the most of this highly powerful modern technology? A distributed technology called a blockchain creates and maintains data records. In order to keep track of how data is shared, modified, or accessed on its peer-to-peer network, it keeps a digital ledger of interconnected "blocks" of data. Any transaction involving a linked device will result in identical blocks being generated by all devices on the same blockchain system.

A block is formed to locally preserve that information on every device if the data on one machine is accessed, altered, shared, or otherwise affected in any way. This makes it simple to spot data changes. Data parity can be achieved using this decentralized method by comparing the blocks of every connected device. The use of "hashing" goes beyond merely logging and comparing data. Every block receives a unique identification by hashing, which varies according to its content. A block's hash would alter if the block's data is changed. This is important since blocks are maintained together in time order and directly relate to the extracting of the block preceding them. Therefore, trying to update the contents in one block might cause the hash to change fast in the following block. This is why connected blocks construct a "kettle" that is safely built in a reliable, autonomous, unchangeable way [1].

Blockchain is an autonomous node network where the data is stored. It is an excellent piece of technology for protecting sensitive data throughout the whole system. With the use of this technology, sensitive information may be shared securely and privately. It is the best option for safely keeping all pertinent paperwork in one location. Blockchain also accelerates the search for

 DOI: 10.1201/9781003466949-9

candidates who satisfy certain clinical trial requirements by using an individual patient storage system. It facilitates trustworthy cooperation since knowledge can be transmitted and preserved by all network users, and an ongoing history of past and present operations is retained. With the use of this technology, several networks may be combined to reveal the benefit of tailored treatment. As a result, it is simple to recognize the immutability and security of blockchain technology. Blocks, nodes, and miners are the three main notions on which blockchain is built. The basic functions of blockchain technology are shown in Figure 9.1. Blockchain, in contrast to previous forms of technology, does not keep any of its data in a single location. Instead, the blockchain is distributed and copied by a network of computers. Every machine connected to the internet updates its blockchain to reflect the addition of a new block. The following research questions (RQ) are answered in this chapter [2]:

RQ1: Look at the applications of distributed ledger technology in the medical field.
RQ2: To ascertain how the distributed ledger could benefit the social fabric of global medical care.
RQ3: To determine and talk about blockchain technology's facilitators for improving medical care services.
RQ4: To decide the work process flow for executing blockchain innovation in the arrangement of medical care conveniences.
RQ5: To discover important blockchains in the prosecution healthcare industry [3].

In this chapter, we discuss the necessity of blockchain in healthcare. Then we discuss the various features and applications of blockchain that support global healthcare culture. Then we talk through some limitations of the uses of blockchain in the healthcare industry. Last, we present the conclusion and some future scope of blockchain in the healthcare industry.

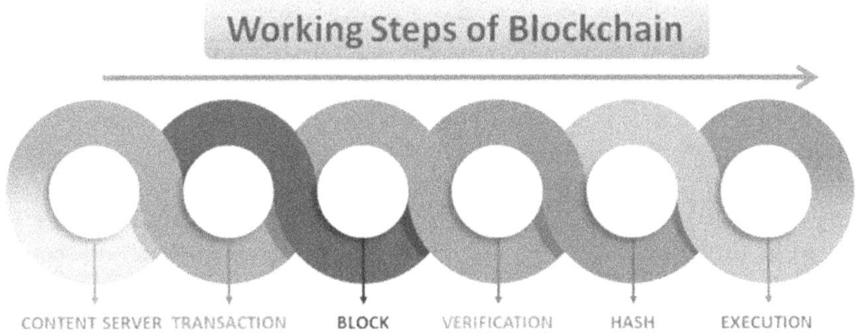

Figure 9.1 Workflow for the blockchain technology

9.2 NECESSITY OF BLOCKCHAIN IN HEALTHCARE

In the field of healthcare, development is growing at ever-increasing rates. Modern healthcare facilities that are equipped with the latest innovations are highly sought after. In this scenario, blockchain would significantly contribute to the transformation of the healthcare industry. Additionally, the structure of the medical industry is changing to accommodate a patient-centered strategy that underlines an essential component: continuous access to the right resources for treatment. The healthcare industry may more efficiently deliver proper patient care and exceptional healthcare providers thanks to blockchain. Health information sharing is another time-consuming, monotonous job that drives up costs in the healthcare sector, but it may be quickly remedied with the use of this technology. Blockchain technology allows for public participation in health research activities [4].

Furthermore, better data exchange and research on community well-being will enhance treatment for many populations. An integrated database is used to handle all businesses and the medical gardening [5].

Data sharing, privacy, and interoperability issues have up until now been the biggest challenges in population health management. Blockchain technology is dependable for solving these issues. When used properly, this innovation enhances mobility, security, data transfer, seamless integration, and integrity. Significant worries exist over data security as well, particularly in the areas of wearable technology and individualized treatment. These issues can be fixed with blockchain technology; recipients and healthcare personnel expect easy, safe ways to capture, send, and consult data via networks without security worries [6].

9.3 BLOCKCHAIN TECHNOLOGY CONCEPTS THAT ENDORSE A GLOBAL MEDICAL SERVICES CULTURE

Blockchain is a technology with many potential uses in the healthcare sector. By allowing safe distribution of client documentation, controlling the medicine distribution system, and managing the secure transmission of patient medical data, ledger advances assist medical researchers in understanding the human genome. Figure 9.2 illustrates the wide range of impact of blockchain in numerous healthcare areas, including medical records protection, governance of genetic material, digital information, seamless integration, and digitalized tracking. Some of the remarkable and scientifically determined factors used to develop and apply blockchain infrastructure include trouble breakout [7]. The blockchain creates transparency throughout the all steps involved in making a medication order, from production to drugstore counters. With the help of IoT and blockchain, it is possible to monitor traffic, goods direction, and speed. It allows the chance to efficiently plan

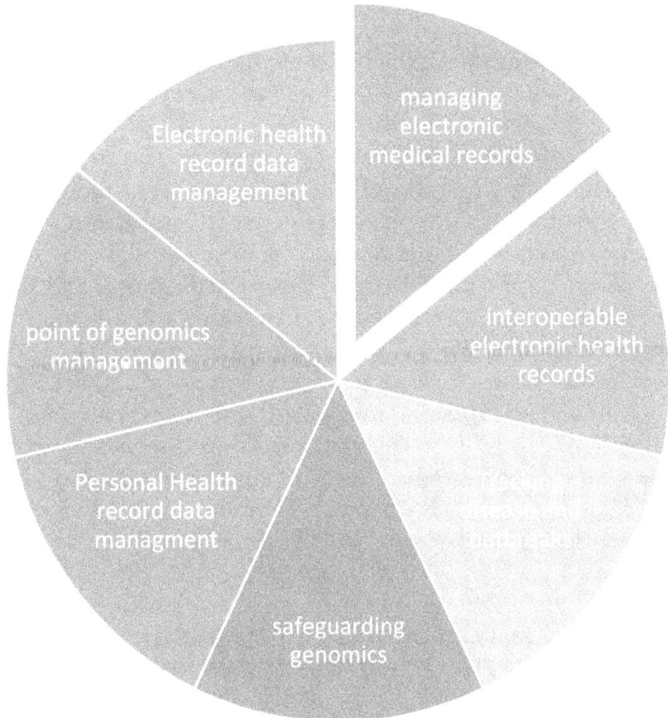

Figure 9.2 Blockchain is having an impact on the healthcare industry

purchases to avoid medication delays and shortages in pharmacies, clinics, and other healthcare institutions [8].

Blockchain-based digital frameworks can be used to help ensure that unauthorized changes to logistics data are avoided. It fosters confidence and inhibits individuals who are interested in obtaining drugs from handling information, funds, and medication in an unauthorized manner. The use of technology can also significantly enhance patients' conditions while keeping costs low. It eliminates obstacles and problems associated with multilevel authenticity. Blockchain is ideal for safeguarding purposes because it can maintain an unalterable, autonomous, and transparent log of all medical data. Furthermore, blockchain maintains the delicate nature of health information by hiding a person's identity beneath complex and secure techniques, making it both readily accessible and private. Thanks to the technology's dispersed structure, patients, medical personnel, and other medical practitioners can quickly and safely exchange information [9].

This increases confidentiality and privacy while giving patients more control over their personal information. Quality management and enforcement measurement and implementation are challenging. Applications of the blockchain in healthcare could resolve any of these technological problems.

Blockchain will help regulatory officials distinguish authentic medications from fake ones while tracing drugs. Blockchain guarantees the exchange of digital transactions including the patient's information between all authorized parties. Patients who switch doctors can exchange all their records by updating a single consent [10].

With the help of blockchain technology, a complex data storage system can be created that keeps track of the full medical dossier of an individual, including diagnoses, analysis, results, previous treatments, and readings from highly sophisticated sensors. Using this approach, a medical professional can easily obtain all the evidence needed to provide precise diagnoses and suggestions for improvement. A single blockchain system stores all the data, protecting it from loss and change. Blockchain can be used to avoid an organization's internal networks. A substantial organization comprising numerous independent participants, with different levels of authority on a blockchain database that is encrypted, can protect organizations from threats and attacks from the outside world. If an accredited medical administration effectively uses a distributed ledger, cyberattacks and other problems, including system malfunction or hardware breakdowns, would be eradicated [11].

9.4 BLOCKCHAIN TECHNOLOGY ENABLERS FOR REVITALIZING HEALTHCARE SERVICES

Figure 9.3 illustrates the wide range of characteristics and essential blockchain concept enablers in numerous healthcare and related areas. Blockchain is used to create updated patient records for physicians at other healthcare providers. New knowledge is frequently repeated and causes time loss, which is a serious patient care problem. Depending on where they are in the supply chain, each person may have access to a variety of rights. Additionally, each block that contained information about a drug would have a hash linking it to another block [12].

Clinical trials are being done in healthcare to evaluate the efficacy of medicines in treating or partially reversing conditions. Researchers can keep track of information on examination findings, flesh counts, and information about patients, as well as other features. Clinical trial data should be verified so that researchers, pharmaceutical companies, and politicians can trust the accuracy of the findings. Blockchain technology may increase accountability and transparency in clinical studies. Blockchain provides excellent recordkeeping for the medical industry because it makes medical treatment accessible for doctors and patients, and the gathering of previous disease data with a comprehension of patient issues. Blockchain is becoming more widely used in the supply chain and is effective for managing pharmaceuticals in the medical sector [13].

Blockchain makes it simple to think ahead about medical professionals' procedures and offerings. This blockchain technology is used in the

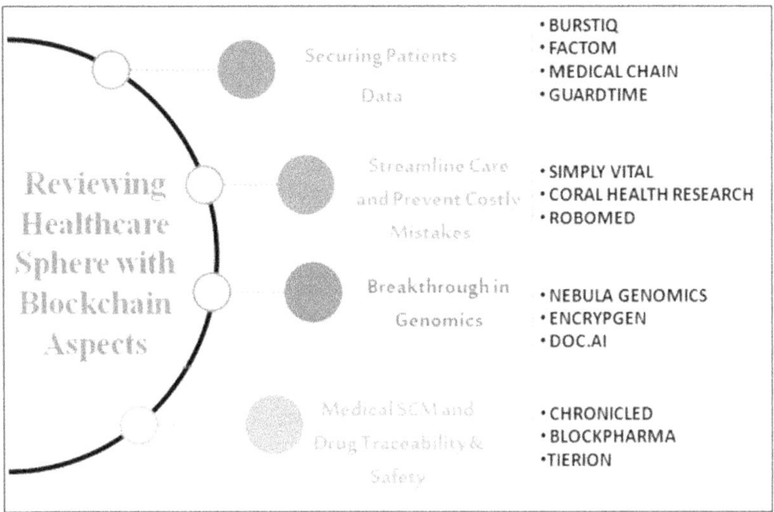

Figure 9.3 Blockchain technology enablers for revitalizing healthcare services

healthcare sector to rapidly process and get approval. Blockchain makes it simple to avoid wasting time waiting in line while enhancing efficiency and productivity. This technology intends to promote individualized treatment, professional guidance, and useful health research. Blockchain could change the healthcare sector and turn it into a solid and reliable electronic directory. Administering patient information, clinical studies, and prescribed drugs are just a few of the difficulties that blockchain technology in healthcare will assist with [14].

Patient voices will now be heard more clearly during the processing of their medical records. As members of the blockchain network, healthcare providers will be permitted to trade data, thus enhancing privacy and control. Long term, a nationwide blockchain network will boost efficiencies and support outcomes that are better for patient health. Blockchain holds a shared, permanent record of transactions generated from linked transactions. It may contain some medical instructions and shipment information [15].

9.5 IMPLEMENTATION OF BLOCKCHAIN TECHNOLOGY WITH A SINGLE WORKFLOW PROCESS IN HEALTHCARE FACILITIES

Primary patient gauge asserts modifications, excelled medical logistics management, seamless integration, and unique and uninterrupted data collection are some of the advantages of blockchain that apply to the healthcare industry. Thanks to distributed network flow, digitalized operations, shared data, and interactive work-process flow (Figure 9.4), blockchain personnel can function more assiduously to enhance the quality and innovation of medical procedures [16].

The fundamentals of distributed ledger technology are quite simple, and they are always developing and growing an ecosystem of blocks that can be tailored to match the various needs and distinctive qualities of the many companies. A more extensive tracking option is provided by the standalone blockchain architecture, which also allows for real-time results modifications. Blockchain will considerably reduce financial failures as well as prevent theft and illegal record transfers. It can fix issues with shifting results and data spying. It makes it possible to permanently transfer timestamped clinical study reports and results, which lowers the likelihood of fraud and errors occurring during clinical trials. Blockchain technology adoption is primarily the responsibility of the health sector [17].

Blockchain technology has an impact on every industry. Blockchain technologies are employed in fields where it is necessary to build trust among many parties and stakeholders. Blockchain has the potential to fundamentally transform the current fragmented process in which patients sign consent for every appointment, clinical procedure, and medical test. Some of the promises made by blockchain for these applications

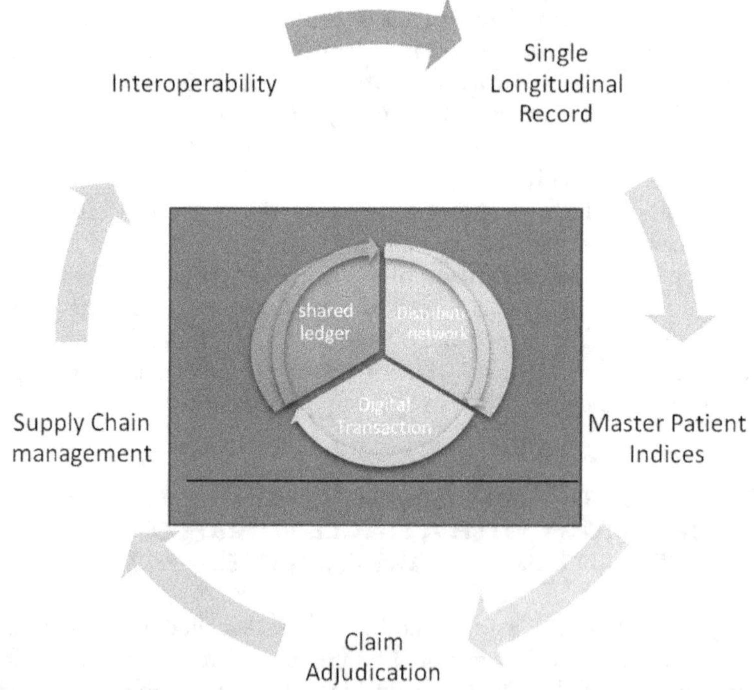

Figure 9.4 Blockchain technology integrated productivity method for medical culture

include the interchange of clinical test data and the potential for uncovering advantages for test subjects. Blockchain has the potential to become a crucial component of healthcare consent management that promotes information sharing [18].

An authenticated blockchain is an isolated network that links to other networks for all users of the system. It is developed and used in enterprises and institutions to make exchanges of data while safeguarding transfers easier. Once the activity has been approved, it is considered as an infallible record and integrated as a new block to the blockchain [19].

Pharmaceuticals are supplied securely, dependably, and quickly thanks to a blockchain-driven method for logistics. It gives the producer the ability to keep the right the composition amalgamates in line with medical norms. Medical devices can verify that the intended patient is receiving therapy, charge for patient data, and communicate procedural information with patients and regulators anonymously. Recent years have seen notable advancements in medical science and high-quality medical treatments. It is a commonly used, open-source digital leader for monitoring transactions that is dispersed and transparent. It is acknowledged for having a considerable impact on several sectors and industries. The existence of this technology addresses problems that cannot be solved by current methods [20].

9.6 DEVELOPING MEDICAL CARE BLOCKCHAIN PROGRAMS

Distributed ledger technology is a recent and constantly developing technology that has found popularity within the healthcare sector and provides innovative uses. Inexpensive medications and leading-edge remedies for numerous ailments depend on adequate data transmission and exchange between all participants and clinicians. Blockchain will speed the expansion of the healthcare industry in the next years. Prospects for blockchain technology in the logistics industry highlight the advantages for the healthcare industry. This is one of the first areas that digital transformation improves and innovates because it immediately affects the quality of life. Additionally gaining prominence is the use of blockchain technology, notably in the sector of finance [21].

9.6.1 Safeguarding Every Patient's Personal Info

Before and after the different investigation phases, health data and details about patients are gathered. Many people have undergone blood tests, cleanliness assessments, estimations, and health surveys. Results may be offered that show that a certain record or document exists. Healthcare professionals may quickly confirm the accuracy of the data by juxtaposing it with the initial information that has been recorded on the blockchain system. Blockchain is constructed on top of cryptographic techniques currently in use, such as the appropriate foundation for data sharing and secure communication [22].

9.6.2 Examine the Results of a Specific Technique

Investigators may successfully investigate any given operation on a group of patients with authenticated access to patient records. Pharmaceutical businesses can use the blockchain framework to gather data instantaneously, allowing them to offer patients a wide range of tailored prescription services and products. Since all the data is in the blockchain, it simplifies the job of pharmacists. Based on these findings, pharmacists can competently counsel patients on how to take medications. With the wearable data obtained in real time, it will inform the professionals of the patient's current state and notify them of any emergencies [23].

9.6.3 Security and Openness

Blockchain offers unparalleled security and full disclosure while enabling clinicians to dedicate additional time to managing patients. It would also make it feasible to sponsor clinical research and therapeutics for any unusual condition. The regulatory structures of a healthcare system can gain from good data transmission across medical solution providers, which can result in precise diagnoses, successful treatments, and networks that are affordable. Businesses in the health ecosystem may communicate and exchange data on an extensively dispersed leader using blockchain, which improves security and transparency. Users don't need to hunt for extra privacy and security solutions while using such a system because they may communicate data, maintain oversight of their unique activities, and observe other users' data interactions [24].

9.6.4 Health Recordkeeping

Blockchain technology is employed for carrying out routine tasks, administering coverage, transmitting medical information, and storing and maintaining digital medical files. Individuals can input their medical data into a blockchain system via an app. Digital ledger agreements make it possible for scanners and sophisticated gadgets to work together. Many healthcare organizations have access to electronic health records. By coordinating all data, blockchain will provide patients access to their medical history. The linking of all data in one place will allow us to see a patient's health state in a new light. Therefore, the blockchain paradigm will ensure the information is accurate and lawful while preserving the anonymity of the users [25].

9.6.5 Trial in Medicine

Clinical trials are using the distributed ledger to solve issues with data breakdown and deceptive results that conflict with the stated objectives of the study. Clinical studies will enjoy greater public support thanks to blockchain. The forces influencing the market are examined by the business analysis tool so that the healthcare sector may anticipate its potential. By leveraging blockchain credibility, the management of medications on the blockchain provides a further opportunity to establish and oversee the line of custody from the producer to the customer [26].

9.6.6 Identifying Fake Information

Blockchain will improve openness and make fraudulent information easier to spot. Research studies should be easy to understand for subjects and clients to ensure their accuracy. The easiest approach to gain permission is through a smart contract that maintains the transparency of the procedure records that have been used and their results. Thanks to technology, the public may now closely observe what occurs in a clinical study. Patients can get immediate, safe access to their medical and insurance information thanks to this system [27].

9.6.7 Patient Observation

Because of the assurance a blockchain offers, medical workers have access to healthcare technology when they need it. Doctors' remote observation of patients and responses to medical emergencies may also be quickened. Blockchain technology in healthcare can help with regulating patient room temperatures, bed utilization, and supply accessibility. A blockchain-based healthcare network integrates blockchain and IoT technology to boost the supply chain's adaptability and traceability, making healthcare logistics more transparent for effective patient monitoring. This provides a trustworthy electronic identification for healthcare institutions and providers [28–30].

9.6.8 Maintaining Hospital Financial Records

One must retain an accurate record of fiscal statements. Clinical studies are set up for effective operation and evaluation. The accounting and reporting procedure has been shortened in this case because of innovations made by blockchain enterprises. Before visiting a medical professional, people can complete the necessary documentation beforehand using the software provided. They won't have to endure standing in queue [31].

9.7 LIMITATIONS OF BLOCKCHAIN

Blockchain technology has been accepted by the healthcare industry, but there are still certain issues that need to be fixed. The biggest problem with employing this cutting-edge technology in hospitals is a lack of competence. Because they are still in their early phases, technological study and analysis of blockchain applications still need to be done. The responsibilities of medical bodies and regulators are also covered.

9.8 CONCLUSION

Blockchain technology offers innovative applications in the healthcare sector because of its built-in encryption and decentralization. It encourages seamless connectivity between healthcare organizations, the commercialization of health data, and the development of anti-counterfeit drug technologies. Additionally, it improves the security of people's electronic medical records. Numerous aspects of the healthcare sector may change as a result of the usage of blockchain technology. Among the most significant applications of blockchain are the digital agreements made possible by intelligent contracts in the healthcare sector. By eliminating middlemen from the payment chain, intelligent contracts will save costs. The potential of blockchain in the healthcare industry is significantly impacted by the uptake of associated cutting-edge technologies in the ecosystem. Clinical trials, drug tracking, health insurance, and system tracking are all included. Hospitals may plan their services utilizing blockchain architecture and device monitoring. The management of patient history might be greatly enhanced by the tracking and insurance mediation procedures, which would speed up therapeutic actions and better preserve data. In general, the usage and management of clinical records by patients and physicians would be considerably improved by this technology, which would ultimately reinvent how this information gets used and handled.

REFERENCES

1. De Novi, G., Sofia, N., Christine, Y. Z., & Ricotta, F. (2023). Blockchain Technology Predictions 2024: Transformations in Healthcare, Patient Identity and Public Health. *Blockchain in Healthcare Today*, 6(2).
2. T. McGhin, K.K. Choo, C.Z. Liu, D. He "Blockchain in healthcare applications: Research challenges and opportunities" *Journal of Network and Computer Applications*, 135 (2019 Jun 1), pp. 62–75.
3. A. Varshney, N. Garg, K.S. Nagla, et al. "Challenges in sensors technology for industry 4.0 for futuristic metrological applications" *MAPAN*, 36(2) (2021), pp. 215–226.
4. A. Farouk, S. Alahmadi, A. Ghose Mashatan "Blockchain platform for industrial healthcare: vision and future opportunities" *Computer Communications*, 154 (2020 Mar 15), pp. 223–235.

5. M. Hölbl, M. Kompara, A. Kamišalić, L. Nemec Zlatolas "A systematic review of the use of Blockchain in healthcare" *Symmetry*, 10(10) (2018 Oct), p. 470.
6. V. Dhillon, D. Metcalf, M. Hooper "Blockchain in Healthcare" *Blockchain-enabled Applications*, Apress, Berkeley, CA (2021), pp. 201–220.
7. M. Mettler "Blockchain technology in healthcare: the revolution starts here" 2016 IEEE 18th International Conference on E-Health Networking, Applications and Services (Healthcom), IEEE (2016 Sep 14), pp. 1–3.
8. J. Chanchaichujit, A. Tan, F. Meng, S. Eaimkhong "Blockchain technology in healthcare" *Healthcare 4.0*, Palgrave Pivot, Singapore (2019), pp. 37–62.
9. G. Tripathi, M.A. Ahad, S. Paiva "S2HS-A Blockchain-based approach for smart healthcare system" *Healthcare*, Elsevier, 8(1) (2020 Mar 1), p. 100391.
10. G. Srivastava, R.M. Parizi, A. Dehghantanha *The Future of Blockchain Technology in Healthcare Internet of Things Security Blockchain Cybersecurity, Trust, and Privacy*, USA, Singapore, Springer, USA (2020), pp. 161–184.
11. E.M. Abou-Nassar, A.M. Iliyasu, P.M. El-Kafrawy, O.Y. Song, A.K. Bashir, A.A. Abd El-Latif "DI Trust chain: Towards blockchain-based trust models for sustainable healthcare IoT systems" *IEEE Access*, 8 (2020 Jun 2), pp. 111223–111238.
12. M. Javaid, A. Haleem, R. Vaishya, S. Bahl, R. Suman, A. Vaish "Industry 4.0 technologies and their applications in fighting COVID-19 pandemic" *Diabetes and Metabolic Syndrome: Clinical Research and Reviews*, 14(4) (2020 Jul 1), pp. 419–422.
13. C. Esposito, A. De Santis, G. Tortora, H. Chang, K.K. Choo "Blockchain: A panacea for healthcare cloud-based data security and privacy" *IEEE Cloud Computing*, 5(1) (2018 Mar 28), pp. 31–37.
14. M.Z. Bhuiyan, A. Zaman, T. Wang, G. Wang, H. Tao, M.M. Hassan "Blockchain and big data to transform healthcare" Proceedings of the International Conference on Data Processing and Applications (2018 May 12), pp. 62–68.
15. R. Abujamra, D. Randall *Blockchain Applications in Healthcare and the Opportunities and the Advancements Due to the New Information Technology Framework Advances in Computers*, vol. 115, Elsevier, USA (2019 Jan 1), pp. 141–154.
16. A.Sharma, S. Bahl, A.K. Bagha, M. Javaid, D.K. Shukla, A. Haleem "Blockchain technology and its applications to combat COVID-19 pandemic" *Research on Biomedical Engineering* (2020 Oct 22), pp. 1–8.
17. U. Qamar Shahnaz, A. Khalid "Using blockchain for electronic health records" *IEEE Access*, 7 (2019 Oct 9), pp. 147782–147795.
18. A.A. Siyal, A.Z. Junejo, M. Zawish, K. Ahmed, A. Khalil, G. Soursou "Applications of blockchain technology in medicine and healthcare: Challenges and future perspectives" *Cryptography*, 3(1) (2019 Mar), p. 3.
19. R. Jayaraman, K. Salah, N. King "Improving opportunities in healthcare supply chain processes via the internet of things and blockchain technology" *International Journal of Healthcare Information Systems and Informatics (IJHISI)*, 14(2) (2019 Apr 1), pp. 49–65.

20. R.B. Fekih, M. Lahami "Application of blockchain technology in healthcare: A comprehensive study" International Conference on Smart Homes and Health Telematics, Springer, Cham (2020 Jun 24), pp. 268–276.
21. K.N. Griggs, O. Ossipova, C.P. Kohlios, A.N. Baccarini, E.A. Howson, T. Hayajneh "Healthcare blockchain system using smart contracts for secure automated remote patient monitoring" *Journal of Medical Systems*, 42(7) (2018 Jul), pp. 1–7.
22. M. Ejaz, T. Kumar, I. Kovacevic, M. Ylianttila, E. Harjula "Health-BlockEdge: Blockchain-edge framework for reliable low-latency digital healthcare applications" *Sensors*, 21(7) (2021 Jan), p. 2502.
23. A. Khatoon "A blockchain-based innovative contract system for healthcare management" *Electronics*, 9(1) (2020 Jan), p. 94.
24. S. Wang, J. Wang, X. Wang, et al. "Blockchain-powered parallel healthcare systems based on the ACP approach" *IEEE Transactions on Computational Social Systems*, 5(4) (2018 Aug 28), pp. 942–950.
25. D. Berdik, S. Otoum, N. Schmidt, D. Porter, Y. Jararweh "A survey on Blockchain for information systems management and security" *Information Processing and Management*, 58(1) (2021 Jan 1), p. 102397.
26. E. Gökalp, M.O. Gökalp, S. Çoban, P.E. Eren "Analysing opportunities and challenges of integrated blockchain technologies in healthcare" *Eurosymposium on Systems Analysis and Design*, Springer, Cham (2018 Sep 20), pp. 174–183.
27. C.C. Agbo, Q.H. Mahmoud "Comparison of blockchain frameworks for healthcare applications" *Internet Technology Letters*, 2(5) (2019 Sep), p. e122.
28. P.P. Ray, D. Dash, K. Salah, N. Kumar "Blockchain for IoT-based healthcare: Background, consensus, platforms, and use cases" *IEEE Systems Journal*, 15(1) (2020 Jan 21), pp. 85–94.
29. K. Kumar, K. Chaudhury, S.L. Tripathi "Future of machine learning (ML) and deep learning (DL) in healthcare monitoring system" *Machine Learning Algorithms for Signal and Image Processing*, IEEE (2023), pp. 293–313. doi: 10.1002/9781119861850.ch17.
30. S.L. Tripathi, M. Mahmud *Explainable Machine Learning Models and Architecture*, Wiley & Scrivener Publishing, 2023. doi: 10.1002/9781394186570.
31. T.A. Syed, A. Alzahrani, S. Jan, M.S. Siddiqui, A. Nadeem, T. Alghamdi "A comparative analysis of blockchain architecture and its applications: Problems and recommendations" *IEEE Access*, 7 (2019 Dec 4), pp. 176838–176869.

Chapter 10

Deep Learning-Based Renal Biopsy Image Analysis for Diagnosing Diabetic Kidney Disease

Saxena Sachin Kumar, Shrivastava Jitendra Nath, and Agarwal Gaurav

10.1 DIABETIC NEPHROPATHY

In India, approximately, 92.973 million adults (20–79 years) will be living with diabetes in 2030; it was 74.194 million adults (20–79 years) in 2021. Mortality attributable to diabetes was 647,831 adults (20–79 years) in 2021. Major complications of diabetes under microvascular are nephropathy (5.9%), retinopathy (0.8%), neuropathy (10.6%), and under macrovascular coronary are artery disease (2.5%), cerebrovascular disease (0.3%), peripheral artery disease (0.0%), and heart failure (0.2%). Diabetes-related health expenditure per person will be USD 138.9 approximately in 2030; it was USD 114.4 in 2021, according to the International Diabetes Federation [1].

Some global findings for Indian Diabetic Patients and their estimated growth are depicted in Figure 10.1. Hypertension is one of the primary factors in the symptoms of diabetes in Indian patients. Microvascular damage, antihypertensive drugs, arterial stiffness, and nephroparenchymal hypertension are some related factors between hypertension and diabetes [2]. Abnormalities of kidney structure or function are defined when albuminuria (ACR $\geq$ 30 mg/g), recent kidney transplantation, or a glomerular filtration rate (GFR) <60 ml/min/1.73 m^2 are present for more than three months. The criteria for diagnosing chronic kidney disease (CKD) are kidney failure when the G5 GFR category is less than 15 ml/min/1.73 m^2, whereas when the G4 GFR category falls between 15 and 29 ml/min/1.73 m^2, CKD is termed as severely decreased. Identification of non-sclerotic and sclerotic glomeruli in renal tissue can be performed using histopathological examination of kidney biopsy samples. Non-sclerotic glomeruli are normal glomeruli, whereas sclerotic glomeruli are thickened and hardened. Segmentation of glomerulosclerosis from digitized images and classification for an end-stage kidney in various human kidney biopsies can be processed using deep learning algorithms. The number of glomeruli and the presence of glomerulosclerosis can be identified by machine learning engineers in the biopsy image dataset obtained from renal magnetic resonance imaging (MRI) reports. Various deep learning engineers have adopted medical

DOI: 10.1201/9781003466949-10

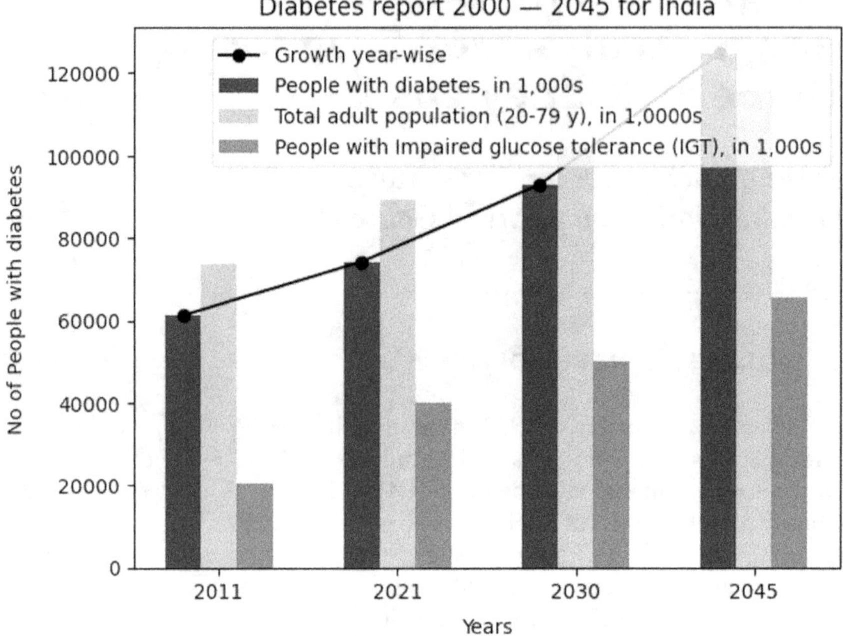

Figure 10.1 Number of people with diabetes, year-wise growth in India

image classification algorithms that incorporate domain-specific techniques for segmenting glomeruli.

This chapter discusses the development of a deep neural network model for classifying sclerotic biopsy images using whole slide imaging contributed by the European project AIDPATH. The model is based on the parametric rectified linear unit (PReLU) activation function and achieved high accuracy, recall, and F1 score for diagnosing diabetic kidney disease (DKD). The researchers also collected an MRI dataset from two hospitals in India for further study and plan to use transfer learning to predict diabetic nephropathy and diagnose acute kidney injury.

The chapter provides details about two datasets used in the study: dataset I and dataset II. Dataset I consists of histopathological images with WSI in SVS format contributed by the European project AIDPATH; while dataset II is from the Institute of Pathology Mannheim, Heidelberg University, Medical Faculty Mannheim. Both datasets were used to deploy deep learning algorithms to classify predefined patterns of glomerular changes in renal biopsy.

The contributions of this chapter are:

1. Proposing a deep neural network model based on the PReLU activation function for classifying sclerotic biopsy images using WSI.

2. Achieving high accuracy, recall, and F1 score for diabetic kidney disease using the proposed model.
3. Collecting an MRI dataset from two hospitals in India for further study and planning to use transfer learning to predict diabetic nephropathy and diagnose acute kidney injury.
4. Providing details about the two datasets used in the study, which can be used by other researchers for glomerular classification.
5. Contributing to the early diagnosis and treatment of kidney diseases, which can lead to better patient outcomes.

10.2 DIABETIC NEPHROPATHY

Anatomical scan and diffusion tensor imaging have emerged as a promising technology in radiology [3]. In recent years, deep neural network (DNN) techniques have gained significant attention in the field of diffusion-weighted renal MRI. Kidney outline and binary masking jobs are very common in anatomical integrity assessment [4]. Deep learning techniques can adaptively optimize the diversification of renal function and diabetic nephropathy based on MR imaging; morphological images are utilized to examine renal functionality [5]. Researchers aim to investigate and evaluate the potential of deep learning algorithm–based segmentation problems, such as kidney cortex and MRI images [6]. However, the glomeruli classification and its efficiency of identification in kidney biopsy remains a critical challenge due to the unavailability of human kidney biopsy datasets [7]. The rapid advancements in eGFR rate in patients led to the observation of mean serum creatinine as 2.9 mg/dl. One crucial aspect of fibrillary glomerulonephritis is the median time to end-stage renal disease has been observed as 24.4 months [8]. A comparative study looked at different cellular diversity in human glomerulonephritis, also associated with kidney disease-associated genes [9]. Researchers have also analyzed the benefits and limitations of tensor imaging preprocessing techniques to segment the kidney regions of interest in the stomach [10]. To investigate the effects of dynamic contrast-enhanced MRI scans on renal parts, it has been concluded that the GFR measurements should be as low as 1.4–2.8 mM [11]. Another study found that in patients with type 2 diabetes (T2D), it was observed that 28% showed no decline in the GFR, while 56% experienced a moderate decline, and 15% developed a severe decline [12]. Descriptive statistics were used to summarize an improved formula for eGFR is 175 × (Serum creatinine)$^{-1.154}$ × (Age)$^{-0.203}$ × (0.742 female) based on chronic kidney participant characteristics [13]. Several studies utilized a randomized controlled trial design to analyze the kidneys of DKD patients for identification of staining in the renal structure [14]. Some potential limitations of the study include the selection of CKD images for analyzing the decline in mGFR based on physical performance [15]. The researchers utilized multiple preprocessing steps on the renal biopsy images to segment a glomerulus with a morphologic appearance of segmental sclerosis [16].

MRI surveillance systems are extensively utilized for diverse applications, including the detection of renal disease symptoms, autosomal dominant polycystic kidney disease, and regional polycystic kidney disease [17]. Clinical sample features are relied upon in traditional microsystem methods, and shallow machine learning is utilized for identifying the amyloid type even in the presence of blood contamination [18]. Other researchers have extensively studied CKD progression to examine the associations between metabolic acidosis, dietary acid load, and kidney disease progression. Kidney disease progression was defined as a 50% reduction in eGFR [19]. Renal biopsy is a procedure that involves obtaining a small sample of kidney tissue for microscopic examination. Table 10.1 shows cases of CKD to avoid unnecessary risks and complications. Real-time processing is critical for investigating kidney damage in diabetic nephropathy, and diagnosing renal failure, nerve damage, and renal scarring [20].

10.3 RELATED WORK AND CONTRIBUTIONS

Marsh et al. [8] explored the use of deep learning algorithms to classify non-sclerotic and sclerotic glomeruli. The study utilized whole slide images (WSIs) acquired from frozen wedge donor biopsies using the Washington University Digital Pathology Exchange (WUPAX) system, which is compliant with regulatory requirements. A total of 48 sample WSIs were selected, representing a wide range of values of globally sclerosed glomeruli. Annotations of glomeruli were manually performed by outlining and labeling all glomeruli in each WSI using an in-house plug-in. Two different

Table 10.1 Exclusion Criteria for Renal Biopsy in Cases of Chronic Kidney Disease (CKD)

Symptoms Suggested by Centers for Disease Control and Prevention
Active infection
Uncontrolled hypertension
Bleeding disorders or use of blood-thinning medications
A solitary kidney or severe CKD, in which a biopsy would not alter management
In cases of severe obesity, obtaining an adequate biopsy sample can be difficult
Inability to remain still during the procedure or to cooperate with post-procedure care
Pregnancy or breastfeeding
An individual of advanced age who has comorbidities that increase the risk of complications
Renal cysts that are likely to make it difficult to obtain an adequate biopsy sample

models were used for glomeruli detection in WSIs: a patch-based model and a fully convolutional model. The patch-based model employed a pretrained VGG16 convolutional neural network (CNN) with modified fully connected layers, and training was performed using a sixfold cross-validation scheme. The fully convolutional model was based on VGG16 and used two 1 × 1 convolutional layers followed by a 64-node 3 × 3 dilated convolution layer. Both models were trained and tested using the categorical cross-entropy loss and Adam optimizer. The patch-based model demonstrated glomerulus differentiation in frozen H&E sections but had limitations when applied to detect glomeruli in WSIs. The fully convolutional model, on the other hand, was able to label WSIs at a higher resolution. Overall, the study presents two different approaches for glomeruli detection in WSIs and provides insights into the challenges and potential solutions for accurate and efficient glomeruli detection in digital pathology. As a comparison table presenting the experiments and results from previous works on glomeruli detection, Table 10.2 lists the comparative accuracy, precision, and recall values of these models.

Wels et al. [31] used patient specimens and raw data obtained from two different pathology institutes in an anonymized manner. The data collection and experiments were conducted in accordance with the ethics commission of Heidelberg University. Glomerulus segmentation and image preprocessing were performed using MATLAB, while machine learning was done using Python with PyTorch. Basal morphologic patterns of glomerular changes were defined for a CNN model-based approach, including normal glomerulus, amyloidosis, nodular sclerosis, global sclerosis, mesangial hypercellularity, mesangial proliferative glomerulonephritis (MPGN), necrosis/crescent, and segmental sclerosis. Three datasets were created for training, validation, and testing, and several classification models were trained using different architectures. The models were trained for 50 epochs with a decay of 0.1 every 7 epochs.

Yao et al. [32] proposed a novel framework and also utilized computer-aided approaches to classify different glomerular lesions, with deep learning algorithms achieving high accuracy in renal pathological findings classification. However, these algorithms often lack generalizability due to their reliance on in-house data, and few studies have developed deep learning approaches for fine-grained classification of globally sclerotic glomeruli. One potential solution to address this challenge is self-supervised learning, particularly contrastive learning, which has shown superior performance in various computer vision tasks. Glomerular detection using deep learning techniques has also shown promising results in accurately detecting and characterizing glomeruli in whole slide images, offering the potential for improved diagnosis and treatment guidance in renal pathology.

For instance, Gallego et al. [29] proposed two methods for glomerulus classification, and a combination of detection using CNNs is presented.

Table 10.2 Comparison Table for Previous Work Experiments and Results for Glomeruli Detection

Reference	*Algorithm*	*Dataset Used*	*Objective*	*Accuracy*
[21]	Mask R-CNN, LSTM, ResNeXt-101	1379 kidney biopsy slides	Glomerulus identification	94.4% F1, 94% accuracy
[22]	CNN architecture (Inception V3)	751 unique images of renal biopsies	Glomerulus classification	92.67% accuracy, 0.8681 kappa
[23]	Proposes a deep convolutional neural network (CNN) and YOLO v4	349 renal biopsy whole slide images (WSIs)	Glomeruli object detection and classification	95.1% accuracy, 0.932 kappa
[24]	Faster R-CNN	46 WSI images form Tokyo Hospital and 42 WSI images form Kitano Hospital	Detection of glomeruli	0.670 mean intersection over union (IoU)
[25]	Fine tunned CNN architecture (Inception V3)	WSIs of 283 renal biopsy cases	Classification of global sclerosis	>0.98 AUC
[26]	Patch-based CNN model, fully convolutional VGG16 model	870 sclerosed and 2997 non-sclerosed glomeruli	Classification of sclerosed and non-sclerosed glomeruli	84.75% F1 non-sclerosed, 64.92% sclerosed
[27]	Active contour method	10 sample images	Segmentation of renal biopsy images	90% SNR, 100% PSNR
[28]	Deep learning–based model	199 WSIs of mice	Assessment of glomerular lesions and structures	58%–93% sensitivity, 72%–100% specificity, and 74%–94% accuracy
[29]	CNN, AlexNet, GoogleNet	700 glomeruli annotations and 700 non-glomeruli	Classification glomerulus and non-glomerulus, detect glomerulus in WSI	93.7% F1 score, 88.1% precision, 100% recall
[30]	Tenfold cross-validation, shallow ANN	428 sclerotic glomeruli and 2344 non-sclerotic glomeruli	Glomerulus classification	95% accuracy, 98.44% precision, 93.1% recall

The method first focuses on achieving correct glomerulus classification into glomerulus/non-glomerulus classes using a CNN configuration, while the second method utilizes the best-performing CNN configuration from the first method to detect glomeruli in WSIs. The proposed method is suitable for PAS samples from different laboratories due to the color normalization process used in data augmentation. The detection is performed using a sliding window approach with overlapping and a majority vote decision for each pixel to reduce false positives. The proposed method achieves a detection score of 93.7%, which improves upon reference methods.

Weis et al. investigated the use of an approach based on a CNN model to classify various patterns of glomerular alterations in kidney biopsies [31]. Eight prototypical patterns of glomerular alterations (patterns 01–08) were identified: normal glomerulus, amyloidosis, nodular sclerosis, global sclerosis, mesangial hypercellularity, mesangial proliferative glomerulonephritis, necrosis/crescent, and segmental sclerosis. An additional category (pattern 09) was designated for extraglomerular structures. Three datasets were created for training, validation, and testing, and multiple published classification models were trained using a stochastic gradient descent optimizer. Transfer learning was employed to retrain the models on a smaller dataset. The study utilized a GPU for calculations and ensured that there were no ancillary studies in routine diagnostics.

There has been a growing interest in deep learning. Lu et al. [33] used EfficientNet-B016 as the backbone model for classification due to its high efficiency in learning large scale images. The model was pretrained on ImageNet17 and customized for the specific tasks by adapting the fully connected layers. The model was trained and tested using fivefold cross-validation, with data split at the subject level. Data augmentation techniques such as horizontal and vertical flipping and random cropping were applied to all experiments. The results showed that the proposed CircleMix augmentation improved the model's performance in terms of balanced accuracy and balanced F1 score compared to the baseline model and CutMix augmentation. Hierarchical training with different combinations also showed promising results.

Hara et al. [34] demonstrated the potential of U-Net, a CNN model, for semantic segmentation. Fine-tuning was performed using the VGG16 model, pretrained on the ImageNet dataset, as the U-Net encoder. The input to the model was image and annotation data, and the output was label information for each pixel. Among several models compared, U-Net exhibited the highest accuracy and relatively clear segmented images. Data augmentation techniques such as contrast adjustment, horizontal flipping, and rotation were applied during training to improve generalization performance. The performance of U-Net was evaluated using the Dice coefficient, and agreement rates were compared between renal pathologists with and without referring to U-Net–segmented images.

Zeng et al. [35] enhanced the transparency of LSTM-GCNet, which is a biomedical image classification approach that combines DenseNet with a long short-term memory (LSTM) layer for fine-grained classification of glomerular cells. The method includes a global context block and squeeze-excitation block for attention focusing, as well as a 2D V-Net with a self-attention module and center channel for identifying intrinsic glomerular cells. Image processing algorithms like marked watersheds are used for glomerular structure detection. The approach is trained and evaluated using renal biopsy specimens from IgAN patients. The proposed method achieved high accuracy (92.8%) and Cohen's kappa (0.91) for glomerulus classification and shows promising results for intrinsic glomerular cell recognition compared to previous approaches.

CNNs have been widely adopted for image analysis tasks, with AlexNet emerging as the winner of the ImageNet Large Scale Visual Recognition Challenge in 2012. In Altini et al.'s study [36], two main approaches based on SegNet and DeepLab v3+ architectures were considered for semantic segmentation in medical imaging. SegNet removes the need for learning the up-sampling process by storing indices used in max pooling, while DeepLab v3+ introduces atrous convolution for a broader field of view. The proposed computer-aided diagnosis (CAD) architecture integrates with Aperio ImageScope software for visualization and annotation of WSIs. The semantic segmentation workflow involves using a CNN for pixel-level classification and object detection to estimate the Karpinski histological score. Preprocessing techniques, such as thresholding and undersampling, are employed to reduce the dimensions of WSIs for efficient deep learning.

The visual evaluation of histopathological WSIs for kidney biopsies is time-consuming, prone to errors, and subjective. To address these challenges, CAD systems based on image processing and machine learning techniques have been proposed. For instance, researchers have utilized a texture-based feature set and support vector machine (SVM) model for glomeruli localization, achieving high precision (>90%) and reasonable recall (>70%). Authors have also introduced a new descriptor, Segmental HOG, for comprehensive detection of glomeruli, showing significant improvements in detection performance. Other authors have focused on analyzing glomeruli's shape and color using different approaches. These advancements in CAD systems aim to improve the accuracy and efficiency of evaluating kidney biopsies for pathological conditions [30].

10.4 DIABETIC PREDICTION

10.4.1 Data Resources

Many researchers have obtained kidney biopsy images from two resources: dataset I [37] and dataset II [38]. Dataset I consists of histopathological images with WSI in SVS format contributed by the European project AIDPATH. For semantic segmentation, biopsy samples were collected with an outer diameter between 100 μm and 300 μm and 20× zoom using a Leica Aperio ScanScope CS scanner. Images containing several kinds of glomeruli were mounted with tissue sections of 4 μm. As far as dataset II is concerned, glomerular morphological patterns were collected from various patients at the Institute of Pathology Mannheim, Heidelberg University, Medical Faculty Mannheim. The purpose of this research data was to deploy deep learning algorithms to classify predefined patterns of glomerular changes in renal biopsy. The nine models are AlexNet, ResNet18-152, Res_Net34, Res_Net50, Res_Net101, Res_Net152, vgg_11, vgg_16, vgg_19, squeez_net, inception, and densenet_121, and downloadable in the .pt format for glomerulus classification. The results of the research for this study will help in various domains such as glomerular disorder, renal glomerulus, and digital pathology.

An evaluation of morphological patterns using diverse numerical values across multiple datasets is shown in Table 10.3. Figure 10.2 shows the histological analysis of kidney biopsy samples from dataset I. Figure 10.3 depicts variations in saturation levels for sclerotic tissues. Figure 10.4 shows artifacts in normal or non-sclerotic tissue samples, whereas Figure 10.5

Table 10.3 Assessment of Various Numbers in Both Datasets for Morphological Patterns

Reference	*Research Data for Convolutional Neural Networks*	*Further Classification*	*Number of Samples Used*	*Type*
Dataset I [37]	Whole slide images (WSIs)	Biopsy sample	31	SVS
	Glomerular morphological patterns	Normal	1170	PNG
	Glomerular morphological patterns	Sclerosed	1170	PNG
Dataset II [38]	Pattern 01 (available for test)	Normal glomerulus	20	TIF, JPG
	Pattern 02 (available for test)	Amyloidosis	20	TIF, JPG
	Pattern 03 (available for test)	Nodular sclerosis	20	TIF, JPG
	Pattern 04 (available for test)	Global sclerosis	20	TIF
	Pattern 05 (available for test)	Mesangial expansion	20	TIF
	Pattern 06 (available for test)	Membranoproliferative glomerulonephritis (MPGN)	20	TIF
	Pattern 07 (available for test)	Necrosis	20	TIF
	Pattern 08 (available for test)	Segmental sclerosis	20	TIF
	Pattern 09 (available for test)	Other structures/ default	20	TIF

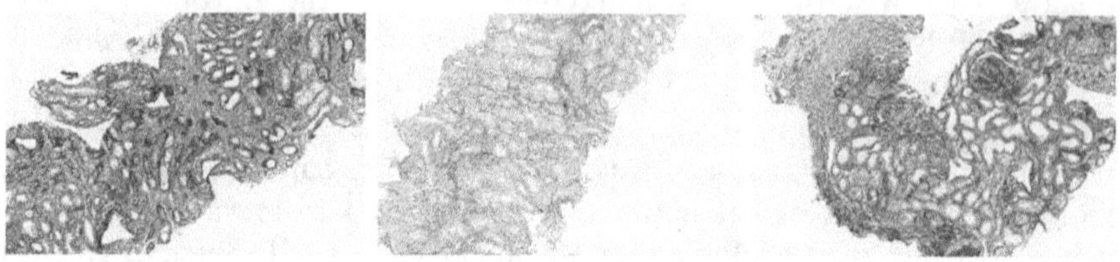

Figure 10.2 Histological processed image samples of kidney biopsy taken from dataset I

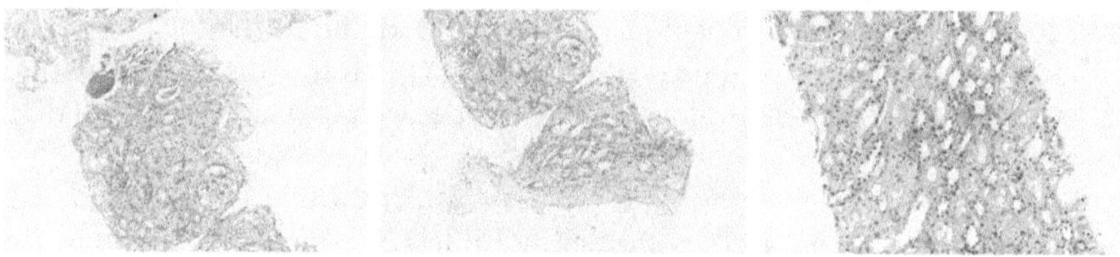

Figure 10.3 Dataset I consists of different saturation levels for sclerotic tissues

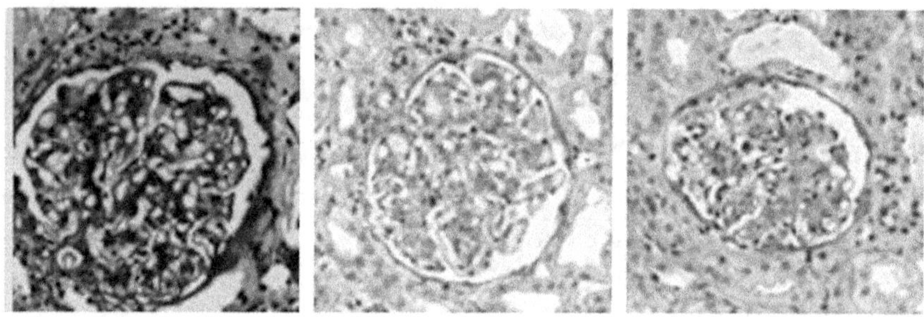

Figure 10.4 Normal or non-sclerotic tissue sample artifacts

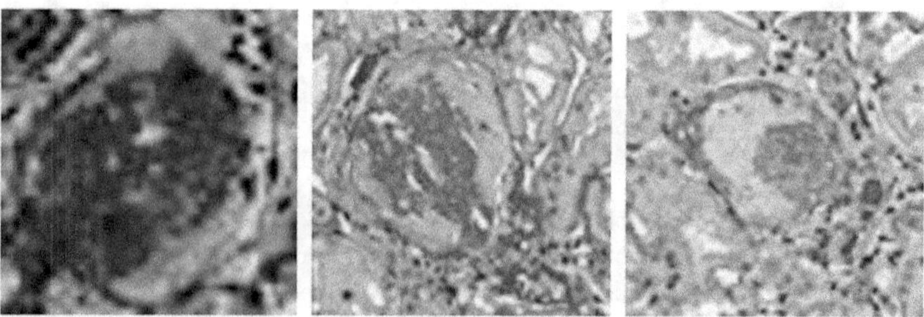

Figure 10.5 Sclerotic sample cropped to glomeruli with complex changes

represents cropped images of glomeruli with complex changes in sclerotic tissue samples. Figure 10.6 shows renal pathology images utilizing a pretrained CNN network and transfer learning for glomerular population feature extraction. Table 10.4 shows the analysis of biopsy images in the dataset.

10.4.2 Data Pathogenesis and Biopsy History of Glomeruli

Various classifiers of machine learning can detect renal imaging biomarkers in diabetic kidney disease and several proposed deep neural networks are helpful to diagnose clinical history of renal diseases [39]. Deep learning has revolutionized the field of computer vision to detect and treat diabetic

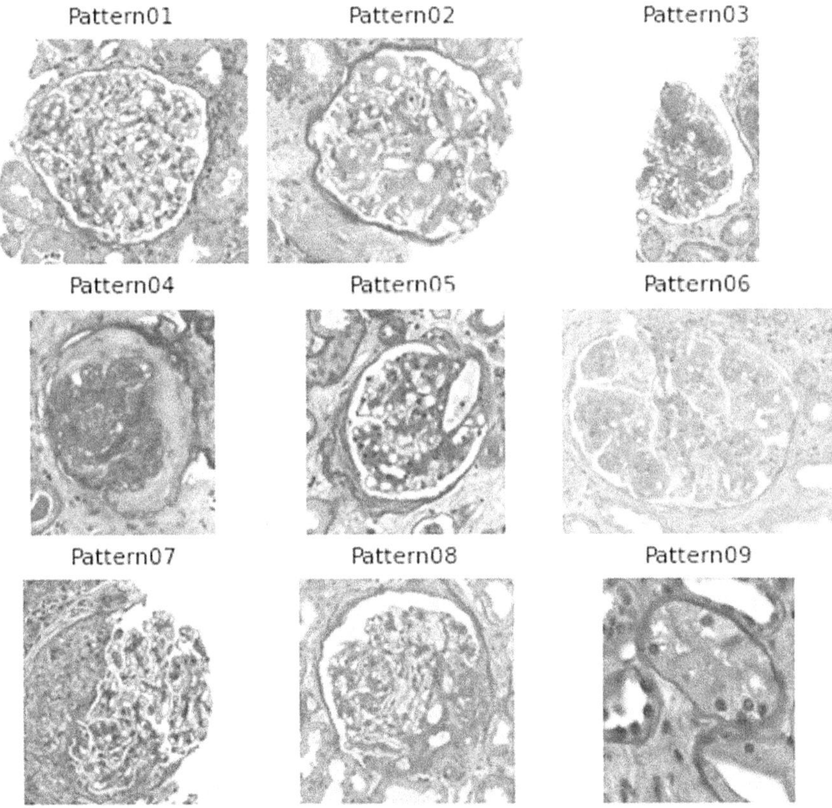

Figure 10.6 Pretrained CNN network or transfer learning is used for feature extraction with glomerulus population; input image patterns are normal glomerulus, amyloidosis, nodular sclerosis, global sclerosis, mesangial expansion, membranoproliferative glomerulonephritis (MPGN), necrosis, segmental sclerosis, other structures/default

Table 10.4 Characteristics of Biopsy Images in Dataset

Parameter	*Value*
Zoom	20×
Image resolution	0.499 microns per pixel
Apparent magnification	20 (equivalent objective)
Type of file	ScanScope Virtual Slide (.svs)
Software used	ImageScope
Size	~33 MB (single .svs file)
Converted file size	~4.13 MB (single .tif file)
Type of converted image	TIF file (.tif)
Resolution of converted file	1496 × 966 px

kidney disease. The presence of fibrosis, fibroblasts, and proteinuria in CKD tubules are the leading global causes of nephropathy [40]. Qezelbash-Chamak et al. conducted a comprehensive comparative study with different machine learning to determine the CKD stages and level of glomerulonephritis [41]. Ayyar et al. experimented with different popular CNN architectures to classify glomeruli in kidney tissue slide images [42]. Feng et al. investigated the performance of these CNNs by analyzing various metrics such as region of interest, glomerular filtration rate, HbAlc, blood oxygenation level dependent, and diffusion tensor imaging [43].

A CAD system to classify histopathological biopsy renal images is established for the glomeruli dataset [30]. Statistical analysis was conducted for the pathological reports and the digital images were processed for identifying glomeruli. The glomerular segmentation and segmentation of capillary openness are tedious tasks for researchers. It is noteworthy that the process of digital images for automatically identifying glomeruli is most often reported [44]. As far as the scientific reports about abdominal MRI images are concerned, the region of the tractography is successfully identified. Apart from the biopsy reports, kidney segmentation alone in MRI images can dramatically affect reproducibility [45].

10.5 METHODOLOGY

Various classifiers of machine learning introduced imaging-based systems in patients with hypertensive nephropathy. The proposed deep neural networks or deep CNNs [46–47] for image classification use the PReLU activation function to classify sclerosed biopsy images and perform testing on dataset I and dataset II. The proposed multilayer deep neural network associated with the CNN architecture is implemented using the Keras library, and the model is trained and evaluated on a dataset of images. During training, the PReLU activation function is utilized in the convolutional layers of the CNN, while other standard layers such as max pooling, dropout, and fully connected (dense) layers are also included. The study was conducted using a large dataset collected from dataset I along with the Adam optimizer with a learning rate of 0.001, beta_1 value of 0.9, and beta_2 of 0.999 for model compilation. The first step in the proposed methodology is to preprocess the data, and later, the model is trained for 50 epochs with a batch size of 40 using data augmentation techniques such as rotation, zooming, and horizontal/vertical flips. Figure 10.7 shows the flowchart required to obtain classification results using CNN models for pathologist reports. The definitive diagnosis of renal tissue biopsy typically necessitates the collection of a physical sample of kidney tissue, which is examined under a microscope. MRI images and reports are insufficient for conducting a biopsy. In this model, the total number of images is 2340, all sized 180 × 180; and the number of x_train, x_test, y_train, and y_test shapes were 1872 of size 180 × 180, 468 with size 180 × 180, 1872 with size 180 × 180, respectively.

10.6 EXPERIMENT DISCUSSION

We proposed deep neural networks with different activation functions for glomerular detection, segmentation, and lesion characterization. The results of this experiment have important implications for nontechnical users aiming for glomerular quantification. This research includes the design and operation of glomerular image classification and identification

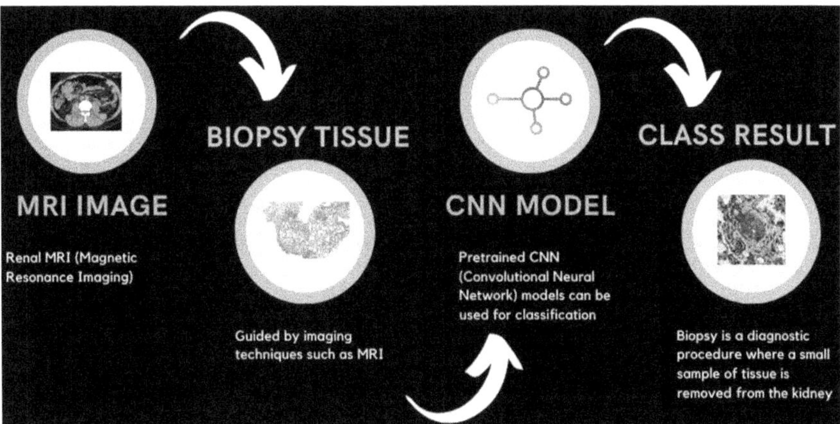

Figure 10.7 Flowchart to classify results using CNN models for pathologist reports. Biopsy of renal tissue typically requires obtaining a physical sample of the kidney tissue for examination under a microscope to make a definitive diagnosis. MRI images and reports alone are not sufficient for a biopsy

of patches with renal glomeruli segmentation. Therefore, strategies such as the classification problem of the glomerulus of interest applied to human renal biopsy samples can be implemented. The findings of this experiment indicate that the DNN model can achieve promising results in the classification problem of sclerotic sample cropped glomeruli. In this experiment, two different types of sclerotic sample cropped glomeruli were selected for testing. Understanding the effects of the activation function on DNN performance is crucial for optimizing the classification problem. Our experimental results reveal that DNNs consistently outperform while classifying glomeruli and will be helpful for renal pathologists. Our findings provide valuable insights into pathological concordance for the count of glomerular biopsy images. Accurate and real-time detection of glomeruli and sclerotic glomeruli is essential for effective detection and segmentation of glomerular boundaries on WSIs. This review aims to contribute to the classification problem of kidney biopsy images that are annotated with two classes. Open research directions in the field of AI have contributed significantly to the glomerular lesion classification problem. Furthermore, this chapter discusses the implications of AI in identifying intrinsic glomerular cells. In recent years, there has been a rapid proliferation of research on deep neural networks along with renal glomeruli classification. Fully convolutional networks have emerged as a transformative technology in various fields, such as glomerulosclerosis image classification and digital pathology.

We next discuss the implications of our findings and compare our results with the compilation of the model with Adam optimizer and categorical cross-entropy loss. We evaluate the model performance using accuracy as a metric. We detail the experimental design used in our study and then discuss the model's performance evaluation using precision, recall, F1 score, and support metrics. The model's accuracy is 0.9465, indicating a high level of accuracy. The recall, which measures the model's ability to correctly identify positive cases, is 0.9358, showing that the model performs well in identifying positive cases. The F1 score, which combines precision and recall, is 0.9375, indicating a good balance between precision and recall. The support, which refers to the number of instances in the dataset, is 468. Overall, the study demonstrates that the model has high accuracy, good recall, and a balanced F1 score, making it a promising approach for the task at hand.

The dataset for further study was collected from two hospitals: the Shri Ram Murti Smarak Institute of Medical Sciences (SRMS IMS) and the Bareilly MRI & CT Scan Centre, both located in Bareilly, Uttar Pradesh, India. The SRMS Institute, established in 1990, offers medical education degrees such as MBBS and postgraduate (MD/MS) programs, and the hospital at SRMS has advanced CT scan and MRI machines with various capabilities. The original private dataset used in this study can be accessed from a Google Drive link, and the raw DICOM images have specific names for each patient, such as DURGA_DATT_JOSHI_72Y_M_42215137 and

RAM_DEVI_65Y_F_42214353. The images were processed using Python scripting language to rename, convert to jpeg, and crop to focus on the kidney feature. Examples are shown in Figure 10.8. and Figure 10.9. The images will help provide additional information for biopsy reports such as localization of glomeruli, assessment of surrounding tissues, and monitoring of glomeruli changes.

The report includes several figures, including Figure 10.8, which shows an MRI scan of the renal structure responsible for blood supply and drainage; Figure 10.9, a cross-sectional MRI of a kidney without metadata; Figure 10.10, graphs depicting the training progress of a deep learning model in terms of accuracy versus epochs; Figure 10.11, showing the convergence of the model in terms of training loss versus epochs; and Figure 10.12, a confusion matrix used to evaluate the performance of the model.

10.7 CONCLUSIONS AND FUTURE WORK

We have applied deep learning pipelining glomerular disease and the identification of glomerular lesions in biopsy images. In this section, we conclude the results of our experiments regarding kidney biopsy image interpretation.

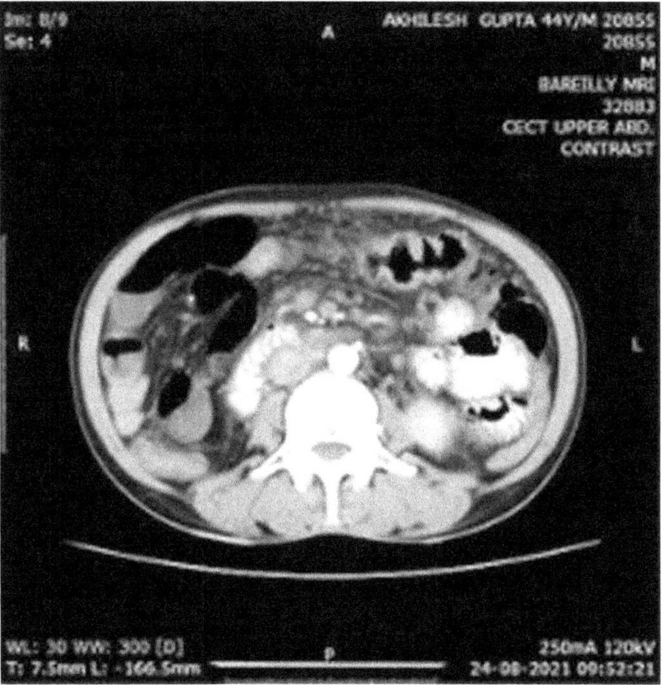

Figure 10.8 MRI scan surrounding the structure of the renal artery, which is responsible for supplying and draining blood from the kidneys

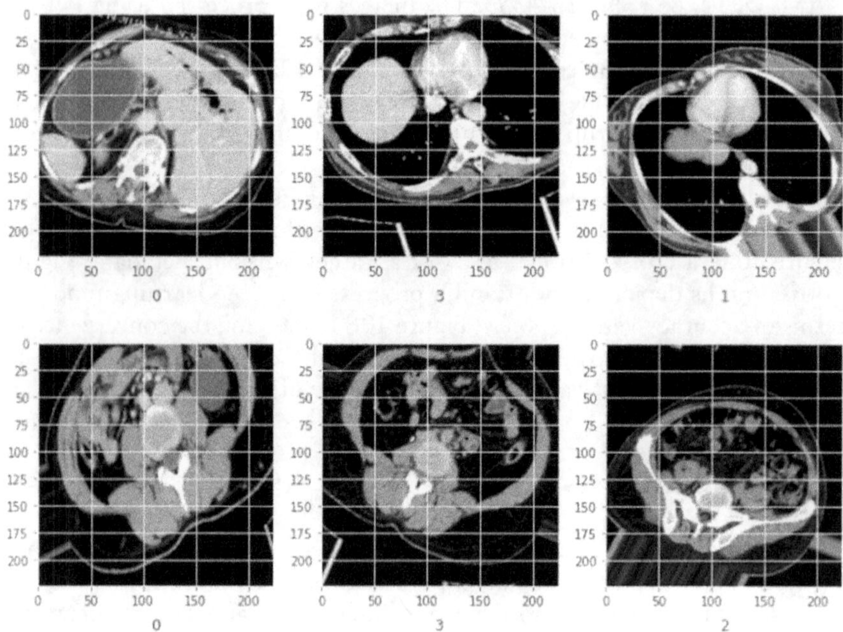

Figure 10.9 Cross-sectional MRI image of a kidney without metadata

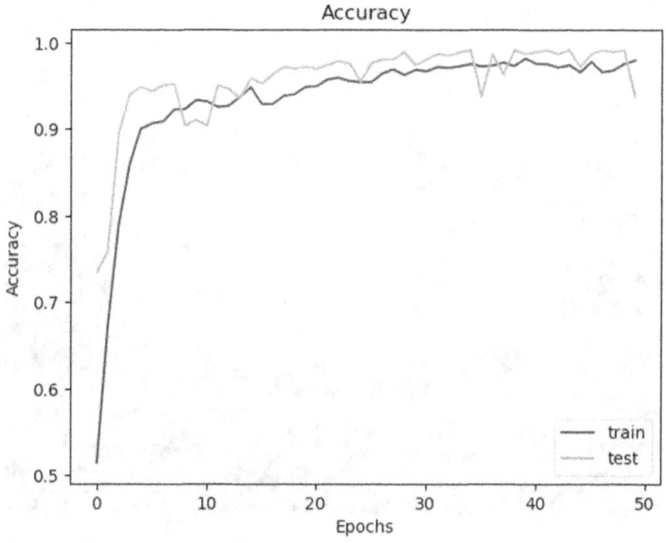

Figure 10.10 Training progress: accuracy versus epochs

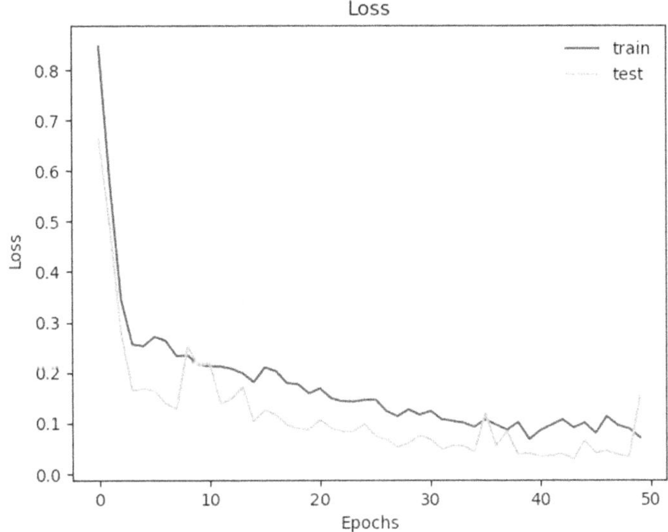

Figure 10.11 Training loss versus epochs: evaluating the convergence of a deep learning model

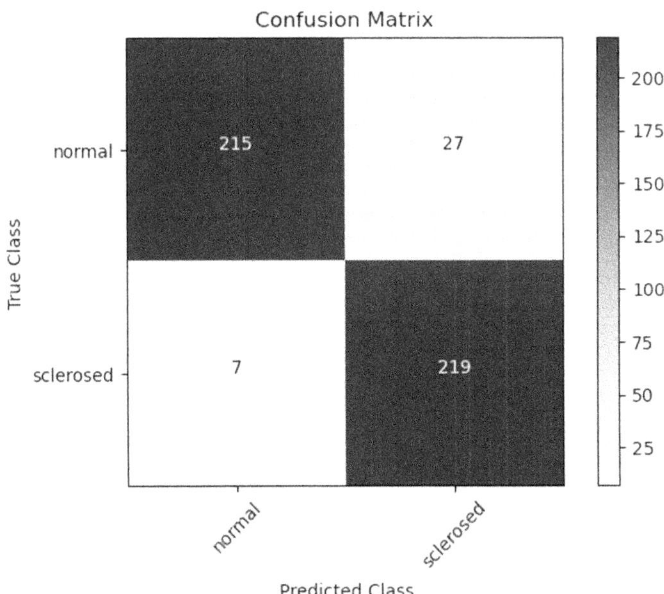

Figure 10.12 Performance evaluation of deep learning model using a confusion matrix

We described the process of feature extraction from imitating nephropathologists' reports on kidney biopsy images collected from open resource datasets. We also provided an overview of the research problem of glomerulus detection and lesion annotations. This chapter aimed to investigate the effects of classifying the glomerular features and glomerular biopsy images detectable by conventional deep learning algorithms. Multiple statistical models were employed to determine the performance of deep learning for tensor imaging of the human kidneys. The relationship between renal functional decline in DKD and comprehensive renal imaging involves multiple measurements. The precision, recall, F1 score, and support for the experiment were 0.9465, 0.9358, 0.9375, and 468, respectively. In the future, we intend to use MRI images for biopsy reports.

ACKNOWLEDGMENTS

The authors express gratitude to God for providing them with the wisdom and resources to create informed content and for enabling human participation in their work. The authors also acknowledge guidance in implementing the prediction model and recognize that under their guidance, they were able to conduct their research with adherence to all ethical standards.

REFERENCES

1. https://diabetesatlas.org/data/en/country/93/in.html
2. Kumar V, Agarwal S, Saboo B, Makkar B (2022) RSSDI Guidelines for the management of hypertension in patients with diabetes mellitus. *Int J Diabetes Dev Ctries* 42:576–605. https://doi.org/10.1007/s13410-022-01143-7
3. Chan RW, Von Deuster C, Stoeck CT, et al. (2014) High-resolution diffusion tensor imaging of the human kidneys using a free-breathing, multi-slice, targeted field of view approach. *NMR Biomed* 27(11):1300–1312. https://doi.org/10.1002/nbm.3190
4. Periquito JS, Paul K, Huelnhagen T, et al. (2019) Diffusion-weighted renal MRI at 9.4 tesla using RARE to improve anatomical integrity. *Sci Rep* 9(1). https://doi.org/10.1038/s41598-019-56184-6
5. Su CH, Hsu YC, Thangudu S, et al. (2021) Application of multiparametric MR imaging to predict the diversification of renal function in miR29a-mediated diabetic nephropathy. *Sci Rep* 11(1). https://doi.org/10.1038/s41598-021-81519-7
6. Jayapandian CP, Chen Y, Janowczyk AR, et al. (2021) Development and evaluation of deep learning–based segmentation of histologic structures in the kidney cortex with multiple histologic stains. *Kidney Int* 99(1):86–101. https://doi.org/10.1016/j.kint.2020.07.044
7. Wu J, Shi Z, Zhang Y, et al. (2021) Native T1 mapping in assessing kidney fibrosis for patients with chronic glomerulonephritis. *Front Med (Lausanne)* 8. https://doi.org/10.3389/fmed.2021.772326

8. Rosenstock JL, Markowitz GS (2019) Fibrillary glomerulonephritis: An update. *Kidney Int Rep* 4(7):917–922.
9. Chen Z, Zhang T, Mao K, et al. (2021) A single-cell survey of the human glomerulonephritis. *J Cell Mol Med* 25(10):4684–4695. https://doi.org/10.1111/jcmm.16407
10. Borrelli P, Zacchia M, Cavaliere C, et al. (2021) Diffusion tensor imaging for the study of early renal dysfunction in patients affected by Bardet-Biedl syndrome. *Sci Rep* 11(1). https://doi.org/10.1038/s41598-021-00394-4
11. Ebrahimi B, Textor SC, Lerman LO (2014) Renal relevant radiology: Renal functional magnetic resonance imaging. *Clin J Am Soc Nephrol* 9(2):395–405. https://doi.org/10.2215/CJN.02900313
12. Mora-Gutiérrez JM, Fernández-Seara MA, Echeverria-Chasco R, Garcia-Fernandez N (2021) Perspectives on the role of magnetic resonance imaging (MRI) for noninvasive evaluation of diabetic kidney disease. *J Clin Med* 10: 120–133.
13. Wei X, Hu R, Zhou X, et al. (2022) Alterations of renal function in patients with diabetic kidney disease: A BOLD and DTI study. *Comput Intell Neurosci* 2022. https://doi.org/10.1155/2022/6844102
14. Guo M, Chen Q, Huang Y, et al. (2023) High glucose-induced kidney injury via activation of necroptosis in diabetic kidney disease. *Oxid Med Cell Longev* 2023. https://doi.org/10.1155/2023/2713864
15. Hellberg M, Höglund P, Svensson P, Clyne N (2019) Randomized controlled trial of exercise in CKD—The RENEXC study. *Kidney Int Rep* 4(7):963–976. https://doi.org/10.1016/j.ekir.2019.04.001
16. Bu L, Chen J, Nelson AC, et al. (2019) Somatic mosaicism in a male patient with X-linked Alport syndrome. *Kidney Int Rep* 4(7):1031–1035. https://doi.org/10.1016/j.ekir.2019.03.005
17. Lanktree MB, Guiard E, Li W, et al. (2019) Intrafamilial variability of ADPKD. *Kidney Int Rep* 4(7):995–1003. https://doi.org/10.1016/j.ekir.2019.04.018
18. Taylor GW, Gilbertson JA, Sayed R, et al. (2019) Proteomic analysis for the diagnosis of fibrinogen Aα-chain amyloidosis. *Kidney Int Rep* 4(7):977–986. https://doi.org/10.1016/j.ekir.2019.04.007
19. Pike M, Stewart TG, Morse J, et al. (2019) APOL1, acid load, and CKD progression. *Kidney Int Rep* 4(7):946–954. https://doi.org/10.1016/j.ekir.2019.03.022
20. Masoumeh Ghoreishi S, Amiri M, Shabestani Monfared A, Hamidi F, Najafzadehvarzi H (2022) Therapeutic effect of antihypertensive drug on diabetic nephropathy: Functional and structural kidney investigation. *Saudi J Biol Sci* 29(8). https://doi.org/10.1016/j.sjbs.2022.103353
21. Yang CK, Lee CY, Wang HS, et al. (2022) Glomerular disease classification and lesion identification by machine learning. *Biomed J* 45(4):675–685. https://doi.org/10.1016/j.bj.2021.08.011
22. Kannan S, Morgan LA, Liang B, et al. (2019) Segmentation of glomeruli within trichrome images using deep learning. *Kidney Int Rep* 4(7):955–962. https://doi.org/10.1016/j.ekir.2019.04.008
23. Zheng Z, Zhang X, Ding J, et al. (2021) Deep learning-based artificial intelligence system for automatic assessment of glomerular pathological findings in lupus nephritis. *Diagnostics (Basel)* 11(11). https://doi.org/10.3390/diagnostics11111983

24. Kawazoe Y, Shimamoto K, Yamaguchi R, et al. (2022) Computational pipeline for glomerular segmentation and association of the quantified regions with prognosis of kidney function in IgA nephropathy. *Diagnostics* 12(12). https://doi.org/10.3390/diagnostics12122955
25. Uchino E, Suzuki K, Sato N, et al. (2020) "Classification of glomerular pathological findings using deep learning and nephrologist-AI collective intelligence approach." *International journal of medical informatics* 141: 104231.
26. Marsh JN, Matlock MK, Kudose S, et al. (2018) Deep learning global glomerulosclerosis in transplant kidney frozen sections. *IEEE Trans Med Imaging* 37(12):2718–2728. https://doi.org/10.1109/TMI.2018.2851150
27. Patil YB. (2017) Analysis of diabetic nephropathy using contour based segmentation of image processing on renal biopsies images. *Int. Multidiscip. J. Pune Res* 3(4).
28. Shen L, Sun W, Zhang Q, et al. (2022) Deep learning-based model significantly improves diagnostic performance for assessing renal histopathology in lupus glomerulonephritis. *Kidney Dis* 8(4):347–356. https://doi.org/10.1159/000524880
29. Gallego J, Pedraza A, Lopez S, et al. (2018) Glomerulus classification and detection based on convolutional neural networks. *J Imaging* 4(1). https:// https://doi.org/10.3390/jimaging4010020
30. Cascarano GD, Debitonto FS, Lemma R, et al. (2021) A neural network for glomerulus classification based on histological images of kidney biopsy. *BMC Med Inform Decis Mak* 21. https://doi.org/10.1186/s12911-021-01650-3
31. Weis CA, Bindzus JN, Voigt J, et al. (2022) Assessment of glomerular morphological patterns by deep learning algorithms. *J Nephrol* 35(2):417–427. https://doi.org/10.1007/s40620-021-01221-9
32. Yao T, Lu Y, Long J, et al. (2022) "Glo-In-One: Holistic glomerular detection, segmentation, and lesion characterization with large-scale web image mining." *Journal of Medical Imaging* 9, no. 5: 052408-052408.
33. Lu Y, Yang H, Zhu Z, et al. (2021) "Improve global glomerulosclerosis classification with imbalanced data using CircleMix augmentation."arXiv preprint arXiv:2101.07654.
34. Hara S, Haneda E, Kawakami M, et al. (2022) Evaluating tubulointerstitial compartments in renal biopsy specimens using a deep learning-based approach for classifying normal and abnormal tubules. *PLOS One* 17(7). https://doi.org/10.1371/journal.pone.0271161
35. Zeng C, Nan Y, Xu F, et al. (2020) Identification of glomerular lesions and intrinsic glomerular cell types in kidney diseases via deep learning. *J Pathol* 252(1):53–64. https://doi.org/10.1002/path.5491
36. Altini N, Cascarano GD, Brunetti A, et al. (2020) Semantic segmentation framework for glomeruli detection and classification in kidney histological sections. *Electronics (Switzerland)* 9(3). https://doi.org/10.3390/electronics9030503
37. https://data.mendeley.com/datasets/k7nvtgn2x6/3
38. https://doi.org/10.11588/data/JWZ2CK
39. Gooding KM, Lienczewski C, Papale M, et al. (2020) Prognostic imaging biomarkers for diabetic kidney disease (iBEAt): Study protocol. *BMC Nephrol* 21(1). https://doi.org/10.1186/s12882-020-01901-x

40. Tillman L, Tabish TA, Kamaly N, et al. (2022) "Advancements in nanomedicines for the detection and treatment of diabetic kidney disease." *Biomater Biosyst* 6: 100047.
41. Qezelbash-Chamak J, Badamchizadeh S, Eshghi K, Asadi Y (2022) A survey of machine learning in kidney disease diagnosis. *Mach Learn Appl* 10:100418. https://doi.org/10.1016/j.mlwa.2022.100418
42. Ayyar M, Mathur P, Ratn Shah R, et al. (2018) "Harnessing AI for kidney glomeruli classification." In *2018 IEEE International Symposium on Multimedia (ISM)*, pp. 17–20. IEEE.
43. Feng YZ, Ye YJ, Cheng ZY, et al. (2020) Non-invasive assessment of early stage diabetic nephropathy by DTI and BOlD MrI. *The British Journal of Radiology*, 93(1105), p.20190562.
44. Sheehan SM, Korstanje R (2018) Automatic glomerular identification and quantification of histological phenotypes using image analysis and machine learning. *Am J Physiol Ren Physiol* 315:1644–1651. https://doi.org/10.1152/ajprenal
45. Borrelli P, Cavaliere C, Basso L, et al. (2019) Diffusion tensor imaging of the kidney: Design and evaluation of a reliable processing pipeline. *Sci Rep* 9(1). https:. https://doi.org/10.1038/s41598-019-49170-5
46. Kumar K, Chaudhury K, Tripathi SL (2023) Future of machine learning (ML) and deep learning (DL) in healthcare monitoring system. In *Machine Learning Algorithms for Signal and Image Processing*, IEEE, pp.293–313. https://doi.org/10.1002/9781119861850.ch17
47. Wijayanto I, Humairani A, Hadiyoso S et al. (2023) Epileptic seizure detection on a compressed EEG signal using energy measurement. *Biomed Signal Process Control* 85:104872. https://doi.org/10.1016/j.bspc.2023.104872

Chapter 11

Blockchain

Evolution and Future Scope

Navneet Kaur, Nidhi Chahal, Ritu Dewan, Shikha Singh, Gautam Bansal, Dikshant Dishu, and Santosh Kumar

11.1 INTRODUCTION

Blockchain can be characterized as a data system that conserves transactional records while promoting decentralization, security, and transparency. Blockchain can also be described as a chain of histories that are held in the form of blocks and managed by numerous authorities. Blockchains are distributed ledgers that are available to everyone on the network. However, once data is placed on a blockchain, it is extremely challenging to change or modify it. Each transaction on a blockchain is protected by an alphanumeric signature that verifies its legitimacy. The information saved on the blockchain is tamperproof and cannot be altered thanks to encryption and digital signatures [1].

BCT enables consensus, which is the process of reaching an agreement among all network users. Each item of data stored on a blockchain is digitally preserved and has a common history that is available to everyone on the network [2, 6]. By doing this, it is possible to avoid using a third party and prevent fraud or transaction duplication.

In simple words, a block is a group of transactions that have been rationally prepared by being grouped together. Its size varies as per the type and layout of the blockchain being employed and is made up of transactions. Unless it's a genesis block, the initial block in a blockchain that was hardcoded when the blockchain was created, the block additionally contains a reference to a preceding block [6]. Depending on the kind and architecture of a blockchain, the structure of a block may vary, but generally speaking, a few properties, including the block header, references to preceding blocks, the transaction counter, transactions, timestamp, nonce, and other properties, are crucial to a block's functionality [2]. Figure 11.1 illustrates the workings of blockchain.

11.2 PHASES OF ADVANCEMENT OF BLOCKCHAIN

An explanation of each stage in the development of blockchain is provided in the following.

 DOI: 10.1201/9781003466949-11

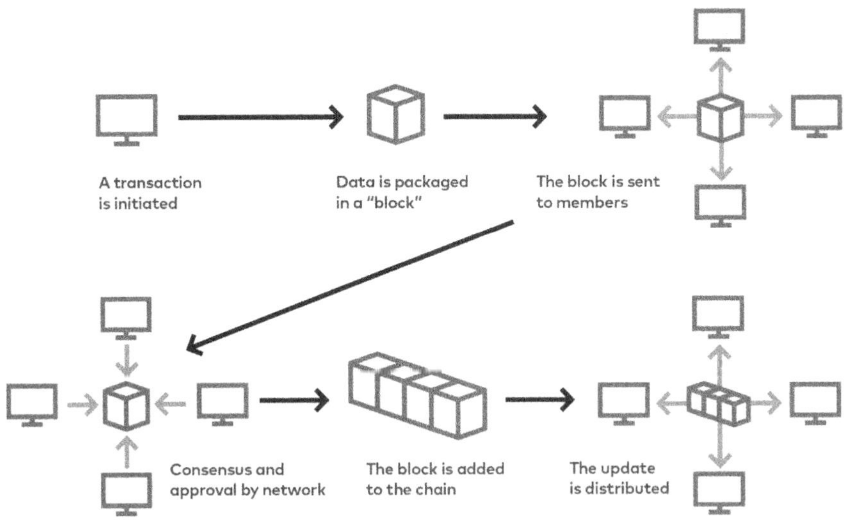

Figure 11.1 Blockchain technology

11.2.1 Phase 1

Blockchain 1.0 (Bitcoin Emergence): 2008–2013. This is the first form of blockchain that supports distributed ledger, Merkle trees, digital currency, proof of work, and blockchain data [19]. It was first presented in 2008 by Satoshi Nakamoto [2, 15, 19]. The first release is version 1.0. It is the most fundamental type and operates on a 16-bit architecture [2, 6, 19].

11.2.2 Phase 2 (Contracts)

2013–2015: Blockchain 2.0 (Ethereum Development). Phases of blockchain are depicted in Figure 11.2.

- Vitalik Buterin began creating what he believed to be an elastic blockchain that could do an array of functions in addition to operating as a peer-to-peer network, because Bitcoin had some limitations [6].
- The 2013 announcement of Ethereum, a new public blockchain with more functionality as compared to Bitcoin [23].
- Vitalik Buterin distinguished Ethereum from the Bitcoin blockchain by enabling users to record assets such as contracts and trademarks in addition to Bitcoin transactions.
- The most recent update added a foundation for creating decentralized apps, expanding Ethereum's capabilities beyond that of a currency [23].

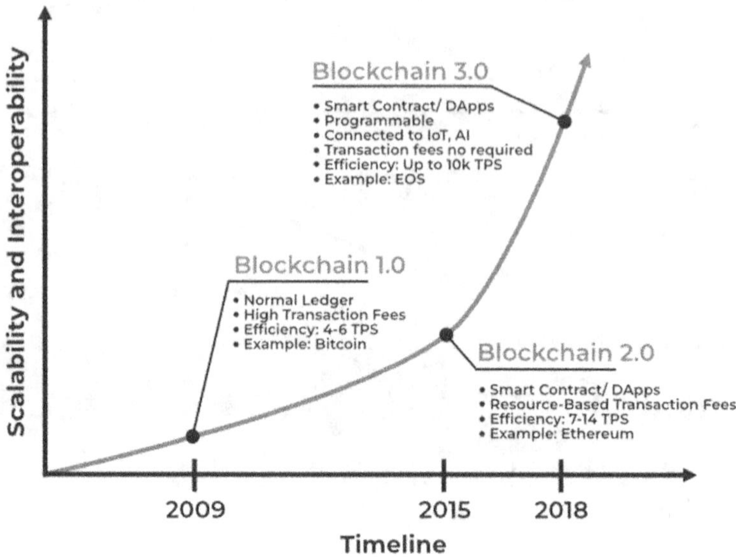

Figure 11.2 Phases of blockchain

- The Ethereum blockchain, which can handle smart contracts, is used to perform a range of activities [6].
- Ethereum BCT has proven effective in uniting a robust developer community, enabling it to create a real ecosystem.
- Most daily transactions occur on the Ethereum BCT, which can manage decentralized apps and smart contracts. The market capitalization of the Bitcoin sector has also dramatically increased [6].

2015: Hyperledger

- It is a combined effort to support the creation of dispersed ledgers [9].
- Hyperledger, led by Brain Behlendorf, aims to advance industry-wide cooperation for the advancement of BCT and distributed ledgers.
- The goal of Hyperledger is to improve the dependability and performance of modern systems to facilitate international business operations [9].

11.2.3 Phase 3 (Applications)

2016–2018: Blockchain 3.0 (dApps): Applications supported by Blockchain 3.0 are scalable, provide a positive user experience, and are interoperable [7].

- Numerous initiatives surfaced to take advantage of the possibilities of BCT.

- Several projects have aimed to fix several issues with Bitcoin and Ethereum in addition to creating novel features that use BCT.
- One of the most recent blockchain uses is NEO, which bills itself as the first open-source, decentralized, and blockchain platform to be published in China [21].
- NEO, which brands itself as the Chinese Ethereum and aims to challenge Baidu's hegemony in the nation, has already received sponsorship from Alibaba CEO Jack Ma [21].
- The cryptocurrency platform promises to offer fee-free transactions and distinctive verification procedures; therefore, it was created for the Internet of Things [7, 21].
- IOTA was urbanized as a result of developers employing BCT to speed the growth of the Internet of Things.
- The Second Generation Blockchain Platform is also creating a stir in the market [21].
- Collaborations like Microsoft appear to be moving in the right direction when considering the new blockchain applications that are being developed in the so-called private, hybrid, and federated blockchains [7].

2017: EOS.IO

- In 2017, a private corporate block published a white paper proposing a novel blockchain system that used EOS as the inhabitant token [22].
- Two examples of traits that EOS tries to imitate are the GPU and CPU. Smart contracts can be used on the decentralized operating system IO.
- Through a self-reliant decentralized organization, the main goal is to encourage the development and adoption of decentralized apps (dApps).
- dApps run their decentralized peer-to-peer networks' backend code [22, 18, 28].
- Just like a typical app, any language that can call its backend may be used to write the user interfaces and frontend blockchain example code for a dApp.

2020: The Future: Blockchain 4.0 (Industry)

Blockchain 4.0 outlines methods and answers that enable BCT to be used for commercial and industrial purposes.

- BCT's future seems bright since so many companies, governments, and other organizations are making significant investments in new innovations and applications.
- Supply management and the cloud computing industries both exist, already heavily utilizing the technology [3, 4].

- Future uses of the technology should incorporate commonplace devices like web search engines.
- According to Gartner Trend Insights, by 2022, at least one BCT-based company will allegedly have a market value of over $10 billion [5].
- According to the research firm, the blockchain digital revolution will cause business value to transcend $3.1 trillion by 2030 and surpass $176 billion by 2025 [5]. Figure 11.3 illustrates the four stages of blockchain.

11.3 BLOCKCHAIN APPLICATIONS

- **Cryptocurrency:** The most widely used use of BCT is cryptocurrency, which uses it to make money transfers secure and decentralized [2, 4, 15]. See Box 11.1.
- **Voting system:** BCT can be used to design a safe and open voting process to prevent or limit tampering and fraud [10].
- **Gaming:** Self-executing contracts, which are transparent, safe, and impenetrable, can be made using BCT [8].
- **Supply chain management:** BCT can be employed to keep track of how items travel across the supply chain and to make a clear record of every action taken [3, 4, 25].
- **Healthcare:** By improving data security, interoperability, and transparency, BCT has the potential to completely transform the healthcare sector [13]. Following are some notable applications of blockchain in healthcare:
    1. Data security and privacy: Since blockchain offers an immutable, decentralized ledger, it is suited for protecting sensitive patient data. The blockchain can be used to hold medical records, data

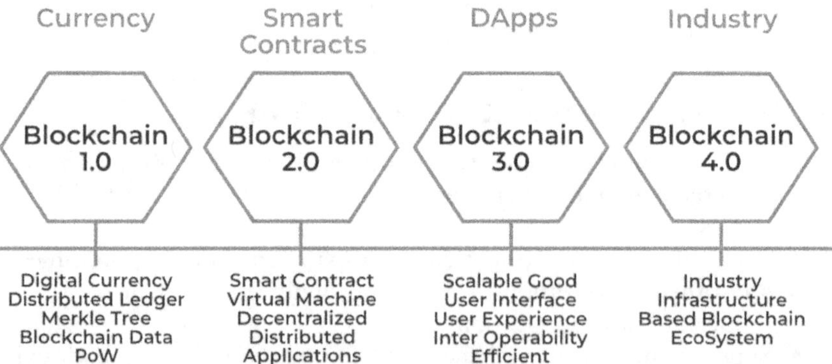

Figure 11.3 Stages of blockchain

from clinical trials, and individual patient health information, protecting privacy and limiting unauthorized access [8, 13].
2. Interoperability: Healthcare systems frequently experience interoperability problems, which make it difficult for patients' data to be shared easily between various providers and organizations [13]. BCT can make it possible for diverse healthcare systems to communicate data in a standardized and secure manner, improving care coordination and continuity [8, 28].
3. Clinical studies and medical research: By securely storing and managing trial data, patient consent, and trial results, blockchain helps streamline the management of clinical studies. Processes may be automated with the use of smart contracts, ensuring compliance and transparency while easing administrative constraints [28].
4. Drug traceability and supply chain management: Blockchain can improve pharmaceutical product traceability by keeping track of all supply chain steps, from manufacturing to distribution [13]. By doing so, the supply chain's integrity is protected and counterfeit pharmaceuticals are less likely to be distributed [25].
5. Health insurance and claims processing: By safely storing contract information, claims data, and information about policyholders, blockchain can simplify and streamline the processes involved in handling health insurance [13, 17]. Claim processing can be automated using smart contracts, which lowers processing times, administrative expenses, and fraud.

- **Smart contracts**: Using BCT, self-executing, transparent, and secure contracts may be made [23].
- **Identity verification**: By building a decentralized and secure system and removing the need for centralized authorities to manage identification information, blockchain can be utilized for identity verification [3, 4].

BOX 11.1 EVOLUTION OF CRYPTOCURRENCY

1. **Bitcoin**: Bitcoin, the first decentralized cryptocurrency, does away with middlemen thanks to its network of peers. The blockchain is a widely used public ledger where transactions for Bitcoin are recorded. In contrast to the existing limit of 21 million Bitcoin tokens in circulation [2].
2. **Litecoin**: Charlie Lee, a former Google employee, invented Litecoin in 2011. He made changes to the Bitcoin protocol that resulted in faster transaction times, lower transaction fees, and a concentration of miners [20].

3. **Ethereum**: In July 2015, Vitalik Buterin unveiled Ethereum. Ethereum is currently the second-largest cryptocurrency by market valuation, just after Bitcoin. Both Solidity, the programming language used by the blockchain network Ethereum, and Ether (ETH), the digital currency it uses, are proprietary [6].
4. **Ripple**: Ripple is a type of cryptocurrency, much like Litecoin or Bitcoin, that operates on an open-source, decentralized infrastructure that makes it simple to transfer money in any format. The currency used by Ripple, XRP, is the name of a blockchain-based protocol and digital payment network.
5. **NEO**: The Chinese-developed cryptocurrency NEO, originally known as Antshares, is actively attempting to surpass other significant competitors in the global cryptocurrency market. It is centered on smart contracts, also known as digital contracts, which enable users to create and execute contracts without the need for an intermediary.
6. **IOTA**: IOTA is an Internet of Things (IoT) application that was created in 2016. There will be 50 billions of devices online by 2025. When conducting daily transactions in an IoT context, elegant devices can exchange data along with payment information with a wide range of other devices. IOTA intends to become the standard for conducting transactions on smart devices in place of other ways.

11.4 RESULTS

- **Enhanced security**: BCT has the ability to significantly affect the way that others see your sensitive and important data. Blockchain creates an immutable, end-to-end encrypted record that stops fraud and criminal behavior. By implementing access restrictions and data anonymization on the blockchain, privacy issues can be handled [12, 26].
- **Greater transparency**: Each company would need to run its own database without blockchain. Blockchain uses a distributed ledger to ensure that information and transactions are recorded consistently worldwide [18]. This allows members to view the complete transaction history, virtually eliminating the potential for fraud.
- **Instant traceability**: Blockchain establishes an audit trail that records the origin of an object at each stage of its travel. In markets where customers are concerned about a product's impact on the environment or human rights, or in markets where there is a high incidence of fraud and counterfeiting, this helps to provide proof [14, 16].

- **Enhanced efficiency and speed:** Traditional paper-based processes require third parties to mediate and are time-consuming, prone to human error, and inefficient. Blockchain-based automation of these procedures may enable more rapid and effective transaction completion [11–14, 24, 27].
- **Automation:** With "smart contracts," transactions may also be automated, boosting your productivity and accelerating the process even further. The following step of a transaction or process is automatically initiated when prespecified requirements are satisfied [11, 23].

11.5 CHALLENGES IN MASS ADOPTION

The following list of BCT difficulties includes real-world examples:

- **Scalability:** As transaction volumes rise, scaling issues with blockchain arise. For instance, the block size and processing capacity of the Bitcoin blockchain are constrained, which causes longer transaction times and higher fees during times of heavy demand [4].
- **Energy consumption:** Some blockchain networks need a lot of processing power and energy, especially those that use proof of work consensus processes. Concerns about sustainability have been raised in light of how energy-intensive blockchains like Bitcoin affect the environment [4, 29–34].
- **Interoperability:** It can be difficult to get multiple blockchain networks to function together. For instance, maintaining data consistency and interoperability between systems or transferring assets between different blockchains can be challenging and impede seamless integration.
- **User experience:** It can be difficult for BCT to gain widespread adoption because users frequently need to manage private keys, wallets, and sophisticated procedures. For greater adoption, it is essential to enhance user experience and provide user-friendly interfaces.
- **Regulatory and legal uncertainty:** BCT frequently works in a legal and regulatory gray area. Laws differ from one jurisdiction to another, and legal systems find it difficult to keep up with the rapid innovation in the blockchain industry. Businesses and users have difficulties in terms of compliance and legal clarity as a result of this uncertainty [7, 18].
- **Security and privacy:** Although blockchain promotes transparency, protecting user privacy might be difficult. It's critical to strike a balance between openness and privacy.
- **Consensus and governance:** Managing consensus mechanisms and decision-making procedures inside blockchain networks can be difficult. It can be difficult to obtain agreement among participants with

divergent interests and to ensure that governance models are functional and meet the various needs of stakeholders [7].

- **Blockchain education and skill gap:** Due to the technology's rapid development, there is a dearth of people with knowledge of blockchain implementation, security, and development. To fully utilize blockchain, the knowledge gap must be closed and a competent workforce must be developed.
- **Legal identity and KYC/AML compliance:** For adherence to legal requirements like know your customer (KYC) and anti-money laundering (AML) laws, blockchain applications frequently require participant identity verification. It is difficult to provide secure, decentralized identity verification solutions while upholding regulatory requirements [7].
- **Resistance to change and adoption:** Traditional industries, well-established institutions, and regulatory authorities frequently oppose the introduction of BCT. It takes educating stakeholders about the advantages, resolving common misconceptions, and showcasing successful use cases to overcome skepticism and promote acceptance [35–37].

These difficulties bring to light some of the challenges that need to be resolved on a practical level for BCT to fulfill its full potential. They will need to be overcome through continued research, innovation, stakeholder cooperation, and regulatory clarity.

11.6 INTERSECTION WITH OTHER TECHNOLOGIES

The future of BCT will be greatly influenced by its intersections with other technologies. The following are some crucial areas where blockchain and other cutting-edge technology interact:

- **Artificial intelligence (AI):** When blockchain and AI are combined, it could lead to the development of useful applications. Blockchain can offer a private and transparent platform for sharing data with AI models while maintaining the integrity of the data. By analyzing massive volumes of data, automating procedures, and boosting decision-making algorithms, AI can improve blockchain systems [3, 38].
- **Internet of Things (IoT):** Blockchain can offer a safe and decentralized framework for IoT gadgets. IoT devices may securely exchange data, carry out transactions, and build trust without relying on a centralized authority by utilizing BCT. New IoT applications like supply chain management, smart cities, and autonomous vehicle networks may be made possible by this integration [39, 40].
- **Cloud computing:** Blockchain and cloud computing can work together to enhance each other. Cloud-based systems' security, privacy, and auditability can all be improved by this technology. However, to

reduce the danger of data breaches and unauthorized access, it can provide decentralized and tamper-proof records of data transfers and transactions. In contrast, cloud computing can deliver the processing strength and storage needed for blockchain networks to scale and function effectively [3, 6].

- **Big data analytics:** Blockchain can make it possible for numerous parties to share information in a secure and auditable manner, enhancing big data analytics. In data sharing networks, BCT can guarantee data integrity, privacy, and consent management. Additionally, it can make it easier to build decentralized marketplaces for data exchange where users can keep control and ownership of their data while still gaining from its value.
- **Cybersecurity:** BCT has the ability to completely change cybersecurity procedures. Blockchain's decentralized and unchangeable structure can improve data security, identity verification, and authentication processes. Blockchain-based cybersecurity solutions can provide a more robust and secure digital infrastructure by preventing data breaches, fraud, and tampering [41, 42].
- **Edge computing:** Blockchain can give edge computing networks a distributed and secure foundation, enabling reliable transactions, data exchange, and device coordination. Peer-to-peer interactions in edge computing environments can be made efficient and safe thanks to this combination.
- **Machine learning (ML):** The combination of blockchain with ML can create new opportunities across a range of industries. Ensuring data provenance, privacy, and auditability, BCT can offer ML models secure and transparent data architecture. A further way that ML algorithms can be employed to improve the effectiveness and intelligence of blockchain systems is by analyzing blockchain data, spotting trends, and making predictions [43–46].

  In addition, deep learning-based applications can be enhanced by considering the main features of deep learning and blockchain [47] as summarized in Table 11.1. Further, various merits resulting from the integration of BCT and deep learning [44] are depicted in Figure 11.4.

11.7 CONCLUSION

In conclusion, BCT is a groundbreaking invention that has the power to completely alter the way we handle data, perform transactions, and secure digital assets. It is a decentralized, open-source system that makes transactions more trustworthy by doing away with the need for middlemen. With the improvement of cryptocurrencies like Bitcoin and Ethereum, blockchain has already had a big impact on the financial industry, and it is predicted that it will have much bigger effects on other sectors.

Table 11.1 Deep Learning along with Blockchain Features That Help in Enhancing Deep Learning-Based Uses

Deep Learning	*Blockchain*	*Outcomes*
Scalable	Immutable	Flexibility in learning strategies
Data intensive	Cybersecurity	Data security can be enhanced
Layered	Transparent	Combined model update
Resource intensive	Integrity	Scalability can be enhanced

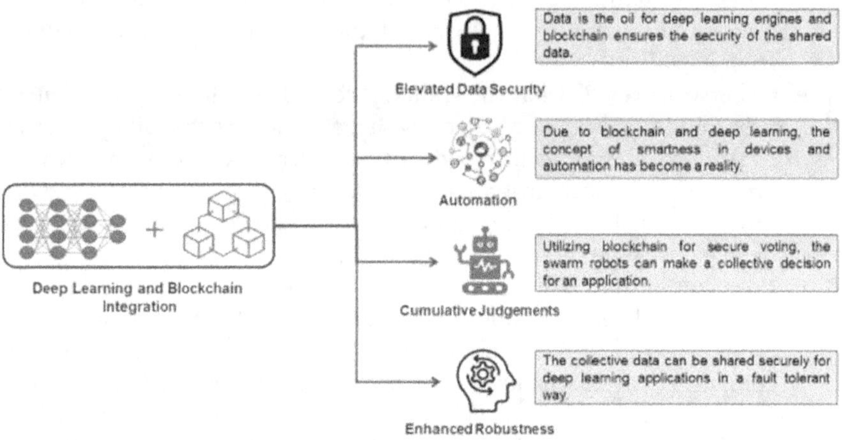

Figure 11.4 Schematics illustration of various merits resulting from the integration of blockchain and deep learning technology

Although the potential advantages of blockchain are obvious, there are still big problems that need to be solved before the technology can be fully utilized. Scalability problems, regulatory obstacles, and energy use issues are a few of these difficulties.

In general, BCT has a bright future, and as it develops further, we may anticipate even more cutting-edge use cases and applications. It will be fascinating to see how BCT evolves and what the future holds for it.

REFERENCES

1. Aster, T., Tasca, P., & Matteo, T. D. (Jan. 2017), "Blockchain technologies: The foreseeable impact on society and industry", *Computer*, 50(9), pp. 18–28.
2. Nakamoto, S. (2008). *Bitcoin: A Peer-to-Peer Electronic Cash System.* Citeseer [Online]. http://bitcoin.org/bitcoin.pdf.
3. Salah, K., Rehman, M. H. U., Nizamuddin, N., & Al-Fuqaha, A. (2019), "Blockchain for AI: Review and open research challenges", *IEEE Access*, 7, pp. 10127–10149.

4. Litke, A., Anagnostopoulos, D., & Varvarigou, T. (Jan. 2019), "Blockchains for supply chain management: Architectural elements and challenges towards a global scale deployment", *Logistics*, 3(1), p. 5.
5. "Forecast: Blockchain Business Value, Worldwide, 2017–2030", *Gartner Research*, p. 2, Mar., 2017.
6. Vitalik Buterin "Ethereum Whitepaper", published 2015 [Online]. https://ethereum.org/en/whitepaper/.
7. Peters, G., Panayi, E., & Chapelle, A. (Nov. 2015), "Trends in cryptocurrencies and blockchain technologies: A monetary theory and regulation perspective", *Journal of Financial Perspectives*, 3(3), pp. 1–25.
8. Al-Jaroodi, J., & Mohamed, N. (2019), "Blockchain in industries: A survey", *IEEE Access*, 7, pp. 36500–36515.
9. "An Introduction to Hyperledger", by Linux Foundation. https://www.hyperledger.org/wp-content/uploads/2018/07/HL_Whitepaper_IntroductiontoHyperledger.pdf.
10. Tripathi, R. C., Singh, H., & Chakravarty, A. "Smart home sensorized security system", *AIP Conference Proceedings*, 247.
11. Zheng, Z., Xie, S., Dai, H.-N., Chen, X., & Wang, H. (2016), "Blockchain challenges and opportunities: A survey", *International Journal of Web and Grid Services*, 14(4), pp. 352–375.
12. Bano, S., Al-Bassam, M., & Danezis, G. (Dec. 2017), "The road to scalable blockchain designs", *USENIX, Login, Magazine*, pp. 1–6.
13. Eklund, J. M., Mahmoud, Q. H., & Agbo, C. C. (Apr. 2019), "BCT in healthcare: A systematic review", *MDPI*, p. 4.
14. Gervais, A., Karame, G. O., Wüst, K., Glykantzis, V., Ritzdorf, H., & Capkun, S. (Oct. 2016), "On the security and performance of proof of work blockchains", in *Proceedings of ACM SIGSAC Conference on Computer and Communications Security*, pp. 3–16.
15. Rana, A., Chakraborty, C., Sharma, S., Dhawan, S., Pani, S. K., & Ashraf, I. (2022), "Internet of Medical Things-based secure and energy-efficient framework for health care", *Big Data*, 10(1), pp. 18–33.
16. Kumar, A., & Sharma, S. (2021), "Internet of robotic things: Design and develop the quality of service framework for the healthcare sector using CoAP", *IAES International Journal of Robotics and Automation*, 10(4), p. 289.
17. Dhawan, S., Chakraborty, C., Frnda, J., Gupta, R., Rana, A. K., & Pani, S. K. (2021), "SSII: Secured and high-quality steganography using intelligent hybrid optimization algorithms for IoT", *IEEE Access*, 9, pp. 87563–87578.
18. Rana, S. K., Kim, H. C., Pani, S. K., Rana, S. K., Joo, M. I., Rana, A. K., & Aich, S. (2021), "Blockchain-based model to improve the performance of the next-generation digital supply chain", *Sustainability*, 13(18), p. 10008.
19. Rana, A. K., & Sharma, S. (2021), "Internet of things based stable increased-throughput multi-hop protocol for link efficiency (IoT-SIMPLE) for health monitoring using wireless body area networks", *International Journal of Sensors, Wireless Communications and Control*, 11(7), pp. 789–798.
20. Kumar, A., Sharma, S., Goyal, N., Gupta, S. K., Kumari, S., & Kumar, S. (2022), "Energy-efficient fog computing in Internet of Things based on routing protocol for low-power and lossy network with Contiki", *International Journal of Communication Systems*, 35(4), p. e5049.

21. Pandit, M., Gupta, D., Anand, D. et al. (2022), "Towards design and feasibility analysis of DePaaS: AI based global unified software defect prediction framework", *Applied Sciences*, 12(1), p. 493.
22. Lilhore, U. K., Imoize, A. L., Lee, C. C. et al. (2022), "Enhanced convolutional neural network model for cassava leaf disease identification and classification", *Mathematics*, 10(4), p. 580.
23. Rana, S. K., Rana, S. K., Nisar, K., Ag Ibrahim, A. A., Rana, A. K., Goyal, N., & Chawla, P. (2022), "Blockchain technology and artificial intelligence based decentralized access control model to enable secure interoperability for healthcare", *Sustainability*, 14(15), p. 9471.
24. Rana, A. K., & Sharma, S. (2019), "Enhanced energy-efficient heterogeneous routing protocols in WSNs for IoT application", *IJEAT*, 9(1), pp. 4418–4415.
25. Rana, A. K., & Sharma, S. (2021), "Industry 4.0 manufacturing based on IoT, cloud computing, and big data: Manufacturing purpose scenario", in *Advances in Communication and Computational Technology*, pp. 1109–1119. Springer, Singapore.
26. Rana, A. K., Krishna, R., Dhwan, S., Sharma, S., & Gupta, R. (Oct. 2019), "Review on artificial intelligence with Internet of Things – Problems, challenges and opportunities", in 2nd International Conference on Power Energy, Environment and Intelligent Control (PEEIC), Vol. 2019, pp. 383–387. IEEE.
27. Rana, A. K., & Sharma, S., 2021, "Contiki Cooja Security Solution (CCSS) with IPv6 routing protocol for low-power and lossy networks (RPL) in Internet of Things applications", in *Mobile Radio Communications and 5G Networks*, pp. 251–259. Springer, Singapore.
28. Hussein, Z., Taher, S. W., Singh, H. K., & Swee, W. C. "Diabetes Care in Malaysia: Problems, new models and solutions", *ScienceDirect*, 81(6), pp. 851–862.
29. Kumar, S. (2022), "Influence of processing conditions on the mechanical, tribological and fatigue performance of cold spray coating: A review", *Surface Engineering*, 38(4), pp. 324–365. https://doi.org/10.1080/02670844.2022.2073424.
30. Kumar, S., & Kumar, R. (2021), "Influence of processing conditions on the properties of thermal sprayed coating: A review", *Surface Engineering*, 37(11), pp. 1339–1372. https://doi.org/10.1080/02670844.2021.1967024.
31. Kumar, S., Handa, A., Chawla, V., Grover, N. K., & Kumar, R. (2021), "Performance of thermal-sprayed coatings to combat hot corrosion of coal-fired boiler tube and effects of process parameters and post coating heat treatment on coating performance: A review", *Surface Engineering*, 37(7), pp. 833–860. https://doi.org/10.1080/02670844.2021.1924506.
32. Gupta, V., Kumar, S., Kumar, S., Kumar, R., & Kumar, R. (2020), "Biodiesel as an alternate energy resource: A study", *Asian Review of Mechanical Engineering*, 9(1), pp. 50–58. https://doi.org/10.51983/arme-2020.9.1.2470.
33. Kumar, R., Kumar, M., Chauhan, J. S., & Kumar, S. (2022), "Overview on metamaterial: History, types and applications", *Materials Today: Proceedings*, 56(5), pp. 3016–3024. https://doi.org/10.1016/j.matpr.2021.11.423.
34. Kumar, R., Kumar, M., Chohan, J. S., & Kumar, S. (2022), "Effect of process parameters on surface roughness of 316L stainless steel coated 3D printed PLA parts", *Materials Today: Proceedings*, 68(4), pp. 734–741. https://doi.org/10.1016/j.matpr.2022.06.004.

35. Jindal, H., Kumar, S., & Kumar, R. (2020), "Environmental pollution and its impact on public health: A critical review", *Asian Review of Mechanical Engineering*, 9(1), pp. 11–18.
36. Kumar, S., Kumar, M., & Handa, A. (2019), "High temperature oxidation and erosion-corrosion behaviour of wire arc sprayed Ni-Cr coating on boiler steel", *Materials Research Express*, 6(12), p. 125533. https://doi.org/10.1088/2053-1591/ab5fae.
37. Bedi, T. S., Kumar, S., & Kumar, R. (2019), "Corrosion performance of hydroxyapaite and hydroxyapaite/titania bond coating for biomedical applications", *Materials Research Express*, 7(1), p. 015402. https://doi.org/10.1088/2053-1591/ab5cc5.
38. Kumar, S., Kumar, M., & Handa, A. (2018), "Combating hot corrosion of boiler tubes – A study", *Engineering Failure Analysis*, 94, pp. 379–395. https://doi.org/10.1016/j.engfailanal.2018.08.004.
39. Jindal, H., Kumar, S., & Kumar, R. (2020), "Environmental pollution and its impact on public health: A critical review", *Asian Review of Mechanical Engineering*, 9(1), pp. 11–18.
40. Jindal, H., Kumar, D., Ishika, S.K., & Kumar, R. (2021), "role of artificial intelligence in distinct sector: A study", *Asian Journal of Computer Science and Technology*, 10(1), pp. 1–12. https://doi.org/10.51983/ajcst-2021.10.1.2696.
41. Tuli, B., Kumar, S., & Gautam, N. (2022), "An overview on cyber crime and cyber security", *Asian Journal of Engineering and Applied Technology*, 11(1), pp. 36–45. https://doi.org/10.51983/ajeat-2022.11.1.3309.
42. Sharma, M., Jindal, H., Kumar, S., & Kumar, R. (2022), "Overview of data security, classification and control measure: A study", *I-Managers, Journal on Information Technology*, 11(1), pp. 17–34. https://imanagerpublications.com/article/18557/13.
43. Jindal, H., Garg, Y., Kumar, S., Gautam, N., & Kumar, R. (2021)."Social media in political campaigning: A Study", *I-Managers Journal on Humanities & Social Sciences*, 16(1), pp. 49–60. https://imanagerpublications.com/article/18266/.
44. Shafay, M., Ahmad, R. W., Salah, K., Yaqoob, I., Jayaraman, R., & Omar, M. (2023), Blockchain for deep learning: Review and open challenges, *Cluster Computing*, 26(1), pp. 197–221. https://doi.org/10.1007/s10586-022-03582-7.
45. Thillaiarasu, N., Lata Tripathi, S., & Dhinakaran, V. (Eds.). (2022). *Artificial Intelligence for Internet of Things: Design Principle, Modernization, and Techniques* (1st ed.). CRC Press, Boca Raton, UK. https://doi.org/10.1201/9781003335801.
46. Kumar, K., Chaudhury, K., & Tripathi, S. L. (2023), "Future of Machine Learning (ML) and Deep Learning (DL) in healthcare monitoring system", in *Machine Learning Algorithms for Signal and Image Processing*, pp. 293–313. IEEE. https://doi.org/10.1002/9781119861850.ch17.
47. Hassan, T., Hassan, B., Akram, M. U., Hashmi, S., Taguri, A. H., & Werghi, N. (2021), "Incremental cross-domain adaptation for robust retinopathy screening via Bayesian deep learning", *IEEE Transactions on Instrumentation and Measurement*, 70, pp. 1–14.

Chapter 12

COVID-19 Detection and Pandemic Prevention System Using Data Science

Abhimanyu Singh Negi, Prakhar Gupta, Rashi Srivastava, and Arun Kumar Rana

12.1 INTRODUCTION

The coronavirus disease of 2019 (COVID-19) had such a profound effect on the entire planet and slowed normal actions of humans in such a rare fashion that it will leave an enduring mark on history. Places worldwide adopted severe measures to combat the life-threatening sickness. The pandemic's contagious nature put conventional medical models of care to the test. Hence, machine learning (ML) and artificial intelligence (AI) present new channels for efficient treatment throughout the pandemic. Designing effective diagnosis procedures and creating disease spread projections are all tasks that AI and ML can help with [1]. These applications rely heavily on real-time patient monitoring and efficient information coordination, where the Internet of Things (IoT) plays a crucial role. Applications like automated drug distribution, answering patient questions, and tracing the origins of disease can all benefit from IoT. The potential use of AI, ML, and IoT technologies in the fight against the COVID-19 pandemic has been thoroughly examined in this research. A thorough overview of the enabling tools and methodologies is given together with an explanation of the current and future applications of AI, ML, and IoT. There is also a critical examination of the dangers and restrictions of the technologies. The COVID-19 pandemic has brought unprecedented challenges to public health, economies, and society as a whole. Effective detection and prediction of COVID-19 cases are crucial in mitigating the spread of the virus and reducing its impact. In recent years, advances in data science and AI have shown great promise in developing systems that can analyze vast amounts of data to identify patterns, predict outcomes, and provide valuable insights.

In this study, we present a comprehensive analysis of the COVID-19 pandemic and propose an early test prediction system using AI and data science. The study aims to provide insights into the patterns and trends of the pandemic, as well as to develop a system that can predict COVID-19 cases at an early stage. The analysis is based on various data sources, including daily case counts, hospitalization rates, mortality rates, and intervention strategies implemented by governments and public health authorities. The study

 DOI: 10.1201/9781003466949-12

also examines the impact of socioeconomic factors, such as income and education, on the spread of the virus. Future research may consider national-level integration of the project and keeping records for future pandemics and widespread diseases by modifying the model. The COVID-19 pandemic is currently affecting countries around the world, making the need for affordable solutions to tackle the pandemic urgent. IoT is a network of mechanical and digitally connected objects that may transmit data over a predetermined network. IoT is a cutting-edge technology that makes it possible for gadgets to link to networks in hospitals and other key locations to improve the fight against COVID-19. To battle the COVID-19 epidemic, this study analyzes and highlights the uses of IoT by providing a perspective roadmap. The use of IoT will assist patients, doctors, healthcare professionals, and hospital management systems in recognizing the signs of infectious disease and managing COVID-19 infections around the world [2, 3].

12.2 LITERATURE SURVEY

The COVID-19 coronavirus outbreak appears to be uncontrollable. As of March 1, 2020, the virus had already infected more than 558,502 individuals worldwide and caused at least 25,251 fatalities [1]. An unknown-cause pneumonia outbreak connected to the Huanan Seafood Market began in Wuhan, China. The genus of the virus beta coronavirus has connections to the viruses that cause severe acute respiratory syndrome (SARS) and Middle Eastern respiratory syndrome (MERS) [3, 4]. Although numerous instances of pneumonia with an unclear origin were found much earlier (December 8, 2019), the World Health Organization (WHO) was first notified on December 31 [5].

The unchecked spread of the disease was facilitated by the tardy declaration of the epidemic and the neglect to promptly notify foreign authorities. The world is currently paying close attention to this outbreak. China extended a lockdown of Wuhan to cover 20 cities and 56 million people to slow the spread of the virus. The viability of this attempt was first questioned by experts, who also cautioned that a repeat of the SARS pandemic posed a threat to the nation [6]. Although much of China has the pandemic under control, criticism of the use of what some have dubbed "draconian" methods to curb its spread endures. The 2019 novel coronavirus epidemic has been given the COVID-19 designation by the WHO. Numerous nations throughout the world are now vulnerable as a result of this extraordinary epidemic. The repercussions of the COVID-19 outbreaks, which were hitherto only experienced by citizens of China, are now causing grave worry for practically all countries around the globe [7, 8, 9].

Due to a shortage of funding to tackle the COVID-19 outbreak and worries about overburdened healthcare systems, the majority of countries are now on partial or complete lockdown. As of April 30, 2020, there have been more than 3 million laboratory-confirmed coronavirus infections recorded, a worrying rise in incidence globally. Numerous fake claims, faulty informational pieces, and unfounded worries about coronavirus have been generated since the COVID-19 epidemic, only making the situation worse. In response to such activities, we provide a comprehensive summary of all the crucial aspects of the COVID-19 pandemic, based on a wide range of reliable sources. This chapter highlights the COVID-19 outbreak's effects on both the global economy and acute health outcomes [10]. We consider how the COVID-19 outbreak might be impacted by technologies such as the Internet of IoT, unmanned aerial vehicles, blockchain, AI, and 5G [11].

12.3 FRAMEWORK

Since this research will include healthcare records and medical jargon, proper consultation with medical professionals will be needed at each step with more of the test-based approach. Incorporating machine learning and IoT makes the model more experience-based. Hence the database will be made for increasing the efficiency of the system [12].

The system will be developed with each phase incorporating some features and testing with real-time scenarios. The study design of the project will be experiment-based as the work in this domain is limited to analysis of the results of each phase. This project has been extensively focused on identifying the diseases more accurately from the symptoms and making the machine learning model more accurate with emphasis on sample collection and increasing the diversity of data. The proposed framework is shown in Figure 12.1.

12.3.1 Variables

Some key variables that will be incorporated during the project are:

1. Age
2. O_2 levels
3. Medical records
4. Temperature
5. Chronic diseases

More variables and parameters can be added in the upcoming phases of development and research [11].

12.3.2 Controls

Controls incorporated during this project are controlling the error-to-accuracy ratio, controlling the machine learning algorithm, and removing

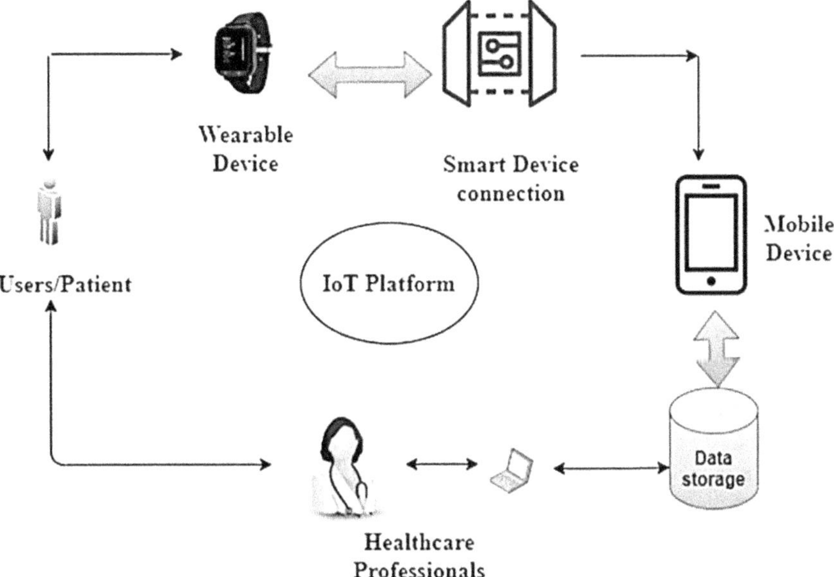

Figure 12.1 Proposed framework

instances of false positives and false negatives by ensuring the proper verification of the test results.

12.3.3 Study Method

The study methods include reading previous research work related to this field and learning about the symptoms of diseases and how disease is spread over a region. Various technologies and methods of data collection that can be used in the project will also studied [6, 13].

12.3.4 Data Collection

Data collection will be done via devices with sensors to measure O_2 levels and body temperature as well as including an assessment of a patient's medical records. Data will then be analyzed and verified for accuracy.

12.3.5 Ethical Clearance

Ethical clearance is the key in this project, as the project works on collecting the sensitive healthcare information of the public, which can be a major concern for security and privacy. In India, this can be solved by getting clearance from the Ministry of Ayush and ensuring the implementation of proper data security protocols. In the context of designing a system related to COVID-19, ethical clearance is crucial to ensure that the system is designed with the highest level of ethical considerations in mind. This includes ensuring that the system is designed in a way that respects individual's privacy rights and does not discriminate against any particular group.

When collecting data for the system, obtaining participants' informed permission and making sure they comprehend the project's goals are crucial in data collection and how it will be used. Additionally, measures must be taken to protect the confidentiality and privacy of the data collected, including appropriate data security measures. Another important ethical consideration is ensuring that the system's design does not perpetuate existing biases or discriminate against any particular group. This can be achieved by ensuring the system was developed using training data that is representative of the community and is varied, and by regularly monitoring the system's performance for any signs of bias or discrimination. Overall, obtaining ethical clearance for a system design related to COVID-19 is essential to ensure that the system is designed in a way that is ethical, respects individual's rights and privacy, and does not perpetuate any existing biases or discrimination.

12.3.6 Algorithm

Density-based spatial clustering of applications with noise (DBSCAN)

Input: CSV file data

Output: Possible positive results

Unsupervised learning uses the data clustering technique density-based spatial clustering of applications with noise (DBSCAN). It is based on the ideas of density-reachability and density-connectivity, which aid in locating groups of points in a dataset that are spaced apart by a specific amount. It is an iterative technique that searches for density-connected locations within a specified radius after beginning at any starting point. A point is included in a cluster of points if it is densely related to another point or points. Until all points have been taken into account, the algorithm searches for points that are densely linked to the cluster. It can locate outliers in datasets and is appropriate for datasets with different densities [14].

The DBSCAN algorithm is a widely used data and machine learning clustering algorithm due to its ability to identify clusters of points in a dataset that have varying densities. It is an unsupervised learning algorithm, meaning it does not require labeled data to operate, and is useful in exploring and analyzing datasets that have no prior knowledge about their internal structure. For the method to function, the dataset must contain core, boundary, and noise points. The epsilon neighborhood, or core points, are points with at least a defined minimum number of other points within a specific radius. Border points are those that are density-reachable from a core point but have fewer points within the epsilon neighborhood than the minimal number. Non-core and non-density-reachable noise points can't be reached from a core point.

DBSCAN iteratively builds clusters by identifying core points and adding them to a cluster along with all their density-reachable neighbors. The algorithm continues to expand the cluster until there are no more density-reachable points. The algorithm then proceeds to identify another core point and repeats the process, building another cluster. The process continues until all the points in the dataset are assigned to a cluster. One of the significant advantages of DBSCAN is its ability to identify outliers or noise points in the dataset. Outliers are points that do not belong to any cluster, and they can be identified as noise points by the algorithm. This ability to identify outliers makes it useful in anomaly detection and fraud detection applications. DBSCAN is also well-suited for datasets with varying densities, as it can identify clusters of different sizes and shapes. However, the selection of parameters, such as the size of the epsilon neighborhood and the bare minimum of points needed to designate a core point, might have an impact on the method. Therefore, careful parameter tuning is required to ensure the optimal performance of the algorithm.

One of the advantages of the DBSCAN algorithm is its ability to handle noise and outliers effectively. Noise points can cause problems for many clustering algorithms, as they may be mistakenly assigned to a cluster, leading to inaccurate results. DBSCAN's ability to identify noise points as separate from clusters allows for more accurate clustering results. DBSCAN is also capable of identifying clusters of different shapes and sizes, such as elongated or irregularly shaped clusters. This is because the algorithm uses densities-reachability and densities-connectivity to determine which points belong to a cluster, rather than relying on the assumption of Euclidean distance between points.

DBSCAN and k-means are two popular clustering algorithms, as shown in Figure 12.2. DBSCAN is especially useful for finding clusters of varying densities in a dataset. It uses a core distance metric to identify clusters in the data. In contrast, k-means is a centroid-based clustering algorithm that finds clusters based on their proximity to a predetermined number of centroids. k-Means is better suited for finding clusters of uniform density. Both algorithms are useful for different types of data and applications, so it is important to choose the right algorithm for your use case. DBSCAN is distinct from other clustering algorithms in that it does not require the user to specify the number of clusters to generate. It also allows for clusters of varying densities and can identify noise and outliers. In contrast, other clustering algorithms such as k-means and hierarchical clustering require the user to specify the number of clusters they want to generate and are unable to identify noise and outliers. Additionally, these algorithms cannot handle clusters of varying densities [15, 16, 17].

12.3.7 Functional Specification of System

The COVID-19 detection and pandemic prevention system is a web-based system that aims to detect suspicious phrases related to COVID-19 in

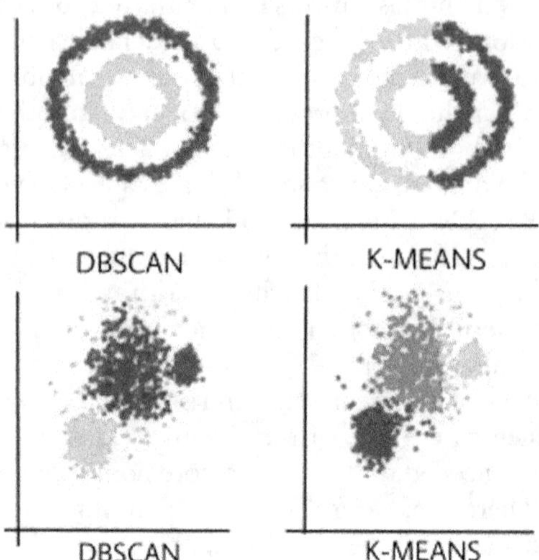

Figure 12.2 DBSCAN versus k-means

real-time instant messaging chats. The system uses OBIE (ontology-based information extraction) and association rule mining to monitor chat sessions and identify suspicious phrases. The system also includes a messaging server; a directory server; and a database to store chat data, code words, ontology information, and short words. The following subsystems make up the COVID-19 detection and pandemic prevention system:

- *Clients and web browser instant messaging system.* The directory server is used to authenticate clients and store their identities, as shown in Figure 12.3. When the chatter starts the next talking session via SMTP, the online messages are transmitted to the messaging server. Suspicious phrases extracted from instant chats sent between chatters using predefined database criteria.
- *Active chat monitoring and suspicious chat detection systems* use OBIE (ontology-based information extraction) and CBA (classification-based association) rules to monitor the system.
- *Information database.* This subsystem includes a message database, code word database, ontology database, and short word database. The message database stores chat data, the code word database stores COVID-19–related keywords, the ontology database stores domain-specific knowledge, and the short word database stores abbreviated words or phrases.
- *System features.* The COVID-19 detection and pandemic prevention system has the following features:
- *Real-time chat monitoring.* The system continuously monitors chat sessions in real-time to detect suspicious phrases related to COVID-19.

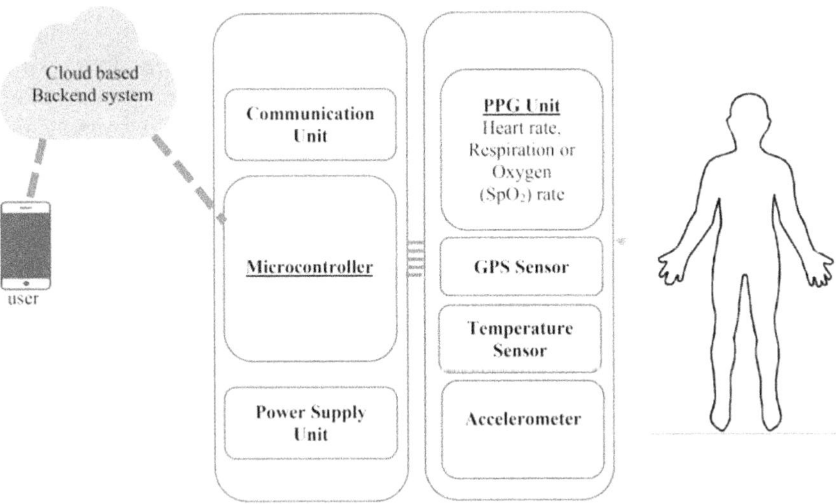

Figure 12.3 Functional specification of system

- *Suspicious phrase detection.* The system uses OBIE and association rule mining to identify suspicious phrases related to COVID-19.
- *User authentication.* The system uses a directory server to authenticate users and ensure secure access to the chat system.
- *Database storage.* The system stores chat data, code words, ontology information, and short words in respective databases for efficient and easy access.
- *Automatic alerting.* The system sends automatic alerts to the designated authorities in case of the detection of any suspicious phrases.

12.4 LIMITATIONS

12.4.1 Model Cannot Be 100% Accurate So It Will Never Replace Medical Testing

It's crucial to remember that while machine learning models have demonstrated great performance in forecasting COVID-19 risk, they are not perfect and cannot take the place of medical diagnostics. There is always a chance that the training data may contain bias or errors, and machine learning models are only as accurate as the data they are trained on. Additionally, rather than relying on specific diagnostic standards, machine learning models are created to generate predictions based on patterns and correlations in the data. As a result, even while a machine learning model may be able to identify those who are more likely to have an illness, it cannot diagnose COVID-19 or provide definitive medical advice. As such, machine learning should be viewed as a complementary tool to traditional medical testing rather than a replacement [18–23]. When used in conjunction with medical tests and clinical expertise, machine learning models can provide valuable insights into COVID-19 risk and help inform public health interventions. However, we must continue to prioritize rigorous testing and accurate diagnosis to ensure the safety and well-being of patients.

12.4.2 Users Must Use Provided Chat Application

Requiring users to use a specific chat application poses both privacy and operational limitations. From a privacy perspective, users may be uncomfortable with sharing personal information through a third-party application, particularly if they are not familiar with the provider's privacy policies or data management practices. This can be particularly concerning if the chat application is hosted on a third-party server, as this raises questions about who has access to user data and how it is being used. Additionally, users may be hesitant to use a chat application that is not compliant with industry-standard privacy regulations or that does not provide end-to-end encryption to protect sensitive information.

From an operational standpoint, mandating the use of a specific chat application can also be limiting. Users may prefer to use another messaging application and requiring them to switch to a different platform can create confusion and extra work. Additionally, users may be reluctant to use a chat application that is not integrated with their existing workflow or that does not support the features they need. This can lead to reduced productivity and frustration among team members [24–27].

Considering these privacy and operational limitations, it is important to carefully consider the decision to mandate the use of a specific chat application. While there may be valid reasons for doing so, such as security concerns or the need for standardized communication channels, it is essential to ensure that users are fully informed about the privacy implications and that the chosen application meets their operational needs. By balancing these considerations and working closely with users, organizations can implement chat applications that are both effective and respectful of users' privacy and preferences.

Furthermore, the implementation of such a system may require significant financial resources, including the cost of data collection, infrastructure, and maintenance. It may also raise privacy concerns, as sensitive health information is being collected and analyzed.

Despite these limitations, the COVID-19 detection and pandemic prevention system using data science has the potential to be a valuable tool in the fight against the pandemic. It can provide early detection of COVID-19 cases, identify hotspots, and enable prompt response and intervention. Therefore, efforts must be made to address these limitations and ensure the ethical implementation of such a system.

12.4.3 Limitations of Machine Learning Algorithms

Although the proposed system's machine learning algorithms have shown good accuracy rates, they might not be able to take into account all the variables that affect the probability of COVID-19 transmission. For example, the system does not take into account the air circulation or ventilation in a given area, which can also affect the spread of the virus.

12.4.4 Need for Human Intervention

While the proposed system is designed to automate the monitoring and tracking of COVID-19 risk in public areas, it still requires human intervention to interpret the data and make decisions about risk. This can be a time-consuming and labor-intensive process, particularly in areas with large crowds or high levels of foot traffic.

12.4.5 Lack of Generalizability

The suggested system was created and examined using a specific dataset and may not be generalizable to other regions or populations. The system's accuracy may also be affected by factors such as cultural norms, socioeconomic status, or public health policies, which can vary widely between different areas or populations. The limitations of the proposed system highlight the importance of considering contextual factors when developing and testing machine learning models. While the system may perform well on the specific dataset it was trained on, its accuracy and generalizability may be affected by a range of contextual factors that are unique to different regions or populations. For example, cultural norms concerning healthcare-seeking behavior may differ among populations, which could affect the accuracy of the system's predictions. Similarly, socioeconomic status can impact access to healthcare and the prevalence of underlying health issues that may influence COVID-19 risk infection and transmission. Public health policies and interventions can also vary widely between regions, which can affect the trajectory of the pandemic and the efficacy of different strategies.

To address these limitations, it is crucial to collect and analyze data from diverse populations and contexts, and to carefully consider the factors that may influence the accuracy and generalizability of machine learning models. This can include factors such as demographics, health outcomes, healthcare utilization, and cultural and social determinants of health. By taking a holistic approach to data collection and analysis, we can develop more accurate and effective machine learning models that are sensitive to the unique needs and characteristics of different populations. Additionally, it is important to continually monitor and evaluate the performance of machine learning models in real-world contexts, and to adapt and refine them as necessary to ensure their ongoing accuracy and usefulness.

It is important to keep these limitations in mind when considering the potential benefits and drawbacks of the proposed system, and to continue exploring new methods and technologies for monitoring and tracking COVID-19 risk in public areas [28–31].

12.5 CONCLUSIONS

The COVID-19 pandemic has affected almost every aspect of life and has caused a significant impact on public health and the global economy. To mitigate the spread of the virus, it is crucial to develop effective strategies for monitoring and predicting the risk of COVID-19 in public areas. This study proposes a novel approach that utilizes machine learning algorithms to analyze temperature, physical separation, and mask usage to assess the risk of COVID-19 in public areas. The results are highly promising, with various machine learning algorithms achieving high accuracy rates. Future work can incorporate additional machine learning methods, such as deep learning strategies, to further enhance the model's accuracy. Furthermore, the proposed system's ability to collect and analyze real-time data can be crucial in mitigating the spread of COVID-19. The insights gained from this study can help policymakers make informed decisions about implementing preventive measures to limit the virus's transmission. In addition, researchers have developed a deep learning framework that incorporates a top-tier activation function for M-LSTM and a set of deep reinforcement learning guidelines to optimize prediction outcomes. This deep learning approach demonstrated remarkable accuracy in forecasting COVID-19 cases and has the potential to transform the way we manage pandemics in the future. Future work in this area can focus on developing a semi-supervised hybrid scheme that can identify COVID-19 suspects and monitor social media sites to stop further spread.

In conclusion, the ongoing COVID-19 pandemic has highlighted the urgent need for innovative and effective approaches to tracking and mitigating the virus's spread. Through the use of machine learning algorithms, IoT sensors, and other emerging technologies, researchers and policymakers have a powerful set of tools at their disposal for understanding and combating the virus. By continuing to explore new approaches and technologies, we can hope to develop even more effective strategies for managing pandemics in the future, and ultimately safeguard public health and well-being.

REFERENCES

1. Wang, P. W., Horby, F. G., Hayden, G. F., & Gao, G. F. (2020). GaoA novel coronavirus outbreak of global health concern. *Lancet*, 395(10223), 470–473 [PMC Free article] [PubMed] [Google Scholar].
2. Tuli, S., Tuli, S., Wander, G., Wander, P., Gill, S. S., Dustdar, S., Sakellariou, R., & Rana, O. Next generation technologies for smart healthcare: Challenges, vision, model, trends and future directions. *Internet Technology Letters*, e145.

3. Sharma, A., Tiwari, S., Deb, M. K., & Marty, J. L. (2020). "Severe acute respiratory syndrome coronavirus-2 (SARS-CoV-2): A global pandemic and treatment strategies." *International journal of antimicrobial agents*, 56(2), 106054.
4. Jang, J., & Jiang, H. (2019). "DBSCAN++: Towards fast and scalable density clustering." In *International conference on machine learning*, pp. 3019–3029. PMLR.
5. Mojjada, R. K., Yadav, A., Prabhu, A. V., & Natarajan, Y. (2020). Machine learning models for Covid, 19 future forecasting. *Materials Today: Proceedings* 81: 597–601.
6. Lal, S., & Singh, V. Techniques to enhance the performance of DBSCAN clustering algorithm in data mining. In 2017 International Conference on Energy, Communication, Data Analytics and Soft Computing (ICECDS) (pp. 1559–1564). IEEE.
7. Manchanda, N. (2014). Nursing officer (BL Kapoor Max) reg. Delhi Nursing Council DNC (Covid, 19 and how to detect it in preliminary stages). New York: Guttmacher Institute, 12–14.
8. Villa, S., Lombardi, A., Mangioni, D., Bozzi, G., Bandera, A., Gori, A., & Raviglione, M. C. (2020). "The COVID-19 pandemic preparedness ... or lack thereof: from China to Italy." *Global Health & Medicine*, 2(2), 73–77.
9. Abir, S. A. A., Islam, S. N., Anwar, A., Mahmood, A. N., & Oo, A. M. T. (2020). Building resilience against COVID-19 pandemic using artificial intelligence, machine learning, and IoT: A survey of recent progress. *IoT*, 1(2), 506.
10. Chakraborty, S., & Nagwani, N. K. (2014). "Analysis and study of incremental DBSCAN clustering algorithm." *International Journal of Enterprise Computing and Business Systems*, 1. arXiv preprint arXiv:1406.4754
11. Drewry, A. M., Hotchkiss, R., & Kulstad, E. (2020). Response to "Body temperature correlates with mortality in COVID-19 patients." *Critical care*, 24, 1–3.
12. Alballa, N., & Al-Turaiki, I. (2021). Machine learning approaches in COVID-19 diagnosis, mortality, and severity risk prediction: A review. *Informatics in medicine unlocked*, 24, 100564.
13. Zhang, Y., Jiang, B., & Yuan, J., & Tao, Y. (2020). The impact of social distancing and epicenter lockdown on the COVID-19 epidemic in mainland China: A data-driven SEIQR model study. *MedRxiv.*
14. Siddiqui, M. K., Menendez, R. M., Gupta, P. K., Hussain, F., Khatoon, K., & Ahmad, S. Correlation between temperature and COVID-19 (suspected, confirmed and death) cases based on machine learning analysis.
15. Tuli, S., Tuli, S., Wander, G., Wander, P., Gill, S. S., Dustdar, S., Sakellariou, R., & Rana, O. (2020). "Next generation technologies for smart healthcare: challenges, vision, model, trends and future directions." *Internet technology letters*, 3(2), e145.
16. Zhang, Y. DBSCAN clustering algorithm based on big data is applied in network information security detection. Department of Information Engineering, Shijiazhuang University of Applied Technology, Shijiazhuang 050081, Hebei, China.
17. A technical survey on DBSCAN clustering algorithm Nidhi Suthar (Department of Compute Engineering, Hashmukh Goswami Collage of Engineering, Vahelal, Gujarat.nidhisuthar2610@gmail.com), Prof. Indr Jeet Rajput (Head of Department of Compute Engineering, Hashmukh Goswami Collage of Engineering, Vahelal, Gujarat.), Prof. Vinit Kumar Gupta (Department of Compute Engineering, Hashmukh Goswami Collage of Engineering, Vahelal, Gujarat).

18. Rana, S. K., Kim, H. C., Pani, S. K., Rana, S. K., Joo, M. I., Rana, A. K., & Aich, S. (2021). Blockchain-based model to improve the performance of the next-generation digital supply chain. *Sustainability*, 13(18), 10008.
19. Rana, A. K., & Sharma, S. (2021). Internet of things based stable increased-throughput multi-hop protocol for link efficiency (IoT-SIMPLE) for health monitoring using wireless body area networks. *International Journal of Sensors, Wireless Communications and Control*, 11(7), 789–798.
20. Kumar, A., Sharma, S., Goyal, N., Gupta, S. K., Kumari, S., & Kumar, S. (2022). Energy-efficient fog computing in internet of things based on routing protocol for low-power and lossy network with Contiki. *International Journal of Communication Systems*, 35(4), e5049.
21. Pandit, M., Gupta, D., Anand, D., Goyal, N., Aljahdali, H. M., Mansilla, A. O., ... Kumar, A. (2022). Towards design and feasibility analysis of DePaaS: AI based global unified software defect prediction framework. *Applied Sciences*, 12(1), 493.
22. Lilhore, U. K., Imoize, A. L., Lee, C. C., Simaiya, S., Pani, S. K., Goyal, N., ... Li, C. T. (2022). Enhanced convolutional neural network model for cassava leaf disease identification and classification. *Mathematics*, 10(4), 580.
23. Rana, S. K., Rana, S. K., Nisar, K., Ag Ibrahim, A. A., Rana, A. K., Goyal, N., & Chawla, P. (2022). Blockchain technology and artificial intelligence based decentralized access control model to enable secure interoperability for healthcare. *Sustainability*, 14(15), 9471.
24. Rana, A. K., & Sharma, S. (2019). Enhanced energy-efficient heterogeneous routing protocols in WSNs for IoT application. *IJEAT*, 9(1), 4418–4415.
25. Rana, A. K., & Sharma, S. (2021). Industry 4.0 manufacturing based on IoT, cloud computing, and big data: Manufacturing purpose scenario. In *Advances in Communication and Computational Technology* (pp. 1109–1119). Springer, Singapore.
26. Rana, A. K., Krishna, R., Dhwan, S., Sharma, S., & Gupta, R. (2019, October). Review on artificial intelligence with internet of things-problems, challenges and opportunities. In 2019 2nd International Conference on Power Energy, Environment and Intelligent Control (PEEIC) (pp. 383–387). IEEE.
27. Rana, A. K., & Sharma, S. (2021). Contiki Cooja Security Solution (CCSS) with IPv6 routing protocol for low-power and lossy networks (RPL) in internet of things applications. In *Mobile Radio Communications and 5G Networks* (pp. 251–259). Springer, Singapore.
28. Yousefzadeh, M., Emrouznejad, A., Saati, S., & Tavana, M. (2020). Machine learning approaches for prediction of COVID-19: A review and appraisal. *Expert Systems with Applications*, 164, 113705.
29. Ayyoubzadeh, S. M., Zahedi, H., Ahmadi, M., & Kalhori, S. R. N. (2020). Predicting COVID-19 incidence through analysis of Google Trends data in Iran: Data mining and deep learning pilot study. *JMIR Public Health and Surveillance*, 6(2), e18828.
30. Lata Tripathi, S., Dhir, K., Ghai, D., & Patil, S. (Eds.) (2021). *Health Informatics and Technological Solutions for Coronavirus (COVID-19)* (1st ed.). CRC Press. https://doi.org/10.1201/9781003161066.
31. Tripathi, S. L., Mendiratta, N., Ghai, D., Avasthi, S., & Dhir, K. (2022). Coronavirus: Diagnosis, detection and analysis. In *Biomedical Engineering Applications for People with Disabilities and Elderly in a New COVID-19 Pandemic and Beyond* (pp.109–117). Elsevier, USA.

Chapter 13

Use of Machine Learning and IoT in Smart Farming

The Future of Agriculture

Tanushree Sanwal, Sandhya Avasthi, Meenakshi Tyagi, Ankita Sharma, Sapna Yadav, and Suman Lata Tripathi

13.1 INTRODUCTION

The agriculture sector is undergoing a major shift due to potential growth in the market and the use of the latest information technology tools. Much research is going on in agriculture, machine learning (ML), Internet of Things (IoT) for optimizing smart farming, and rationalization of the use of natural resources and good sustainable practices. With the growth in IoT-based applications and data analysis, agro-industrial and smart farming systems are largely altered, and using these information technology tools to optimize resources in the agriculture sector is taking place (Figure 13.1).

This chapter also discusses the IoT-based solutions that are used in agriculture to monitor soil condition and soil moisture. The ML model provides the most accurate prediction for the optimal fertilizer application for a crop. Drones are used for monitoring fields and crops, spraying pesticides, and drip irrigation, which is another beneficial IoT-based application. The chapter discusses drones that employ an AI-powered water irrigation method that is trained on weather patterns and reduces water waste in trickle irrigation. Further, the chapter also discusses the harvesting of crops with AI-enabled robotics and the use of IoT-based sensors for livestock management.

13.1.1 Machine Learning and Its Use in Agriculture

The number of people in this world will increase to approximately 10 billion by the end of the year 2050, so the demand for food will increase. However, due to urbanization, available resources for agriculture are diminishing. Agriculture is confronted with many challenges, including rising food consumption due to global population growth, climate change [1, 2], natural resource diminution [2, 3], changing dietary predilections [3, 4], and safety and well-being issues [5, 6]. There is a crucial need to increase agricultural efficiency while reducing environmental impact to address the challenges, which put pressure on the agricultural sector. These two factors have augmented agriculture's shift to precision agriculture. This modernization of

DOI: 10.1201/9781003466949-13

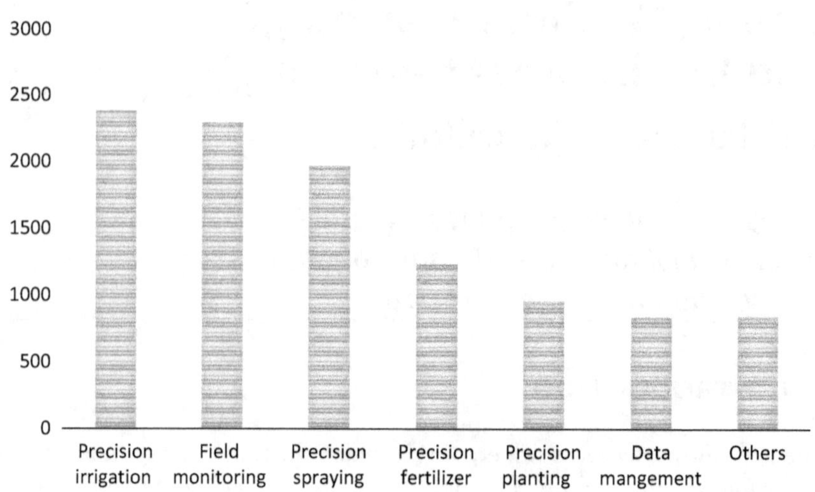

Figure 13.1 Growth market for various applications in smart farming

agriculture has the potential to significantly improve sustainability, productivity, and environmental health [5]. To meet increasing demand, smart farming is built on four key pillars: (a) natural resource management, (b) efficient use of natural resources, (c) application of modern technologies, and (d) expansion of suitable services [6]. The most populated country will be India by the year 2050, and the country is already falling short of meeting its current demand for food.

The adoption of information and communications technology (ICT) is an unavoidable requirement of modern agriculture, as urged by governments all over the world. Farm management information systems, wireless sensor networks, cameras, drones, humidity and soil sensors, low-cost satellites, accelerometers, internet services, and automated guided vehicles are examples of information technology [7].

Additionally, enormous storage space is required for editing, analyzing, and interpreting the massive amounts of data generated by digital technologies, which is frequently referred to as "big data." The latter has the potential to have a sizable positive impact on society, the environment, and policymakers [8]. On the other hand, big data presents challenges as a result of the "5 Vs": (a) value, (b) variety, (c) veracity, (d) velocity, and (e) volume [9]. Outdated data dispensation methods are not able to keep up with the ever-increasing needs of smart farming, posing a barrier to extracting needful information from field data [10]. Machine learning, a subset of AI, was developed to accomplish this goal as a consequence of the exponential progress in processing power capacity [11].

Agriculture has numerous applications for ML. A recent review of the literature from 2004 to 2018 revealed four distinct categories, according to

Liakos et al. [12] (Figure 13.2): crop, water, soil, and livestock/animal management. Crop management articles accounted for the majority of articles (61% of total articles) and were further classified as follows:

- Crop quality
- Prediction of yield
- Disease identification
- Detection of weeds
- Crop identification

13.1.2 Agriculture Machine Learning Problems That Haven't Been Solved

This academic subject has been subjected to numerous evaluations because of the breadth of ML applications in agriculture. Detection of crop disease [13–16], detection of weeds [17, 18], prediction of yield [19, 20], crop recognition [21, 22], water management [23, 24], animal welfare [25, 26], and livestock production [27, 28] have been the primary topics of these studies. Another study looked at the practice of machine learning technologies in major grain harvests, examining a variety of factors such as quality and disease detection [29]. Finally, large-scale data analysis using machine learning has gained popularity in identifying real-world challenges related to modern farming [30] or methods for analyzing data [31].

Even though machine learning has made tremendous progress in agriculture, certain points remain unresolved. The primary barriers to sensor deployment on farms are high ICT costs, old practices, and a deficiency of information [23, 24, 28, 32]. Additionally, the existing datasets do not replicate accurate conditions, as they are generated by individuals collecting specimens over a short time span and from a small area [15, 21–23].

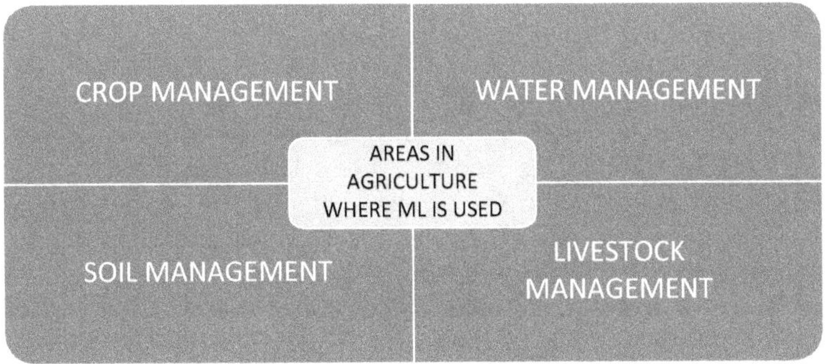

Figure 13.2 Four groups in agriculture that are used by machine learning algorithms, as mentioned by Liakos et al. [12]

Thus, a higher number of datasets are needed [18, 20]. Also, the requirement for additional and efficient machine learning approaches and scalable computer architectures, which can aid in data processing speed, has been recognized [18, 22, 23, 31]. Lighting changes [16, 29], camera blind spots, ambient noise, and concurrent vocalizations have all been identified as barriers to obtaining audio and video recordings. Also, most farmers aren't experts in machine learning, so they can't see the patterns that algorithms find. This is an important problem that needs to be addressed. Thus, more intuitive systems are required. Simple, easy-to-use solutions, such as a visualization device with a user-friendly edge for proper data presentation [25, 30, 31], would be extremely beneficial. Given farmers' increasing comfort with cell phones, smart mobile phone applications are seen as a potential solution to the aforementioned challenge [15, 16, 21]. Finally, and perhaps most important, the development of effective machine learning techniques based on professional knowledge from stakeholders should be encouraged as a means of constructing accurate solutions, particularly in agriculture, computing science, and the private sector [19, 22, 24, 33]. As highlighted by Liakos et al. [12], current efforts are concentrated on individual solutions that are rarely related to decision-making processes, as demonstrated in other areas.

13.1.3 Use of IoT in Agriculture and AI

In 1956, John McCarthy invented the term "AI," which he defined as the study of creating intelligent machines with human-like intellect. Such AI-based machines can learn, understand, and imitate a given situation. Some subfields of AI are machine learning, computer vision, expert systems, text mining, and machine translation. In various real-life situations, AI-based applications have been in use. In the sectors of agriculture, robotics, healthcare, finance, e-commerce, and automation, intelligent AI systems are being extensively investigated. Samsung, Apple, and other electronics leaders have stated that they will soon include this technology in every item they create.

Another emerging technology is the Internet of Things, which connects smart sensors and devices over the internet. Farming uses IoT-based solutions for monitoring soil condition and soil moisture, such collected data can be used in training ML models. The ML model provides the best prediction for the optimum use of fertilizers for a crop. Another useful IoT-based application comes from drones. They are used to monitor fields and crops, spray pesticides, and drip irrigation. In drip irrigation, drones use AI-powered water irrigation methods trained on weather patterns to reduce the wastage of water. The use of AI-enabled robots in harvesting crops is fast-paced and performs tasks in large volumes. IoT-based sensors are being used in livestock management for monitoring the health of cattle.

13.2 PURPOSE OF THE RESEARCH

As previously stated, numerous review journals have recently been published in response to the uses of ML in agriculture. However, the majority of these studies are narrow in scope, focusing exclusively on one component of agricultural productivity. Figure 13.2 summarizes the categories described by Liakos et al. [12]. A complete bibliographic analysis is offered on the spectrum of these categories. Machine learning improvements, increased worldwide interest, and the potential impact on a wide range of agricultural fields all served as impetuses for this project. A new viewpoint on machine learning applications in agricultural systems is provided by focusing on material released from 2018 to 2020. With the same inclusion criteria, this study represents a continuation of the work of Liakos et al. Several critical features can be used to accurately capture current progress and trends, such as (a) the areas that are most attractive to machine learning in agriculture, (b) efficient machine learning models, (c) the most employed features and technology, and (d) the most researched yields and animals.

The quantity of journal articles published in the last few years has increased by 745% [12], indicating the necessity for an innovative review on the subject. Crop managing was also the most researched sector, with a variety of machine learning algorithms used to manage the heterogeneous data supplied by agricultural areas. In comparison to Liakos et al. [12], a broader range of agricultural and animal species have been explored, with a diverse set of input parameters derived primarily from remote sensing techniques such as satellites and drones. Furthermore, researchers from a variety of scientific disciplines have applied machine learning to agriculture, contributing to the field's remarkable success.

13.3 OVERVIEW OF ML TECHNIQUES

In general, machine learning algorithms, as shown in Figure 13.3, try to improve how well a task is done by using examples or past data. Machine

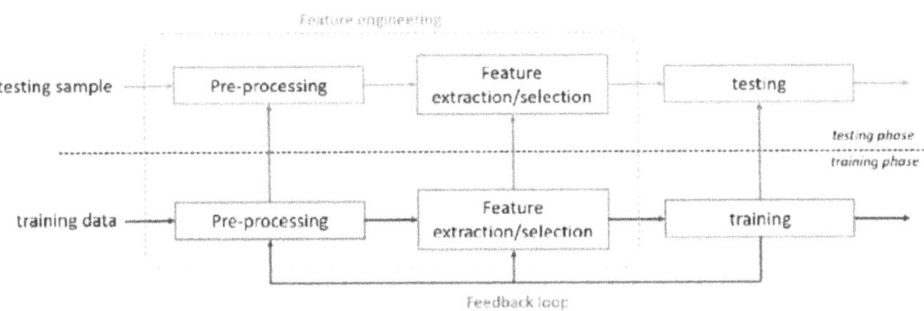

Figure 13.3 Example of the machine learning system in its entirety

learning, for example, can be used to optimize data input relationships and reconstruct a knowledge architecture. The more data there is, the better machine learning performs and the data-driven process, which is equivalent to the degree to which a human performs a task well as their experience grows [34]. The prime result of machine learning is a measure of generalizability, which is the machine learning algorithm's ability to produce accurate predictions when new data is presented using previously learned rules derived from similar data [35]. The term "data" refers to a set of characteristics that describe a collection of samples, which are sometimes referred to as features. In general, machine learning systems use two processes: learning (for training) and testing. These features are frequently merged into a feature vector, which can be binary, numeric, ordinal, or nominal [36]. During the learning phase, this vector is used as an input. In summary, during the learning period, the computer gains experience performing the task by relying on training data. It's over when the student's performance in learning is good enough (as measured by mathematical and statistical relationships). After the model has been trained, it can be used to sort, group, or predict data.

To convert the collected data to a usable state, preprocessing is compulsory. When multiple data sources are used, (a) data cleansing to eliminate inconsistencies, missing objects, and noise; (b) data transformation, such as normalization and discretization; and (c) data integration are frequently required [37]. During the training phase, the extraction/selection feature is used to generate or recognize the informative subset of structures that will be used to implement the learning model [38]. As shown in Figure 13.3, the feedback loop is used to modify the feature extraction/selection unit as well as the preprocessing unit, thereby improving the learning model's overall performance. Previously unknown bugs are discovered throughout the testing phase.

The trained model, sometimes referred to as a feature vector, is fed samples. Finally, the model makes an appropriate decision depending on the features of each sample (classification or regression, for example). Deep learning, a field of machine learning, delegates the duty of converting raw data into features to the learning system (feature engineering). By doing away with the feature extraction/selection unit, we are left with a trainable system that starts with unstructured input and ends with the desired output [39, 40]. Figure 13.3 depicts a distinctive machine learning system. Based on the type of learning, machine learning may be grouped into the following categories, according to the associated research [41, 42]:

- Supervised learning: Given the input and output, the machine attempts to find the shortest path between them.
- Unsupervised learning: Without labels, unsupervised learning requires the learning system to generate structure from the data on its own.

- Semi-supervised learning: Semi-supervised learning is a sort of machine learning in which both labeled and unlabeled data are accepted as input.
- Reinforcement learning: Rather than relying solely on trial and error and a delayed outcome, decisions are made to determine which behaviors will result in a more favorable outcome.

To name a few applications, these include image recognition [43], speech recognition [44], independent driving [45], fraud detection of credit cards [46], stock market forecasting [47], fluid mechanics [48], malware filtering, spam and email [49], medical diagnosis [40], detection of contamination in city water networks [50], and recognition of activity [51].

13.4 MACHINES LEARNING AND IOT IN SMART AGRICULTURE

13.4.1 Crop Management

Crop management is a wide term that refers to different characteristics that result from a mixture of agricultural practices aimed at regulating the crop's biological, chemical, and physical situations to achieve quantitative and qualitative areas and goals [52]. Using modern crop management techniques such as prediction of yield, disease diagnosis, weed identification, crop recognition, and crop quality results in increased production and, as a result, financial benefit. Precision agriculture's primary objectives are as described earlier. Figure 13.4 illustrates various smart agriculture domains and smart farming solutions in each one of them.

13.4.2 Prediction of Yield

Yield estimation becomes the utmost critical and hardest if a major portion of agriculture depends on monsoon. For instance, an exact model can aid farm owners in making informed management decisions about yield and market demand [20]. However, this is not a simple task; it necessitates several steps. Numerous variables, like environmental conditions, management practices, and crop characteristics, have an impact on harvest forecast. As a result, an understanding of the relationship between these interacting characteristics and yield is required. Machine learning helps to establish such relationships and necessitates large datasets and complex algorithms [53].

13.4.3 Detection of Disease

Agricultural production systems are under threat from crop diseases, which can reduce the quality and quantity of crops produced as well as their shelf

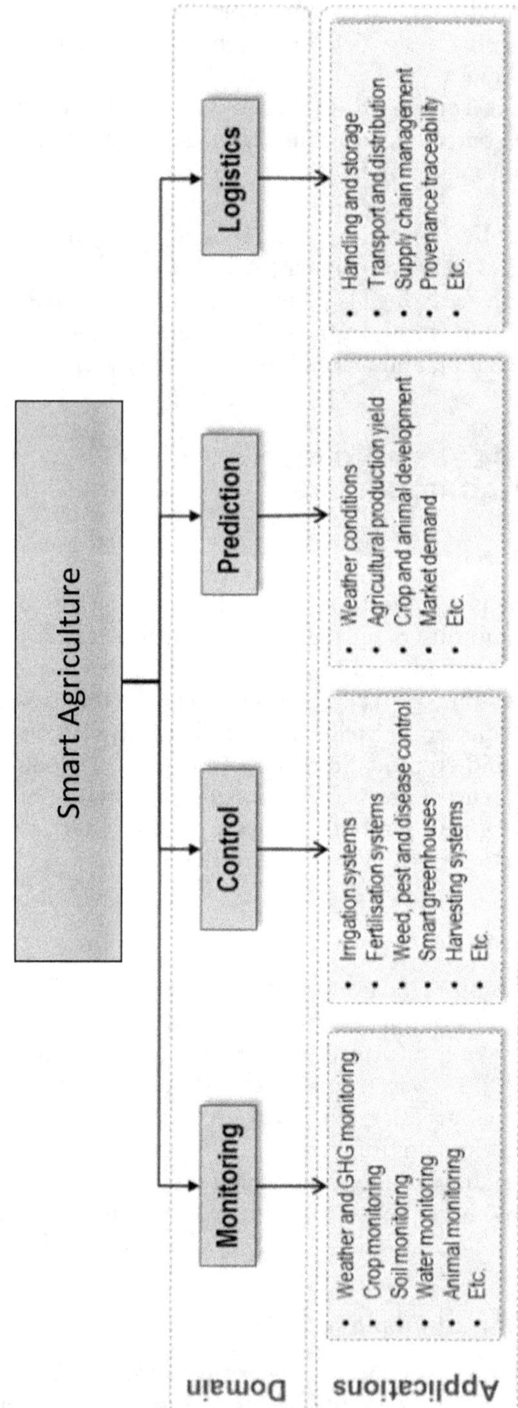

Figure 13.4 Smart agriculture domain and various solutions for smart farming

life and transportation costs. Plant disease-related output losses are frequently reported by farmers [54]. A substantial threat to global food security is posed by crop diseases, as well. Early detection and management of plant diseases are crucial. Plant infections can be caused by a variety of organisms, including bacteria, fungi, parasites, and viruses. Weeds, withering leaves and fruits, leaf curling, and other disease symptoms are all physical signs of pathogens and phenotypic changes in plants. Professional agronomists have always carried out field reconnaissance to identify diseases. It's a laborious process that relies on visual judgment and takes a lot of time. Commercially available sensor systems that can detect unhealthy plants before symptoms appear have been made possible thanks to recent technological advances. It's worth noting that computer vision has made considerable strides recently due mostly to the application of deep learning [55]. As proven by Zhang et al. [56], utilizing deep learning to recognize cucumber leaf diseases is useful to decrease the background before model training due to the shifting environmental context. For accurate disease detection image classifiers, a huge library of healthy and diseased plant photos is also necessary. Automatic approaches can be used in large-scale farming with autonomous vehicles to detect problems sooner and build maps of the plant disease's spatial distribution, indicating the zones of infection in vast farms [57].

13.4.4 Weed Detection

Weeds generally proliferate and spread invasively across large areas of a field as a result of their productive production and long life span, competing with crops that need resources such as space, sun, nutrients, and water. Furthermore, weeds emerge earlier than crops and lack natural enemies, which hurts crop growth [18]. Weed control, whether mechanical or chemical, is critical for preventing agricultural yield decline. Since mechanical treatment is time-consuming and inefficient if done incorrectly, the application of herbicides is the most commonly used method. Using huge quantities of herbicides, however, can be both costly and environmentally damaging, especially when applied consistently without regard for the spatial distribution of weeds. Surprisingly, long-term pesticide use is likely to breed weed resistance, making weed control more difficult and expensive. Based on smart agriculture, significant progress has been made in recent years in distinguishing weeds from crops. Sensors attached to satellites and unmanned vehicles along with aerial and ground vehicles can be used to achieve this differentiation. Converting data collected by unmanned aerial vehicles into useful information remains a difficult task, as collection and classification of data require time and effort [58]. Combining machine learning algorithms with imaging technology or non-imaging spectroscopy enables real-time weed differentiation and localization, enabling precise herbicide application to specific zones rather than spraying entire fields [59–62] and path planning for weeding.

13.4.5 Crop Identification

Automatic recognition of crops has sparked significant interest in a wide range of scientific fields, including botanical gardens, plant taxonomy, and the discovery of new species. Plant organs and parts can be used to identify and categorize species. The most common technique appears to be leaf-based plant recognition, which involves assessing specific leaf characteristics such as color, shape, and texture. Classification of crops using remote sensing has become common as unmanned aerial vehicles and satellites have been used to collect data on crop properties more extensively. As with the previously mentioned subcategories, advancements in computer software and image processing technologies, combined with machine learning, have led to advancements in the automatic recognition of crops and their classification.

13.4.6 Managing the Quality of Crops

Crop quality has a substantial market influence and is determined by a variety of elements, including soil and climatic conditions, cultivation procedures, and crop features. When farmers offer high-quality agricultural products at a higher price, they make more money. The most often used harvesting markers for fruit quality, are flesh hardness, soluble solids content, and skin color. In both high-value crops (such as grapes, vegetables, and herbs) and arable crops, the harvesting date has a considerable impact on the quality of harvested products. As a result, establishing decision support systems can assist farmers in making better management decisions, which will result in higher-quality food. Selective harvesting is a management strategy that can dramatically improve product quality. Crops of poor quality also result in food waste, posing a new difficulty for contemporary agriculture, as crops that do not meet the acceptable shape, quality, color, or size may be rejected. As seen in the prior section, combining machine learning algorithms with picture technology might yield intriguing outcomes.

13.4.7 Water and Rainfall Management

The agriculture industry is the world's largest consumer of readily available freshwater, as plant development is dependent on the accessibility of water. Given the rapid reduction of many aquifers with little or no replenishment, more effective water management is critical for achieving long-term crop production. Proper water management can lead to good water quality as well as a reduction in pollution and health issues. Variable-rate irrigation has the potential to save water, according to recent precision agricultural research. Rather than implementing irrigation at a continual rate across the field, this can be accomplished by implementing irrigation at rates that vary based on field variability and the unique water requirements of discrete management zones. Variable-rate irrigation's performance and viability are influenced by agronomic considerations.

When attempting to save water while optimizing yields, topography, soil properties, and their effect on soil water are all factors that must be considered. Irrigation scheduling and water management can be improved by closely monitoring soil water levels, crop development conditions, temporal and spatial trends, and weather monitoring and forecasting. Remote sensing is one of the ICTs that can provide pictures that show how the soil is wet and how crops are growing so that water can be managed well [33]. In dry areas, it is hard to manage water because irrigation needs groundwater and rainfall only meets a small part of crop evapotranspiration needs. A good way to manage water resources and figure out how bad floods are is to be able to accurately predict rain.

13.4.8 Soil Management

Soil, as a varied natural resource, implies a plethora of systems and processes. Accurate regional soil knowledge is critical for better soil management that is compatible with land potential and, more broadly, for sustainable agriculture [5]. Land degradation, soil nutrient imbalance (as a result of excessive fertilizer use), and erosion of soil (as a result of excessive vegetation cutting, unbalanced crop rotations, livestock overgrazing, etc.) are all issues that must be addressed. Texture, organic matter, and nutrient concentration are just a few of the beneficial soil properties. Traditional soil evaluation methods frequently involve soil sampling and laboratory analysis, which are both expensive and time-consuming. On the other hand, remote sensing and soil mapping sensors can give a low-cost and straightforward method for researching soil spatial variability. When conventional data analysis techniques are used, data fusion and management of such diverse big data can provide substantial challenges. Machine learning approaches have the potential to provide a dependable, low-cost solution for this activity.

13.4.9 Management and Production of Livestock

It is putative that livestock production techniques have been enhanced in terms of productivity per animal. This strengthening includes social concerns about animal welfare and human health, which may influence consumer perceptions of food safety, security, and sustainability. To optimize production processes, it is critical to consider both animal welfare and total productivity. All of the aforementioned domains are part of precision livestock farming, which aims to increase early-stage output by utilizing engineering methodologies to observe animal health in real time and recognize danger signals. Precision livestock farming is becoming increasingly important in assisting livestock owners in making decisions and redefining their roles. It can also help with product traceability and monitoring product quality and animal living conditions, as specified by policymakers. Noninvasive sensors such as cameras, radio-frequency identification systems, and optical or temperature sensors are used in precision livestock husbandry [25]. Sensors in the IoT monitor temperature, sound, humidity, and other variables using physical quantities. IoT sensors, for example, can notify users in real time if a variable physical quantity is unusually high or low, providing critical information on specific animals. As a result, the cost of examining each animal on a regular and laborious basis can be reduced. To use massive amounts of data, machine learning techniques have become ingrained in modern livestock husbandry. Models capable of specifying how a biological system works, relying on causal relationships, and using this biological understanding to make predictions and suggestions can be created.

Sensor technologies combined with advanced machine learning algorithms have the potential to significantly increase the efficiency of cattle production. Given the impact of animal management practices on productivity, livestock owners are becoming more conservative in their investment decisions. However, as livestock herds grow larger, it becomes increasingly difficult to care for each animal. From this vantage point, the aforementioned farmer assistance through precision livestock farming is a positive step toward economic efficiency and the creation of sustainable workplaces with a smaller environmental footprint. Numerous animal production methods have been used in the past, with the majority of them aimed at increasing the efficiency with which animals are raised and fed. However, machine learning techniques are required due to the massive amounts of data involved.

13.5 METHODOLOGIES

Various secondary literature was used to identify studies that examined machine learning about various aspects of agricultural management. Furthermore, the term "machine learning" was associated with the following terminologies: "crop management," "water management," "soil management," and "livestock management." The authors aimed to conduct a literature search using the same methods as Liakos et al. [12], but just for the period 2018–2020.

13.6 CHALLENGES IN SMART FARMING AND USE OF INFORMATION TECHNOLOGY TOOLS

As a means of supplying the world's growing population with food, AI holds great promise. A number of obstacles to its widespread use in the agricultural sector have been described as follows:

- According to a recent survey conducted by the Indian government, the literacy rate of Indian farmers is extremely low, making it difficult to close the technological gap between farmers and technology.
- Farmers have a lower level of motivation to learn new digital skills in order to improve their farming practices.
- Rural areas tend to be home to the majority of agricultural land. It is difficult to implement IoT architecture and a wireless sensor network (WSN) in rural locations without dependable internet connectivity since cloud services are required for data storage and processing.
- It is challenging to make accurate predictions and classifications using computers' cognitive abilities when the geographical conditions differ.
- The initial setup of digital farming, which involves both hardware and software, necessitates a significant financial commitment.
- When smart sensors and other electrical gadgets are installed, they consume a lot of power.
- To create an intelligent harvesting system, an accurate training dataset is essential.
- Farmers lose money if their harvesting is delayed or rejected because of an inaccuracy in the system's detection of ripe or overripe crops.

13.7 CONCLUSIONS

Information and communications technology (ICT) combined with machine learning appears to be the most effective strategy for addressing new challenges. Given the present rate of data acquisition and the emergence of numerous technologies, farms will need to implement customized decision support systems (DSSs) to advance their management practices. These DSSs employ algorithms capable of handling a greater number of cases while taking into consideration a vast quantity of data that would be difficult for farmers to manage. The majority of ICT requires advanced fees, such as substantial infrastructure investment costs, and many farmers are hesitant to adopt these technologies. This is an urgent issue, especially in developing nations where agriculture plays a crucial economic role. The visible impact is a long-term objective that requires effort. All stakeholders must adopt a new way of thinking in order to cultivate innovative skills, which requires an understanding of the benefits of processing large quantities of data and the assertion of adequate financial resources. Due to the increasing use of AI in agriculture, machine learning will unquestionably become a facilitator for the development of agriculture that is both productive and sustainable. Scientists, policymakers, engineers, ICT system developers, manufacturers, and farmers are all anticipated to reap the benefits of the current systematic endeavor, which is anticipated to result in more systematic machine learning research in agriculture.

13.8 DISCUSSION

The current systematic review study focuses on machine learning in agriculture, which is becoming increasingly popular as new technologies are developed around the world. To achieve this goal, Liakos et al. [12] showed an all-inclusive assessment of the current situation of the four groupings described in their previous research. Plant, water, soil, and livestock management are all included. As a result, after reviewing relevant literature from the previous three years (2018–2020) and applying the findings, various elements were analyzed using an integrated approach. Finally, the following key findings can be drawn from this research:

- Crop management accounted for the vast majority of journal publications, with the other three broad topics accounting for roughly equal shares of the total. Using Liakos et al. [12] as a reference study, it is possible to conclude that this has remained largely unchanged, except for a decrease in the percentage of articles about livestock from 19% to 12% in favor of articles about crop management, which has increased from 1% to 2%. This, however, only depicts one side of the picture. When the massive surge in the number of related journals published in the last three years is considered, it is estimated that 400% more publications on livestock management were discovered. Another significant discovery was an increase in interest in crop identification research.
- To deal with the heterogeneous data collected from agricultural areas, several machine learning techniques have been developed. These algorithms can be divided into ML model families, which can then be further subdivided. In a similar vein to Liakos et al. [12], artificial neural networks (ANNs) were discovered to be the most efficient ML models. There has been a shift in emphasis away from Liakos et al. [12] and toward ensemble learning (EL), which can aggregate predictions from a variety of models. Support vector machines (SVM) complete the collection of the three most precise machine learning models in agriculture due to a variety of advantages, including their excellent performance when working with image data.
- When it comes to the most extensively researched crops, maize and, later, wheat, rice, and soybean have all been thoroughly investigated using ML techniques. Cattle, sheep, and goats were the most extensively studied animals in livestock management, accounting for approximately 85% of all research. More species have been added since Liakos et al.'s review [12], but wheat and rice, as well as cattle, remain important specimens for machine learning applications.
- The visualization of the input data used in the ML algorithms, as well as the sensors that provided the data for the algorithms, was a significant outcome in the current review study. RGB images were the most

common, which explains the widespread use of convolutional neural networks (CNNs), which have a greater capacity for dealing with this type of data due to their superior processing speed. A wide range of indicators for climatic, soil, water, and crop quality conditions were also included in the study. Remote sensing, like images from satellites, unmanned aerial vehicles, and unmanned ground vehicles, was the most common way to get data for ML applications, but measurements were also taken in the field and a lab. As was already mentioned, unmanned aerial vehicles are steadily gaining ground on satellites because they are more flexible and can take high-resolution photos in any weather. Satellites, on the other hand, can give information about large areas over time. Lastly, animal welfare research relied a lot on technology like accelerometers to find out what the animals were doing, while livestock production research relied a lot on the animals' core physical and growth characteristics to figure out how happy they were.

- The use of machine learning applications to facilitate many aspects of agricultural management is a major concern on a global scale, as evidenced by the geographical distribution and the wide range of research topics. Indeed, due to its adaptability, it is an excellent choice for convergence research. While convergence research is a relatively new method, it is based on a shared understanding among researchers from various fields and has the potential to benefit the general public. Reduced environmental impact and human health protection are two examples of what is meant by this phrase. In this regard, the application of machine learning in agriculture holds a lot of promise for value generation.
- It is also worth noting that as a result of the study's findings, there is a growing interest in subjects related to machine learning in agricultural applications. When comparing 2018 and 2019, the total number of relevant studies increased by approximately 26%, according to Figure 13. When comparing the findings from 2018 to 2020, the equivalent increase increased by 109%, for a total increase of 164%. A variety of factors, including significant advances in agricultural information and communication technology systems, are contributing to the increased interest in machine learning in agriculture. Enhancing the competence of agricultural practices while reducing their environmental impact is also critical. To present a complete picture of agricultural processes, it is necessary to use both precise measurements and data management techniques capable of handling massive amounts of data. The current technological revolution has the potential to significantly boost agriculture in the direction of improving food security and meeting rising consumer demands. This is particularly true in agriculture.

To summarize, ICT combined with machine learning, seems to be the best option for dealing with new challenges. Given the current rate of data acquisition and the development of numerous technologies, farms will need to advance their management practices by implementing DSSs personalized to the needs of each agricultural system. These DSSs employ algorithms capable of dealing with a greater number of cases while taking into account a huge amount of data that farmers would find difficult to manage. Even though most ICT requires upfront fees, such as high infrastructure investment costs, many farmers are hesitant to use these technologies. This will be a pressing problem, particularly in developing countries where agriculture plays a significant economic role. Having a visible impact, on the other hand, is a long-term goal that necessitates hard work. To develop innovative skills, we must be aware of the profits of processing large amounts of data and assert appropriate financial resources, all stakeholders must adopt a new way of thinking. ML will undoubtedly become a behind-the-scenes enabler for the development of agriculture which is productive and sustainable due to the increasing use of artificial intelligence in agriculture. Scientists, policymakers, engineers, ICT system developers, manufacturers, and farmers are all expected to benefit from the current systematic effort, which is expected to result in more systematic machine learning research in agriculture.

REFERENCES

1. Thayer, A.; Vargas, A.; Castellanos, A.; Lafon, C.; McCarl, B.; Roelke, D.; Winemiller, K.; Lacher, T. Integrating agriculture, and ecosystems to find suitable adaptations to climate change. *Climate* 2020, 8(1), 10.
2. Nassani, A.A.; Awan, U.; Zaman, K.; Hyder, S.; Aldakhil, A.M.; Abro, M.M.Q. Management of natural resources and material pricing: Global evidence. *Resour. Policy* 2019, 64, 101500.
3. Conrad, Z.; Niles, M.T.; Neher, D.A.; Roy, E.D.; Tichenor, N.E.; Jahns, L. Relationship between food waste, diet quality, and environmental sustainability. *PLoS One* 2018, 13(4), 102–114.
4. Benos, L.; Bechar, A.; Bochtis, D. Safety, and ergonomics in human-robot interactive agricultural operations. *Biosyst. Eng.* 2020, 200, 55–72.
5. Lampridi, M.; Sørensen, C.; Bochtis, D. Agricultural sustainability: A review of concepts and methods. *Sustainability* 2019, 11(18), 5120.
6. Zecca, F. The use of internet of things for the sustainability of the agricultural sector: The case of climate-smart agriculture. *Int. J. Civ. Eng. Technol.* 2019, 10, 494–501.
7. Sørensen, C.A.G.; Kateris, D.; Bochtis, D. ICT innovations and smart farming. In *Communications in Computer and Information Science*. Springer, Berlin/Heidelberg, 2019, Volume 953, pp. 1–19.
8. Sonka, S. Big data: Fueling the next evolution of agricultural innovation. *J. Innov. Manag.* 2016, 4(1), 114–136.
9. Meng, T.; Jing, X.; Yan, Z.; Pedrycz, W. A survey on machine learning for data fusion. *Inf. Fusion* 2020, 57, 115–129.

10. Evstatiev, B.I.; Gabrovska-Evstatieva, K.G. A review on the methods for big data analysis in agriculture. In *Proceedings of the IOP Conference Series: Materials Science and Engineering*. Borovets, Bulgaria, 26–29 November 2020; IOP Publishing Ltd., Bristol, 2020, Volume 1032, p. 012053.
11. Helm, J.M.; Swiergosz, A.M.; Haeberle, H.S.; Karnuta, J.M.; Schaffer, J.L.; Krebs, V.E.; Spitzer, A.I.; Ramkumar, P.N. Machine learning and artificial intelligence: Definitions, applications, and future directions. *Curr. Rev. Musculoskelet. Med.* 2020, 13(1), 69–76.
12. Liakos, K.; Busato, P.; Moshou, D.; Pearson, S.; Bochtis, D. Machine learning in agriculture: A review. *Sensors* 2018, 18(8), 2674.
13. Abade, A.; Ferreira, P.; Vidal, F. Plant diseases recognition on images using convolutional neural networks: A systematic review. arXiv 2020, arXiv:2009.04365.
14. Yashodha, G.; Shalini, D. An integrated approach for predicting and broadcasting tea leaf disease at early stage using IoT with machine learning—A review. *Mater. Today Proc.* 2020, 12.
15. Yuan, Y.; Chen, L.; Wu, H.; Li, L. Advanced agricultural disease image recognition technologies: A review. *Inf. Process. Agric.* 2021, 13, 7–22.
16. Mayuri, K. Role of image processing and machine learning techniques in disease recognition, diagnosis and yield prediction of crops: A review. *Int. J. Adv. Res. Comput. Sci.* 2018, 9, 788–795.
17. Wang, A.; Zhang, W.; Wei, X. A review on weed detection using ground-based machine vision and image processing techniques. *Comput. Electron. Agric.* 2019, 158, 226–240.
18. Su, W.-H. Advanced machine learning in point spectroscopy, RGB- and hyperspectral-imaging for automatic discriminations of crops and weeds: A review. *Smart Cities* 2020, 3(3), 767–792.
19. Chlingaryan, A.; Sukkarieh, S.; Whelan, B. Machine learning approaches for crop yield prediction and nitrogen status estimation in precision agriculture: A review. *Comput. Electron. Agric.* 2018, 151, 61–69.
20. Van Klompenburg, T.; Kassahun, A.; Catal, C. Crop yield prediction using machine learning: A systematic literature review. *Comput. Electron. Agric.* 2020, 177, 105709.
21. Pushpanathan, K.; Hanafi, M.; Mashohor, S.; Fazlil Ilahi, W.F. Machine learning in medicinal plants recognition: A review. *Artif. Intell. Rev.* 2021, 54(1), 305–327.
22. Wäldchen, J.; Rzanny, M.; Seeland, M.; Mäder, P. Automated plant species identification—Trends and future directions. *PLoS Comput. Biol.* 2018, 14(4), e1005993.
23. Virnodkar, S.S.; Pachghare, V.K.; Patil, V.C.; Jha, S.K. Remote sensing and machine learning for crop water stress determination in various crops: A critical review. *Precis. Agric.* 2020, 21(5), 1121–1155.
24. Sun, A.Y.; Scanlon, B.R. How can big data and machine learning benefit environment and water management: A survey of methods, applications, and future directions. *Environ. Res. Lett.* 2019, 14(7), 73001.
25. Li, N.; Ren, Z.; Li, D.; Zeng, L. Review: Automated techniques for monitoring the behaviour and welfare of broilers and laying hens: Towards the goal of precision livestock farming. *Animal* 2020, 14(3), 617–625.

26. García, R.; Aguilar, J.; Toro, M.; Pinto, A.; Rodríguez, P. A systematic literature review on the use of machine learning in precision livestock farming. *Comput. Electron. Agric.* 2020, 179, 105826.
27. Ellis, J.L.; Jacobs, M.; Dijkstra, J.; van Laar, H.; Cant, J.P.; Tulpan, D.; Ferguson, N. Review: Synergy between mechanistic modelling and data-driven models for modern animal production systems in the era of big data. *Animal* 2020, 14(S2), s223–s237.
28. Lovarelli, D.; Bacenetti, J.; Guarino, M. A review on dairy cattle farming: Is precision livestock farming the compromise for an environmental, economic and social sustainable production? *J. Clean. Prod.* 2020, 262, 121409.
29. Patrício, D.I.; Rieder, R. Computer vision and artificial intelligence in precision agriculture for grain crops: A systematic review. *Comput. Electron. Agric.* 2018, 153, 69–81.
30. Cravero, A.; Sepúlveda, S. Use and adaptations of machine learning in big data—Applications in real cases in agriculture. *Electronics* 2021, 10(5), 552.
31. Ang, K.L.-M.; Seng, J.K.P. Big data and machine learning with hyperspectral information in agriculture. *IEEE Access* 2021, 9, 36699–36718.
32. Jose, A.; Nandagopalan, S.; Venkata, C.M.; Akana, S. Artificial intelligence techniques for agriculture revolution: A survey. *Ann. Rom. Soc. Cell Biol.* 2021, 25, 2580–2597.
33. Jung, J.; Maeda, M.; Chang, A.; Bhandari, M.; Ashapure, A.; Landivar-Bowles, J. The potential of remote sensing and artificial intelligence as tools to improve the resilience of agriculture production systems. *Curr. Opin. Biotechnol.* 2021, 70, 15–22.
34. Avasthi, S.; Chauhan, R.; Acharjya, D.P. Techniques, applications, and issues in mining large-scale text databases. In *Advances in Information Communication Technology and Computing* (pp. 385–396). Springer, Singapore, 2021.
35. Avasthi, S.; Sanwal, T.; Sareen, P.; Tripathi, S.L. Augmenting mental healthcare with artificial intelligence, machine learning, and challenges in telemedicine. In *Handbook of Research on Lifestyle Sustainability and Management Solutions Using AI, Big Data Analytics, and Visualization* (pp. 75–90). IGI Global, Springer, 2022.
36. Avasthi, S.; Chauhan, R.; Acharjya, D.P. Information extraction and sentiment analysis to gain insight into the COVID-19 crisis. In *International Conference on Innovative Computing and Communications* (pp. 343–353). Springer, Singapore, 2022.
37. Anagnostis, A.; Papageorgiou, E.; Bochtis, D. Application of artificial neural networks for natural gas consumption forecasting. *Sustainability* 2020, 12(16), 6409.
38. Zheng, A.; Casari, A. *Feature Engineering for Machine Learning: Principles and Techniques for Data Scientists.* O'Reilly Media, Inc., Sebastopol, CA, 2018.
39. LeCun, Y.; Bengio, Y.; Hinton, G. Deep learning. *Nature* 2015, 521(7553), 436–444.
40. Kokkotis, C.; Moustakidis, S.; Papageorgiou, E.; Giakas, G.; Tsaopoulos, D.E. Machine learning in knee osteoarthritis: A review. *Osteoarthr. Cartil. Open* 2020, 2(3), 100069.

41. Simeone, O. A Very Brief Introduction to machine learning with applications to communication systems. *IEEE Trans. Cogn. Commun. Netw.* 2018, 4(4), 648–664.
42. Choi, R.Y.; Coyner, A.S.; Kalpathy-Cramer, J.; Chiang, M.F.; Peter Campbell, J. Introduction to machine learning, neural networks, and deep learning. *Transl. Vis. Sci. Technol.* 2020, 9(2), 14 [PubMed].
43. Cheng, Q.; Zhang, S.; Bo, S.; Chen, D.; Zhang, H. Augmented reality dynamic image recognition technology based on deep learning algorithm. *IEEE Access* 2020, 8, 137370–137384.
44. Anvarjon, T.; Mustaqeem; Kwon, S. Deep-net: A lightweight CNN-based speech emotion recognition system using deep frequency features. *Sensors* 2020, 20(18), 5212.
45. Fujiyoshi, H.; Hirakawa, T.; Yamashita, T. Deep learning-based image recognition for autonomous driving. *IATSS Res.* 2019, 43(4), 244–252.
46. Rai, A.K.; Dwivedi, R.K. Fraud detection in credit card data using unsupervised machine learning based scheme. In *Proceedings of the International Conference on Electronics and Sustainable Communication Systems (ICESC)*, Coimbatore, 2– 4 July 2020; Institute of Electrical and Electronics Engineers Inc., Piscataway, NJ, 2020, pp. 421–426.
47. Carta, S.; Ferreira, A.; Podda, A.S.; Reforgiato Recupero, D.; Sanna, A.; Multi, D.Q.N. An ensemble of deep Q-learning agents for stock market forecasting. *Expert Syst. Appl.* 2021, 164, 113820.
48. Sofos, F.; Karakasidis, T.E. Machine learning techniques for fluid flows at the nanoscale. *Fluids* 2021, 6(3), 96.
49. Gangavarapu, T.; Jaidhar, C.D.; Chanduka, B. Applicability of machine learning in spam and phishing email filtering: Review and approaches. *Artif. Intell. Rev.* 2020, 53(7), 5019–5081.
50. Lučin, I.; Grbčić, L.; Carija, Z.; Kranjčević, L. Machine-learning classification of a number of contaminant sources in an urban water network. *Sensors* 2021, 21, 245.
51. Yvoz, S.; Petit, S.; Biju-Duval, L.; Cordeau, S. A framework to type crop management strategies within a production situation to improve the comprehension of weed communities. *Eur. J. Agron.* 2020, 115, 126009.
52. Khaki, S.; Wang, L. Crop yield prediction using deep neural networks. *Front. Plant Sci.* 2019, 10, 621.
53. Harvey, C.A.; Rakotobe, Z.L.; Rao, N.S.; Dave, R.; Razafimahatratra, H.; Rabarijohn, R.H.; Rajaofara, H.; MacKinnon, J.L. Extreme vulnerability of smallholder farmers to agricultural risks and climate change in Madagascar. *Philos. Trans. R. Soc. B Biol. Sci.* 2014, 369(1639).
54. Jim Isleib Signs and symptoms of plant disease: Is it fungal, viral or bacterial? Available online. https://www.canr.msu.edu/news/signs_and_symptoms_of_plant_disease_is_it_fungal_viral_or_bacterial (accessed on 19 March 2021).
55. Anagnostis, A.; Tagarakis, A.C.; Asiminari, G.; Papageorgiou, E.; Kateris, D.; Moshou, D.; Bochtis, D. A deep learning approach for anthracnose infected trees classification in walnut orchards. *Comput. Electron. Agric.* 2021, 182, 105998.

56. Zhang, J.; Rao, Y.; Man, C.; Jiang, Z.; Li, S. Identification of cucumber leaf diseases using deep learning and small sample size for agricultural Internet of Things. *Int. J. Distrib. Sens. Netw.* 2021, 17(4), 1–13.
57. Islam, N.; Rashid, M.M.; Wibowo, S.; Xu, C.-Y.; Morshed, A.; Wasimi, S.A.; Moore, S.; Rahman, S.M. Early weed detection using image processing and machine learning techniques in an Australian chilli farm. *Agriculture* 2021, 11(5), 387.
58. Slaughter, D.C.; Giles, D.K.; Downey, D. Autonomous robotic weed control systems: A review. *Comput. Electron. Agric.* 2008, 61(1), 63–78.
59. Zhang, L.; Li, R.; Li, Z.; Meng, Y.; Liang, J.; Fu, L.; Jin, X.; Li, S. A quadratic traversal algorithm of shortest weeding path planning for agricultural mobile robots in cornfield. *J. Robot.* 2021, 6633139.
60. Thillaiarasu, N.; Lata Tripathi, S.; Dhinakaran, V. (Eds.). *Artificial Intelligence for Internet of Things: Design Principle, Modernization, and Techniques* (1st ed.). CRC Press, Boca Raton, 2022. https://doi.org/10.1201/9781003335801.
61. Goyal, N.; Sharma, S.; Kumar Rana, A.; Tripathi, S.L. (Eds.). *Internet of Things: Robotic and Drone Technology* (1st ed.). CRC Press, Boca Raton, 2022. https://doi.org/10.1201/9781003181613.
62. Sharma, K.; Gupta, A.; Sharma, B.; Tripathi, S.L. (Eds.). *Intelligent Communication and Automation Systems* (1st ed.). CRC Press, Boca Raton, 2021. https://doi.org/10.1201/9781003104599.

Chapter 14

Comprehensive Analysis of Blockchain Frameworks and Their Usability in Various Applications

Harish Kumar, Rajesh Kumar Kaushal, Naveen Kumar, and Praveen Kumar Malik

14.1 INTRODUCTION

Blockchain has emerged as a disruptive force with the potential to revolutionize an extensive range of industries, from finance to healthcare to supply chain management. Blockchain is a sophisticated data structure composed of a developing list of records called blocks [1]. The primary structure of the blockchain is shown in Figure 14.1 [2]. At its core, blockchain is a decentralized, distributed ledger that allows for secure, stable, transparent, and tamper-resistant transactions without the necessity for intermediaries [3]. This technology is built upon cryptography and consensus algorithms, which allow trust and collaboration among participants in a network. One of the significant advantages of blockchain is its capability to facilitate trust between parties that may not have prior interactions or shared history. According to Böhme et al. [4], blockchain has the potential to cope with the demanding situations of trust and transparency in supply chain management, as well as lower costs and enhanced performance. The blockchain can enhance the safety and privacy of financial transactions, as well as reduce the risk of fraud [5]. One of the specific traits of blockchain is its use of a consensus mechanism to validate and affirm the transactions on the network, which guarantees that each one of the nodes of the network agrees on the state of the ledger even in the presence of malicious actors [6].

A block in a blockchain network incorporates four elements: information, the hash of the contemporary block, the hash of the previous block, and a timestamp, in which every new block is linked to its predecessor.

Several types of blockchain technologies have been developed to address different use cases and applications. Following are some of the most common types.

- Public blockchains: These are open and decentralized blockchains that anyone can join and participate in. Anyone can create transactions, mine new blocks, and verify the network. Examples include Bitcoin and Ethereum.

DOI: 10.1201/9781003466949-14

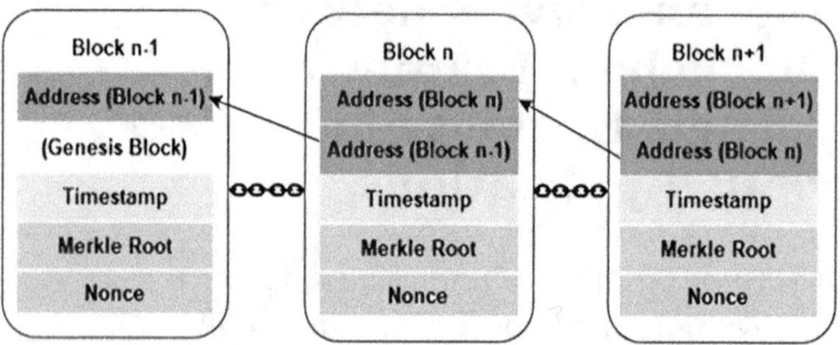

Figure 14.1 Blockchain structure

- Private blockchains: These are permissioned blockchains that restrict access to specific users or organizations. The users are identified and authorized to access the network, and the consensus mechanism is controlled by a small group of participants. Examples include Hyperledger Fabric and Corda.
- Hybrid blockchains: These are a combination of public and private blockchains that provide the benefits of both. The public blockchain provides transparency and security, while the private blockchain provides control and privacy. Examples include Dragonchain and Quorum.

Each type of blockchain has its advantages and disadvantages, and the choice of the blockchain type depends on the specific use case and requirements of the application. A brief description of the key features of blockchain technology is discussed next.

- Decentralization: Blockchain technology is decentralized, meaning no central authority or intermediary controls the network. Transactions are validated and recorded by a network of nodes that are connected [6].
- Distributed ledger: Blockchain technology uses a distributed ledger, meaning that the ledger is replicated and stored on multiple nodes in the network. This makes it difficult for any single node or actor to control or manipulate the ledger [7].
- Cryptography: Blockchain technology uses advanced cryptography to secure transactions and prevent unauthorized access to the ledger. Each transaction is digitally signed and verified by the network, ensuring that only authorized parties can participate in the network [3].
- Immutability: Once a transaction is recorded on the blockchain, it cannot be changed or deleted. This ensures that the data on the blockchain is permanent and tamper-proof [7].

- Consensus mechanism: Blockchain technology uses a consensus mechanism to ensure that all nodes in the network agree on the state of the ledger. This helps to prevent fraud and double-spending [6].
- Transparency: Blockchain technology allows for transparent and auditable transactions, as all transactions are recorded on the public ledger. This can help to increase trust between parties and reduce the risk of fraud [4].
- Security: Blockchain technology provides a prominent level of security using cryptography and distributed storage. This makes it difficult for hackers or malicious actors to compromise the network [7].

Blockchain technology represents a substantial technological advancement with the potential to disrupt an extensive range of industries and allow new applications. However, the adoption of blockchain isn't always without its challenges. One of the primary challenges is scalability, as the current blockchain architecture can only control a restrained quantity of transactions per second. Kumar et al. [8] proposed that combining blockchain with other technologies such as the Internet of Things (IoT) and artificial intelligence (AI) could overcome this challenge and create new enterprise models. Another challenge is the regulatory environment, as blockchain's legal and regulatory frameworks are still evolving. For example, the European Union's General Data Protection Regulation (GDPR) poses demanding situations to use blockchain in certain applications due to its necessity for records protection and privacy. There are still enormous challenges that have to be addressed, which include scalability, power consumption, and regulatory and legal issues [3].

14.2 OBJECTIVES

One objective of this study is to provide a comprehensive analysis of various blockchain frameworks used in IoT systems. Another objective is to analyze the trade-offs among different blockchain framework features, highlight their strengths and weaknesses, and identify the most effective of them in IoT healthcare systems.

14.3 METHODOLOGY

To complete the research work, this study took a structured approach following the PRISMA (Preferred Reporting Items for Systematic Reviews and Meta-Analysis) technique applied in Google Scholar, ResearchGate, ScienceDirect, and IEEE library using search keywords and strings (blockchain [title/abstract] or blockchain framework [title/abstract] or blockchain smart contract [title/abstract], or consensus mechanism, blockchain and IoT use cases [title]). Only papers in English with at least two citations published in journals with an impact factor ≥1 or papers from conferences with at least one citation from the publications (2014–2023) with content relevant to blockchain use cases in various sectors and specifically in a constrained network environment related to the healthcare sector and with the availability of full-text papers were considered.

During the initial search based on the considered criteria, a total of 491 articles were found, and after the filter and reviewing by title and abstract, excluding duplicate papers and inaccessible papers, a total of 40 papers were considered for this research work. Figure 14.2 shows the PRISMA chart exhibiting the whole process.

14.4 LITERATURE REVIEW

A blockchain framework is a set of software tools and components that developers use to build decentralized applications (dApps) and blockchain networks. These frameworks provide a programming environment for developers to create, evaluate, and deploy smart contracts, which are self-executing computer programs that run on the blockchain. These frameworks typically consist of several components, including a consensus mechanism, a virtual machine, a peer-to-peer network, and a data storage

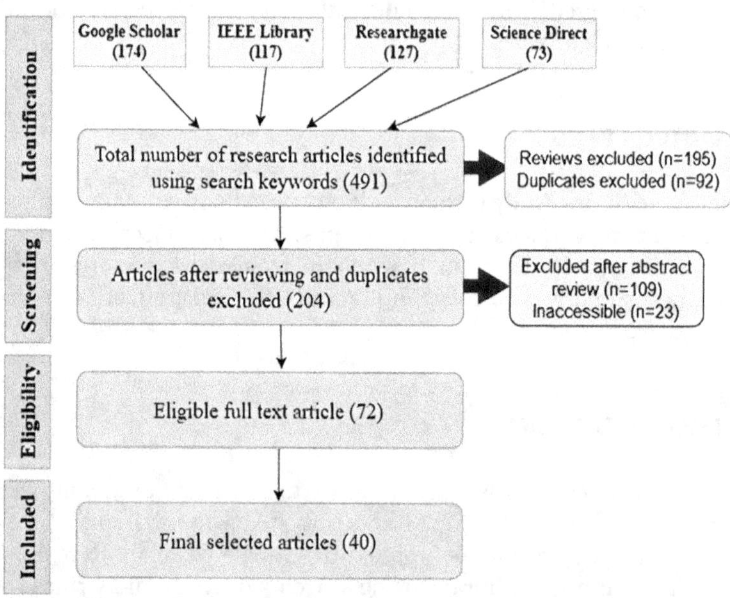

Figure 14.2 Prisma flow diagram

layer. These components work together to ensure that the blockchain network is secure, reliable, and tamper-proof.

When a user initiates a transaction on a blockchain network, the transaction is validated by the network's nodes using the consensus mechanism. Once validated, the transaction is recorded on the blockchain and becomes a part of the immutable ledger. Smart contracts are the backbone of blockchain applications, as they enable the execution of automated, self-executing code on the blockchain. Smart contracts can be used for a wide range of applications, such as tokenization, supply chain management, voting systems, and many sectors. Following are some of the most used blockchain frameworks.

14.4.1 Hyperledger Fabric

Hyperledger Fabric is an open-source blockchain framework designed to build permissioned blockchain networks. It evolved via the Linux Foundation's Hyperledger project, a collaborative effort aimed at advancing blockchain technologies for firms. Hyperledger Fabric provides an extraordinarily modular and configurable structure that lets developers construct steady, scalable, and privacy-preserving blockchain networks. It is a distributed ledger technology (DLT) platform that offers a modular structure to create and set up blockchain-based solutions for industries. Hyperledger Fabric consists of nodes where the membership service provider manages the identities of individuals (nodes) in the network and verifies and validates the authenticity of every node and their transactions in which a peer node continues a copy of the ledger and executes chain code, and a client interacts with the network by submitting transactions and querying the ledger [9]. Ordering service nodes manage the formation of blocks, which include the transaction information, and the ordering of these blocks in the ledger [10]. A ledger is a distributed database that stores all the transaction data and the current state of the system. The architecture of transaction processing in Hyperledger Fabric is depicted in Figure 14.3 [11]. Hyperledger Fabric supports multiple

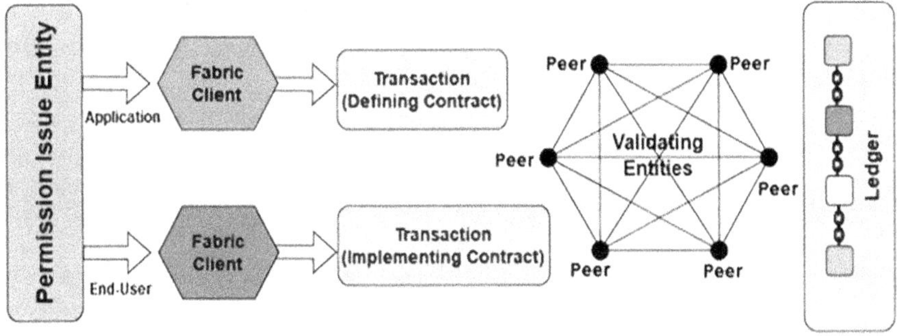

Figure 14.3 Transaction processing with Hyperledger Fabric

consensus algorithms, such as Kafta and Raft, which allow nodes to agree on the state of the ledger. Its smart contracts support allows developers to write smart contracts using the Go programming language, which is also known as chaincode [9]. These contracts are executed in a secure and isolated environment within the network. Chaincode refers to smart contracts that are deployed on the network [10]. No mining and expensive calculations are required in Hyperledger Fabric to ensure transactions.

Iftekhar et al. [12] used Hyperledger Fabric in a large-scale IoT system and presented an experimental approach to characterize the performance (latency and throughput) and scalability of Hyperledger Fabric with a varying number of nodes and workloads. Honar Pajooh et al. [13] introduced Hyperledger Fabric in IoT applications to provide privacy to the application.

IBM has introduced its private blockchain framework named IBM Watson, which is based on Hyperledger Fabric and specifically designed for small-scale networks and resource-constrained IoT networks for IoT networks proposed by IBM.

Features of Hyperledger Fabric

1. Modular architecture: Hyperledger Fabric has a highly modular architecture, which allows developers to build customized blockchain networks tailored to their specific needs. Developers can choose the consensus mechanism, identity management, and other components to build a network that meets their requirements.
2. Permissioned network: Hyperledger Fabric is a permissioned blockchain network, which means that only authorized participants can access and interact with the network. This provides enhanced security and privacy compared to public blockchain networks like Bitcoin and Ethereum.
3. Scalability: Hyperledger Fabric can process thousands of transactions per second, which makes it highly scalable [14]. It achieves this by dividing the workload into smaller components called "channels," which can process transactions in parallel.
4. Flexibility: Hyperledger Fabric supports a wide range of programming languages, including Java, Go, and Node.js. This makes it easy for developers to integrate existing applications with blockchain networks.
5. Privacy and confidentiality: Hyperledger Fabric provides built-in privacy and confidentiality features, such as private channels and confidential transactions. These features allow participants to transact on the blockchain network while keeping their data private and secure.

14.4.2 Ethereum

Ethereum is an open-source blockchain-based platform that allows developers to build and install dApps. It was developed in 2015 by Vitalik

Buterin. The Ethereum blockchain framework is based on a decentralized, peer-to-peer community that allows for the creation of smart contracts, which are self-executing code with the terms of the agreement between client and seller, written into code [15]. Smart contracts can be used to automate complex monetary transactions, vote-casting systems, and other applications that require trust and protection. Ethereum has its native cryptocurrency called Ether (ETH), which is used to pay transaction expenses and reward miners for validating transactions [16]. Ether is the second largest cryptocurrency in the world with the aid of marketplace capitalization after Bitcoin. Initially, Ethereum became a public permissionless blockchain platform that implements the Ethash consensus protocol, which follows proof-of-work (PoW) [3]. Due to the security issues with PoW, Ethereum presently implements the Clique consensus protocol (proof-of-authority). Moreover, Ethereum supports smart contracts and Ethereum Virtual Machine (EVM), which enables any node to execute code of any programming language.

Some researchers used Ethereum smart contracts for IoT applications to manage attributes-based access control policies. The architecture of Ethereum is shown in Figure 14.4 [17]. To check the feasibility of the proposed framework, Yutaka et al. constructed four smart contracts and conducted experiments to test the monetary and time costs [18].

Features of Ethereum

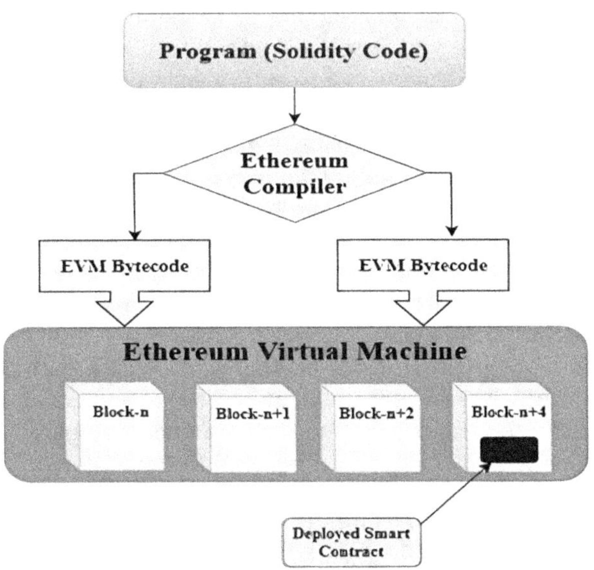

Figure 14.4 Basic architecture of Ethereum

1. Flexibility: Ethereum is a flexible blockchain framework that allows developers to create custom blockchain applications tailored to their specific needs.
2. Decentralization: Due to its decentralized architecture, there is no central authority, which makes it more resilient to censorship and manipulation [15]
3. Smart contracts: Ethereum's smart contracts are self-executing contracts that are stored on the blockchain. They allow for the automation of complex transactions without the need for intermediaries.
4. Community: Ethereum has a large and active community of developers and users, which helps to promote innovation and development on the platform.
5. Interoperability: Ethereum can interact with other blockchains and decentralized applications, which allows for greater interoperability and functionality.

14.4.3 Corda

Corda is a DLT platform specifically designed for businesses. It was created by the consortium R3 in 2015 and is an open-source blockchain framework, which means there is no central authority or intermediary in the network. Each node on the network is responsible for validating and processing its own transactions [19]. This makes Corda more efficient, scalable, and secure than traditional centralized systems.

Its architecture is primarily based on the idea of smart contracts, which are programmable agreements that are executed automatically when certain situations are met. Corda smart contracts are known as "Corda contracts," and they're written in the Kotlin or Java programming language. Corda contracts are designed to be well-matched with existing legal frameworks, making it simpler for organizations to apply them alongside traditional contracts. Corda additionally makes use of a unique data model referred to as "States" to control data, which is a data object that represents a fact or an agreement between two parties and is related to a set of policies and constraints that outline how it may be used and updated [20]. The Corda States may be shared and updated securely between parties, which allows for real-time collaboration and transparency. Additionally, Corda has numerous safety features that make it more secure than conventional systems. These include secure and stable messaging, secure key control, and the capacity to restrict access to data on a need-to-know basis. Corda allows a huge range of identities, from institutions to people, to participate in transactions. In Corda, an identity is represented by a certificate signed by an appropriate authority and representing a named real-world actor. Participants are expected to safeguard the private keys linked with their Corda identities, and transactions signed with a user's key are legally binding on that participant [19].

Features of Corda

1. Transaction finality: Corda guarantees transaction finality, meaning that once a transaction is committed to the ledger, it cannot be reversed. This provides a high degree of certainty and reduces the risk of fraud.
2. Interoperability: Corda is designed to be interoperable with existing financial systems. This makes it a suitable platform for financial institutions as it can easily integrate with their existing system.
3. Scalability: Corda is designed to be scalable and can handle up to 20,000 transactions per second, making it suitable for large-scale applications.
4. Data privacy: It is a permissioned blockchain as it shares data only with the parties involved in the transaction.
5. Security: With Corda, security is never an issue. Each entity must be tied to a legal entity and granted access to join the network.
6. Regulatory compliant: Its architecture enables it to address several challenges facing the financial industry, including regulatory compliance, which is a crucial factor for financial institutions.
7. Sustainability: Transactions do not have to be consecutive, which ensures that the system is extremely efficient and consumes significantly less energy than a public PoW or PoS (proof-of-stake) blockchain.

14.4.4 EOSIO

The EOSIO framework was designed and developed by Block.one. It was designed to provide developers with the tools and techniques to develop more scalable, flexible, and easy-to-use decentralized applications. It also enables them to execute decentralized applications on a blockchain network, and it also provides the support to build and deploy smart contracts. The framework is designed to handle a high volume of transactions per second, making it well-suited for applications that require fast, real-time processing. EOSIO achieves this scalability through its use of a delegated proof-of-stake (DPoS) consensus mechanism, which allows for faster transaction processing than other consensus mechanisms like PoW or PoS [21, 22].

It provides developers with a high degree of flexibility in terms of designing and deploying their dApps. This includes the ability to customize the network parameters, choose the consensus mechanism, and define the governance structure. EOSIO is designed to have low transaction latency, which means that transactions can be processed quickly and efficiently [22]. This is important for applications that require fast processing times, such as gaming or social media platforms. Its framework is designed to be easily upgradable, which allows for new features and capabilities to be added to the network without disrupting existing applications [23]. It includes a built-in governance mechanism that allows stakeholders to participate in the decision-making process for the network. This helps to ensure that the network is managed in a fair and transparent manner. EOSIO is designed to be interoperable with other blockchain networks and systems. This makes it possible for developers to build applications that can interact with other networks and platforms.

14.4.5 Quorum

Quorum was designed for enterprise use cases that require high performance, confidentiality, and flexibility. It is based on the Ethereum blockchain but has been modified to meet the needs of enterprise users [24]. It was developed by J.P. Morgan in 2016 as an open-source project. It was designed to address the limitations of the Ethereum blockchain, which was originally designed for public use cases. Quorum uses a modified version of the EVM that supports private transactions and confidential contracts [24]. It also supports the creation of permissioned networks, where only authorized parties can participate in the network. One of the key features of a Quorum is its support for private transactions.

In the original Ethereum blockchain, all transactions are public and visible to all network participants. This is not suitable for enterprise use cases, where confidentiality is often required. Quorum supports confidential contracts, which are useful for enterprise use cases where the contract logic contains sensitive information that should not be visible to all network participants. A Quorum network can be deployed with three different consensus algorithms: Raft [25], Clique proof-of-authority (PoA) [26], and Istanbul Byzantine Fault Tolerant (IBFT) [27]. Quorum also includes several performance optimizations that make it suitable for enterprise use cases. These include a faster consensus algorithm (IBFT) and a more efficient data storage format (RocksDB). It has achieved significantly higher transaction throughput compared to the original Ethereum blockchain.

Features of Quorum

1. Privacy and confidentiality: Quorum supports private transactions and confidential contracts. This is achieved using a privacy layer, which encrypts the transaction data and restricts access to authorized parties. This is particularly useful for enterprise use cases, where confidentiality is often required.
2. Permissioned networks: Quorum supports the creation of permissioned networks, where only authorized parties can participate in the network. This contrasts with public blockchains like Bitcoin and Ethereum, where anyone can participate in the network. Permissioned networks are useful for enterprise use cases where confidentiality and control are important [28].

3. High performance: Quorum includes several performance optimizations that make it suitable for enterprise use cases. These include a faster consensus algorithm (IBFT) and a more efficient data storage format (RocksDB). Quorum has been shown to achieve significantly higher transaction throughput compared to the original Ethereum blockchain.
4. Interoperability: Quorum is compatible with the Ethereum blockchain, which means that applications developed for the Ethereum blockchain can be easily ported to Quorum. This makes it easier for developers to build applications on top of the Quorum framework.

14.4.6 IOTA

IOTA is a distributed ledger technology specifically designed for IoT. It uses a directed acyclic graph (DAG) data structure-based unique consensus algorithm called Tangle, which is designed to be more energy efficient and scalable than traditional blockchain algorithms. IOTA is also designed to support microtransactions, making it well-suited for IoT devices that need to exchange small amounts of value [29]. Tangle works by having each new transaction validate two previous transactions, effectively creating a mesh network of interdependent transactions [30]. This eliminates the need for miners, as each user is responsible for verifying two other transactions before their own transaction can be validated. This also results in faster transaction times and no transaction fees.

Features of IOTA

1. No transaction costs: There is no need to pay for gas or reward miners to complete transactions. IOTA is a fee-free data and value transfer protocol.
2. Faster transaction capability: Conventional blockchain frameworks mostly experience bottlenecking because of the time required to create new blocks. The Bitcoin blockchain manages approximately five transactions per second (TPS), however, this may vary with the conditions. Ethereum manages around 14–15 transactions per second, and IOTA can manage up to around 1,000 TPS [31].
3. Energy efficiency: IOTA easily accommodates devices like sensors that operate in a low-energy or constrained environment. IoT devices, like toasters with limited computing power, can also write to IOTA's Tangle.
4. Adaptability: Large corporations may adopt IOTA for individual use cases. Its open-source framework enables access to control systems where a car owner can allow someone to remotely access their vehicles [31].
5. Decentralization: IOTA's new version (v.2.0) is fully decentralized.

6. Highly scalable: Unlike other blockchain frameworks, IOTA uses a DAG data structure that allows transactions to be added in parallel [29].
7. Distributed: Its distributed network makes it more resilient and robust against attacks [28].

14.5 SMART CONTRACT

A smart contract is a self-executing computer program that is deployed on a blockchain network. It is a set of rules and conditions that define the terms of an agreement between two or more parties. Once the conditions of the contract are met, the smart contract automatically executes the agreed-upon actions. Smart contracts are stored and executed on a decentralized blockchain network, which makes them secure, transparent, and tamper-proof.

The code of the contract is publicly available, which means that all parties can verify the terms and conditions of the contract [32]. One of the key benefits of smart contracts is their ability to automate and streamline business processes. They can be used for a wide range of applications, such as supply chain management, real estate transactions, insurance claims, and digital identity management. The basic structure of a smart contract is shown in Figure 14.5 [33].

14.6 SMART CONTRACT VERSUS TRADITIONAL CONTRACT

A smart contract is a set of rules and conditions that define the terms of an agreement between two or more parties, while a traditional contract requires manual execution by intermediaries. Table 14.2 shows the key differences between a smart contract and a traditional contract.

14.7 CONSENSUS

Consensus refers to the process by which the network of nodes in a blockchain system reaches an agreement on the validity of transactions and the state of the ledger. In a blockchain system, each node has a copy of the ledger, and all nodes work together to validate transactions and add new blocks to the chain. Consensus mechanisms ensure that all nodes agree on the contents of the blockchain and prevent any malicious actors from manipulating the system.

There are several consensus mechanisms used in blockchain frameworks, including PoW, PoS, DPoS, and BFT (Byzantine Fault Tolerance). Each of

Table 14.1 Feature-Wise Comparison of Blockchain Frameworks

Feature Comparison	*Hyperledger Fabric*	*Ethereum*	*Corda*	*EOSIO*	*IOTA*	*Quorum*
Type of network	Permissioned	Permissionless	Permissioned	Permissioned	Permissionless	Permissioned
Consensus algorithm	Practical Byzantine Fault Tolerant (PBFT)	Proof-of-work (PoW), Proof-of-stake (PoS)	Pluggable consensus algorithm	Delegated proof-of-stake (DPoS)	Tangle	Istanbul BFT
Smart contract language	Go, Java, JavaScript	Solidity	Kotlin, Java	C++, WebAssembly	Solidity	Solidity
Ledger type	Chain	Chain	Database	Chain	DAG	Chain
Scalability	Can manage hundreds of transactions per second	Limited scalability, can manage around 15 transactions per second	Can manage hundreds of transactions per second	Can manage thousands of transactions per second	Can manage thousands of transactions per second	Can manage hundreds of transactions per second
Transaction finality	Immediate finality	Finality in a few minutes	Finality in a few minutes	Finality in a few seconds	Finality in a few seconds	Finality in a few seconds
Privacy	Supports private transactions	Not inherently private, but can implement private transactions	Supports private transactions	Supports private transactions	Public ledger with no inherent privacy	Supports private transactions
Use cases	Enterprise applications, supply chain, financial services	Decentralized applications, smart contracts, cryptocurrency	Financial services, trade finance, healthcare	Decentralized applications, social media, gaming	IoT, supply chain, data integrity	Financial services, supply chain

(*Continued*)

Table 14.1 (Continued) Feature-Wise Comparison of Blockchain Frameworks

Feature Comparison	*Hyperledger Fabric*	*Ethereum*	*Corda*	*EOSIO*	*IOTA*	*Quorum*
Supported programming languages	Go, Java, JavaScript	Solidity, Vyper	Kotlin, Java	C++	JAVA, Solidity, Python	Solidity
Node type	Peer nodes, orderer nodes	Full nodes, light nodes	Notary nodes, regular nodes	Producer nodes, validator nodes	Full nodes, light nodes	Full nodes, light nodes
Data storage	LevelDB, CouchDB, and others	Ethereum World State, other databases	Corda Vault, others	RocksDB, others	Tangle	RocksDB, others
Token support	Can be used to represent assets	Native cryptocurrency (Ether), can create custom tokens	Can represent assets	Can represent assets	IOTA	Native cryptocurrency (Quorum Token), can create custom tokens

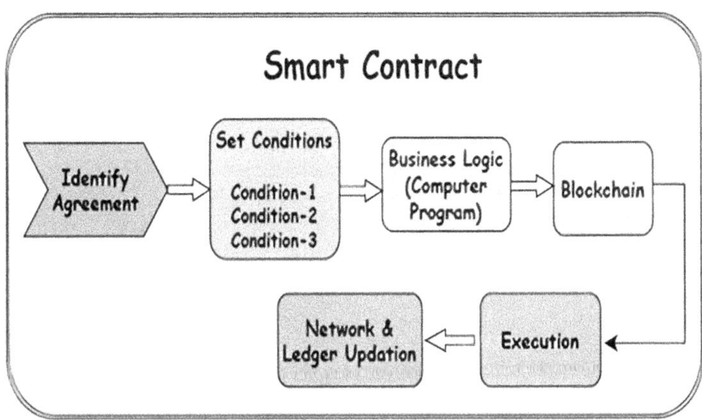

Figure 14.5 Basic structure of the smart contract

Table 14.2 Smart Contract versus Traditional Contact

Feature	*Smart Contract*	*Traditional Contract*
Execution	Self-executing and automated	Manual execution by intermediaries
Transparency	Stored on a public blockchain network, transparent	Typically, not transparent, known only to the parties involved
Security	Stored on a decentralized blockchain network, tamper-proof	Susceptible to fraud and tampering
Flexibility	Highly flexible and programmable	Rigid and difficult to modify once signed
Cost	Can reduce transaction costs by eliminating intermediaries	Can be expensive due to manual execution and processing
Efficiency	Can automate complex business processes, faster and more efficient	Often slow and require manual intervention
Trust	Designed to be trustless, do not rely on trust between parties	Require trust between parties, difficult to enforce in case of dispute

these mechanisms has advantages and disadvantages in terms of security, scalability, and energy efficiency.

In PoW, nodes compete to solve a cryptographic puzzle to validate transactions and add new blocks to the chain. This mechanism is used in Bitcoin and other early blockchain systems but has been criticized for its high energy consumption [34].

In PoS, nodes are chosen to validate transactions based on the amount of cryptocurrency they hold, rather than their computational power. This mechanism is used in newer blockchain systems such as Ethereum 2.0 and aims to be more energy efficient than PoW.

In DPoS, a smaller group of nodes is chosen to validate transactions on behalf of the larger network, making the consensus process more efficient [35]. This mechanism is used in blockchain systems such as EOS and Tron.

In BFT, nodes communicate with each other to reach a consensus on the state of the ledger, even if some nodes are faulty or malicious. This mechanism is used in enterprise blockchain systems such as Hyperledger Fabric [36].

14.8 BLOCKCHAIN AND IOT

Blockchain technology has the potential to bring significant benefits to IoT applications and projects across various sectors. It has revolutionized the way we connect and communicate with IoT devices. There are more than 20 billion active smartphones and IoT devices [37]. IoT devices have become an important component of most sensor-based networks, providing remote monitoring. IoT-based applications of healthcare include patient monitoring (body sensing and disease diagnosis), and for industrial automation, security and surveillance play great roles. However, this also introduces some challenges, specifically related to privacy and security, especially in sensitive information sharing.

By combining blockchain with the IoT, we can expect secure communication. In healthcare, IoT devices such as wearables, smart sensors, and medical devices generate large amounts of sensitive data. By leveraging blockchain's distributed and decentralized nature, IoT devices can securely and transparently share data and execute transactions without intermediaries [38]. One of the main benefits of using blockchain in IoT is increased security. Using blockchain to store and secure IoT data makes it much harder for malicious actors to tamper with or steal sensitive information. Additionally, blockchain can help establish trust between IoT devices and their owners, as all data and transactions are recorded and verified on an immutable ledger.

Numerous industries, as depicted in Figure 14.6 [39], can benefit from combining IoT and blockchain, including healthcare, supply chain management, agriculture, energy management, transportation, and smart cities. By providing a secure and transparent platform for sharing data between different parties, blockchain can help improve efficiency, reduce costs, and improve the quality and safety of products and services.

However, there are also some challenges associated with integrating blockchain and IoT. For example, the energy and computational requirements of blockchain can be a bottleneck for resource-constrained IoT devices. Additionally, there may be challenges around standardization and interoperability between different blockchain and IoT systems. Overall, the

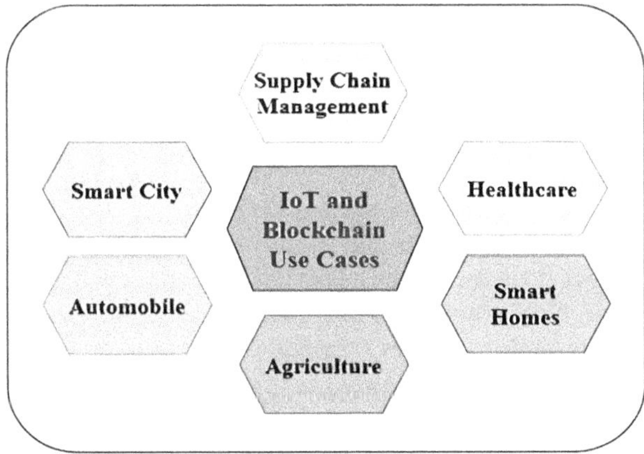

Figure 14.6 IoT and blockchain use cases

combination of blockchain and IoT has the potential to transform how we interact with and manage connected devices and could lead to new use cases and business models in various industries.

14.9 COMPARISON OF VARIOUS BLOCKCHAIN FRAMEWORKS

Using the literature review and information from various online sources, feature-wise and various important parameters like consensus algorithm, smart contract, privacy, use cases, and scalability of blockchain frameworks are discussed in Table 14.1, which compares important aspects of these frameworks used in a variety of projects.

14.10 CONCLUSION

Blockchain technology has the potential to revolutionize IoT by providing a secure and decentralized way for devices to communicate and exchange data. In terms of comparison, each of these blockchain technologies has strengths and weaknesses. As per the literature review, we found that the Hyperledger Fabric, Ethereum, Corda, Quorum, IOTA, and EOSIO are the blockchain frameworks that are used in various projects. Ethereum is more flexible and supports a wide range of dApps, but it can be slower and more expensive than other blockchain technologies. IOTA is specifically designed for IoT and has a unique consensus algorithm that is well-suited for IoT use cases, but security is the main concern with this framework. The EOSIO framework is good at handling high transaction volumes with a fast processing time with low latency, but it has many other issues related to its governance model, security concerns, and technical complexity.

Hyperledger Fabric, Ethereum, and Corda are the most popular among these blockchain frameworks. Hyperledger Fabric and Corda are both designed for use in enterprise environments and allow for the creation of private, permissioned blockchain networks, but they may be a little more complex to use and require more technical expertise. Corda is specifically designed for the financial sector and is not suitable for resource-constrained IoT networks. Most of the studies say that Hyperledger Fabric is the most popular and effective framework for decentralized applications and also good for resource-constrained IoT networks, as far as our literature review is concerned. In most of the studies, the authors suggested that throughput and latency are good in Hyperledger Fabric and scalability is also good.

The best blockchain technology for an IoT use case will depend on the specific requirements and goals of the project.

REFERENCES

1. B. Shah, N. Shah, S. Shakhla, and V. Sawant, "Remodeling the healthcare industry by employing blockchain technology," in *2018 International Conference on Circuits and Systems in Digital Enterprise Technology (ICCSDET)*, pp. 1–5.
2. GeeksforGeeks, "Blockchain structure," Nov. 16, 2022. https://www.geeksforgeeks.org/blockchain-structure/ (accessed Mar. 10, 2023).
3. M. Swan, *Blockchain: Blueprint for a New Economy.* O'Reilly Media, Inc., USA, 2015.
4. R. Böhme, N. Christin, B. Edelman, and T. Moore, "Bitcoin: Economics, technology, and governance," *Journal of Economic Perspectives*, vol. 29, no. 2, pp. 213–238, 2015.
5. T. A. Syed, A. Alzahrani, S. Jan, M. S. Siddiqui, A. Nadeem, and T. Alghamdi, "A comparative analysis of blockchain architecture and its applications: Problems and recommendations," *IEEE Access*, vol. 7, pp. 176838–176869, 2019.
6. Z. Zheng, S. Xie, H. Dai, X. Chen, and H. Wang, "An overview of blockchain technology: Architecture, consensus, and future trends," in *2017 IEEE International Congress on Big Data (BigData Congress)*, 2017, pp. 557–564.
7. H. Pervez, M. Muneeb, M. U. Irfan, and I. U. Haq, "A comparative analysis of DAG-based blockchain architectures," in *2018 12th International Conference on Open Source Systems and Technologies (ICOSST)*, 2018, pp. 27–34.
8. S. Kumar, W. M. Lim, U. Sivarajah, and J. Kaur, "Artificial intelligence and blockchain integration in business: Trends from a bibliometric-content analysis," *Information Systems Frontiers*, pp. 1–26, 2022.
9. C. Cachin and others, "Architecture of the Hyperledger blockchain fabric," in *Workshop on Distributed Cryptocurrencies and Consensus Ledgers*, 2016, pp. 1–4.

10. J. Polge, J. Robert, and Y. le Traon, "Permissioned blockchain frameworks in the industry: A comparison," *ICT Express*, vol. 7, no. 2, pp. 229–233, 2021.
11. E. Tarasenko, "Transaction processing: Hyperledger fabric," Feb. 10, 2023. https://merehead.com/blog/benefits-of-blockchain-hyperledger-fabric/ (accessed Mar. 10, 2023).
12. A. Iftekhar, X. Cui, Q. Tao, and C. Zheng, "Hyperledger fabric access control system for internet of things layer in blockchain-based applications," *Entropy*, vol. 23, no. 8, p. 1054, 2021.
13. H. Honar Pajooh, M. A. Rashid, F. Alam, and S. Demidenko, "Experimental performance analysis of a scalable distributed hyperledger fabric for a large-scale IoT testbed," *Sensors*, vol. 22, no. 13, p. 4868, 2022.
14. C. Gorenflo, S. Lee, L. Golab, and S. Keshav, "FastFabric: Scaling hyperledger fabric to 20 000 transactions per second," *International Journal of Network Management*, vol. 30, no. 5, p. e2099, 2020.
15. M. Schäffer, M. di Angelo, and G. Salzer, "Performance and scalability of private Ethereum blockchains," in *Business Process Management: Blockchain and Central and Eastern Europe Forum: BPM 2019 Blockchain and CEE Forum, Vienna, Austria, September 1–6, 2019, Proceedings 17*, 2019, pp. 103–118.
16. V. Buterin, "A next-generation smart contract and decentralized application platform," *White Paper*, vol. 3, no. 37, pp. 1–2, 2014.
17. Paul, "Ethereum architecture," Nov. 21, 2022. https://www.edureka.co/blog/ethereum-tutorial-with-smart-contracts/ (accessed Mar. 10, 2023).
18. M. Yutaka, Y. Zhang, M. Sasabe, and S. Kasahara, "Using Ethereum blockchain for distributed attribute-based access control in the internet of things," in *2019 IEEE Global Communications Conference (GLOBECOM)*, 2019, pp. 1–6.
19. M. Benji and M. Sindhu, "A study on the Corda and Ripple blockchain platforms," in *Advances in Big Data and Cloud Computing, Proceedings of the ICBDCC18*, 2019, pp. 179–187.
20. R. G. Brown, "The corda platform: An introduction," *Retrieved*, vol. 27, p. 2018, 2018.
21. D. Lee and D. H. Lee, "Push and pull: Manipulating a production schedule and maximizing rewards on the Eosio blockchain," in *Proceedings of the Third ACM Workshop on Blockchains, Cryptocurrencies and Contracts*, 2019, pp. 11–21.
22. Y. Huang, B. Jiang, and W. K. Chan, "EOSFuzzer: Fuzzing Eosio smart contracts for vulnerability detection," in *Proceedings of the 12th Asia-Pacific Symposium on Internetware*, 2020, pp. 99–109.
23. N. He et al., "Understanding the evolution of blockchain ecosystems: A longitudinal measurement study of Bitcoin, Ethereum, and EOSIO," *arXiv preprint arXiv:2110.07534*, 2021.
24. A. Baliga, I. Subhod, P. Kamat, and S. Chatterjee, "Performance evaluation of the quorum blockchain platform," *arXiv preprint arXiv:1809.03421*, 2018.
25. D. Ongaro and J. Ousterhout, "In search of an understandable consensus algorithm," in *2014 {USENIX} Annual Technical Conference ({USENIX} {ATC} 14)*, 2014, pp. 305–319.
26. P. Szilagyi, "Clique proof-of-authority consensus protocol, Ethereum improvement proposals," Mar. 1, 2017. https://eips.ethereum.org/EIPS/eip-225 (accessed Mar. 07, 2023).

27. H. Moniz, "The Istanbul BFT consensus algorithm," *arXiv preprint arXiv:2002.03613*, 2020.
28. M. Mazzoni, A. Corradi, and V. Di Nicola, "Performance evaluation of permissioned blockchains for financial applications: The ConsenSys Quorum case study," *Blockchain: Research and Applications*, vol. 3, no. 1, p. 100026, 2022.
29. IOTA Dev, Team, "Introduction to IOTA," Sep. 28, 2022. https://wiki.iota.org/learn/about-iota/an-introduction-to-iota/ (accessed Mar. 7, 2023).
30. S. Popov, "The tangle," Apr. 30, 2018. https://assets.ctfassets.net/r1dr6vzfxhev/2t4uxvsIqk0EUau6g2sw0g/45eae33637ca92f85dd9f4a3a218e1ec/iota1_4_3.pdf (accessed Mar. 7, 2023).
31. R. Conti and B. Curry, "What is IOTA & how does it work," Jan. 30, 2023. https://www.forbes.com/advisor/investing/cryptocurrency/what-is-iota/ (accessed Mar. 07, 2023).
32. R. Agrawal and N. Gupta, *Transforming Cybersecurity Solutions Using Blockchain*. France: Springer, 2021.
33. B. K. Mohanta, S. S. Panda, and D. Jena, "An overview of smart contract and use cases in blockchain technology," in *2018 9th International Conference on Computing, Communication and Networking Technologies (ICCCNT)*, 2018, pp. 1–4.
34. D. Mingxiao, M. Xiaofeng, Z. Zhe, W. Xiangwei, and C. Qijun, "A review on consensus algorithm of blockchain," in *2017 IEEE International Conference on Systems, Man, and Cybernetics (SMC)*, 2017, pp. 2567–2572.
35. M. S. Ferdous, M. J. M. Chowdhury, M. A. Hoque, and A. Colman, "Blockchain consensus algorithms: A survey," *arXiv preprint arXiv:2001.07091*, 2020.
36. G.-T. Nguyen and K. Kim, "A survey about consensus algorithms used in blockchain," *Journal of Information Processing Systems*, vol. 14, no. 1, pp. 101–128, 2018.
37. Statista, "Internet of Things (IoT) Connected devices installed base Worldwide from 2015 to 2025 (in Billions)," 2018. https://www.statista.com/statistics/471264/iotnumber- of-connected-devices-worldwide/ (accessed Mar. 08, 2023).
38. A. S. Rajawat, R. Rawat, K. Barhanpurkar, R. N. Shaw, and A. Ghosh, "Blockchain-based model for expanding IoT device data security," *Advances in Applications of Data-Driven Computing*, pp. 61–71, 2021.
39. D. Pavithran, K. Shaalan, J. N. Al-Karaki, and A. Gawanmeh, "Towards building a blockchain framework for IoT," *Cluster Computing*, vol. 23, May 2020, doi: 10.1007/s10586-020-03059-5.

Chapter 15

IoT and Healthcare

Development, Architecture, Security, and Its Applicability in Healthcare

Mohit Lalit, Gaurav Bathla, Surender Singh, and Shiraz Khurana

15.1 INTRODUCTION TO IOT

In this digital age, the internet has become ubiquitous, connecting almost everyone, and giving rise to the Internet of Things (IoT). This advancement allows us to control nearby physical objects through handheld devices, expanding mobile-to-mobile and mobile-to-business interactions to unprecedented levels. The present moment presents a prime opportunity to fully tap into the potential of IoT applications across various domains, including health, agriculture, smart cities, smart grids, and automated workplaces. While the exact impact and coverage of IoT in these fields are challenging to measure, its advantages and influence on human life are evident.

To develop effective IoT applications, a secure and standardized architecture is essential to deliver high-quality services. Ensuring seamless communication between physical devices, employing various methods like audio and wireless handheld devices, is a crucial part of the process. However, this data transfer requires protection against potential malicious attacks that may attempt to steal information or modify intended instructions. Past efforts have used various approaches to safeguard data in wireless sensor networks, and newer technologies like machine learning and blockchain are being developed to identify attack patterns based on historical records.

In today's world, we are surrounded by an ever-increasing number of computing devices, and to fully utilize their capabilities, we require parallel communication technology. It is predicted that over 50 billion mobile devices will be operational by 2021, and this number is expected to grow rapidly [1]. The field of IoT has experienced rapid development, driven by innovations in various technological domains like machine learning, big data, artificial intelligence, cloud computing, fog computing, augmented reality, and virtual reality.

15.1.1 Development of IoT

Initially, computer communication was developed to ensure the secure transfer of valuable data and virtual assets. As technology advanced, a

DOI: 10.1201/9781003466949-15

five-step model emerged, revolutionizing the internet's impact and adaptability among people with each step [2]. This five-step model eventually led to the realm of IoT, as depicted in Figure 15.1. These are the following footprints of the development of IoT:

(i) Initially, individuals relied on offline computers with wired connections to transfer their valuable virtual assets.
(ii) In the second step, we entered the era of the internet with the World Wide Web.
(iii) The third step saw people connecting to the internet through their mobile phones.
(iv) The fourth step involved connecting through social media websites and mobile applications.
(v) Finally, in the fifth step, we unlock the door to IoT, harnessing the internet's full potential by enabling handheld devices to wirelessly operate objects around us.

IoT empowers individuals to establish connections between any object, regardless of time or location, utilizing diverse data services across networks. Within the realm of IoT, novel ideas are emerging, such as the Social Internet of Things (SIoT), linking human entities with social networks [3]. Equally notable is the rise of the Industrial Internet of Things (IIoT), geared toward revolutionizing manufacturing systems into intelligent, self-operating entities endowed with autonomous decision-making capabilities.

15.1.2 Application Areas of IoT

IoT has gained significant prominence in the global market due to its extensive and diverse applications. Researchers constantly strive for innovations and developments to enhance human life and address the challenges posed by urbanization and resource scarcity in metropolises. Various researchers have conducted impactful research in IoT, focusing on their interests, and its profound impact on society and human life can be observed in its various application areas, as shown in Figure 15.2.

One major advancement is the implementation of smart home systems (SHS), making appliances autonomous and ensuring steady and reliable power management [4]. Another notable achievement is the smart

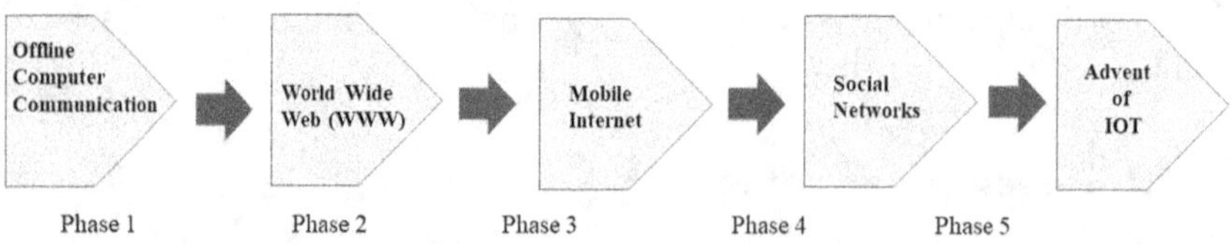

Figure 15.1 Development phase of IoT

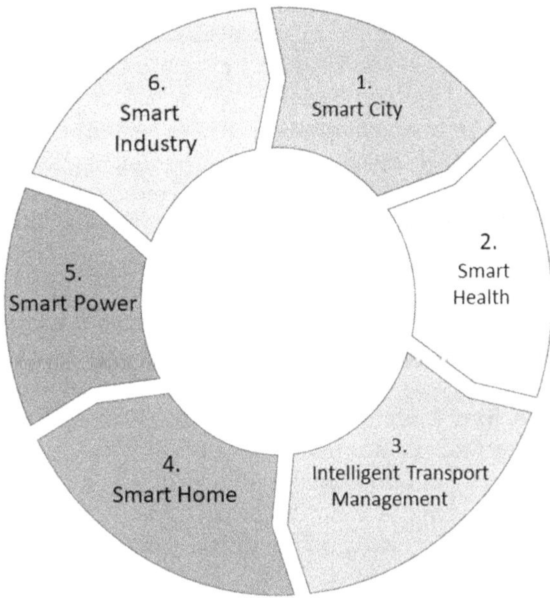

Figure 15.2 Potential IOT application areas

management of health, enabled by the installation of smart sensors to monitor health indoors and outdoors. This allows for easy tracking of calories burned, sugar levels, blood pressure, and more [5, 6]. Furthermore, IoT has positively impacted the lives of disabled and physically challenged individuals, with researchers and developers tirelessly working to introduce new features that can improve their lives at minimal costs [7].

Additionally, IoT has brought about significant changes in the transportation sector by offering smart transportation solutions through the installation of smart sensors in vehicles. This provides real-time information about heavy traffic routes through car GPS systems. IoT also facilitates intelligent traffic signal management using drones and other sensors near traffic lights [8].

15.1.3 Architecture of IoT

IoT has evolved from being just a term to a well-established concept within society, offering optimistic applications that enhance human life and comfort. By 2025's conclusion, forecasts anticipate a staggering count of around 75.44 billion IoT-enabled devices, translating to an average of 10 intelligent devices per individual [3]. The key to IoT's success lies in its ability to connect heterogeneous devices through the internet. To facilitate the connection of diverse devices, a layered architecture is essential. The OSI (Open Systems Interconnection) layered architecture was initially considered, but it proved insufficient. In recent times, various architectures have been proposed, but researchers have not yet reached a consensus on a unified architecture that can effectively meet the execution requirements of IoT applications [9]. In the IoT framework, data is collected through actuators at the perception layer, and then the raw information undergoes further processing through the network layer, which involves selecting suitable routing protocols and paths. Finally, the processed information is delivered to the relevant users or devices through the application layer, as shown in Figure 15.3.

While the five-layer architecture shares some common layers with the three-layer architecture, it also includes additional layers with specific objectives to enhance the overall model. The middleware layer plays a crucial role by evaluating the ubiquitous information received from the network layer [10]. Its primary function is to refine the complex data received in rough form before sending it to the application layer. Furthermore, the five-layer architectural framework introduces the inclusion of a business layer, tasked with formulating business models, graphs, and charts using data derived from the application layer. This specialized layer plays a pivotal role in converting information obtained from the application layer into visually informative graphs and charts.

The next section of the chapter dissects the vulnerabilities faced at various layers of IoT systems. It breaks down security attacks and corresponding preventive strategies for perception, network, and application layers. IoT's impact in the healthcare realm is profound and multifaceted. Section 15.3 elucidates the specific applications within healthcare. It showcases the contributions of smart medical devices such as wearables, remote patient monitoring, and data analytics for proactive care. In conclusion, this chapter encapsulates the transformative potential of IoT in various domains,

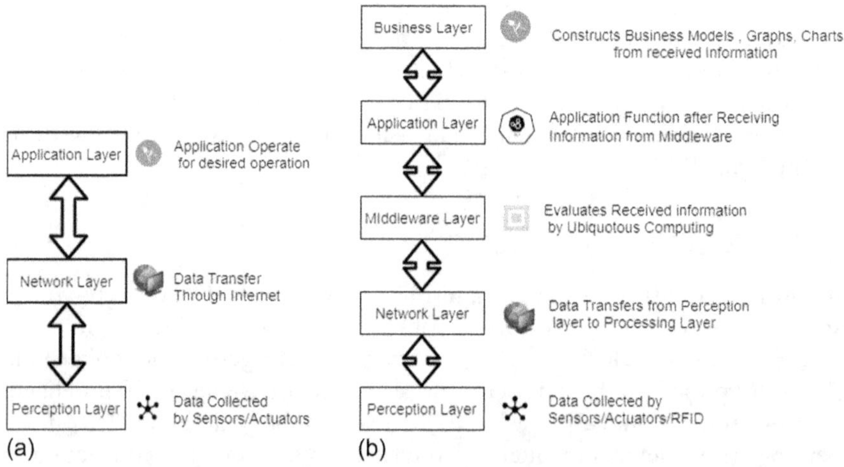

Figure 15.3 (a) Three-layer architecture, (b) five-layer architecture

particularly healthcare. It recaps the key points presented throughout the chapter, highlighting the significance of a unified architecture and strong security measures for successful IoT implementation. Looking ahead, the chapter contemplates the trajectory of IoT and its potential impact on future healthcare advancements, underscoring the ongoing importance of this dynamic technology.

15.2 IOT SECURITY

The expanding realm of IoT embraces an extensive array of application domains, spanning from smart city and smart home environments to smart transportation, smart logistics, smart health, smart agriculture, smart hospitality, smart fleet, and smart grid systems. These applications harness the considerable benefits of the internet, underscoring the fact that there remains untapped potential within the internet, guaranteeing its ongoing significance for the foreseeable times ahead.

However, the widespread use of the internet for communication and data transfer in IoT applications poses significant challenges for researchers. Handling such complex systems and high-end technologies while ensuring the secure transfer of sensitive information among devices is a major concern. Past incidents, such as the Mirai malware attack in 2016, have exposed the vulnerabilities in wireless printers, micro monitors, internet protocol (IP)-based CCTVs, and gateways, highlighting the importance of communication security in IoT. One of the challenges lies in the unrestricted connectivity of devices through the internet, which lacks proper access mechanisms. Additionally, the absence of standardized security protocols that can universally protect all IoT devices adds to the complexity of ensuring data security in IoT applications. It is imperative to tackle these security concerns to fully unleash the potential of IoT and facilitate its secure and dependable integration across diverse sectors.

15.2.1 Attacks and Prevention in IoT

IoT encompasses objects with diverse properties, and each device has its unique way of communication. Security plays a crucial role in ensuring the safety of data transfer, providing a bundle of services such as protecting against tampering, ensuring authenticity, preserving privacy, authorizing access, and preventing information leakage [11]. However, due to the lack of a uniform architecture for all devices in IoT, ensuring security during data transfer becomes a significant challenge.

IoT extends its services to various application areas, including smart cities, smart homes, smart health, and transportation, as depicted in Figure 15.2. Dealing with such sensitive applications makes security a major concern in IoT.

As illustrated in Figure 15.4, data is collected and processed at three major levels in the IoT architecture. At the perception layer, data is collected through various devices such as radio-frequency identification (RFID), actuators, sensors, and Bluetooth. This data is then transferred through the network layer to cloud services in the background, and finally, the requested data is sent to the respective applications through the application layer. Unfortunately, these multilayer platforms are vulnerable to security breaches at different levels. At the device or perception layer, attacks like tracking, robustness, eavesdropping, spoofing, information gathering, node supervision, and false node messages can easily occur [12, 13]. The network level is susceptible to attacks like bluejacking, denial-of-service (DOS) attacks, corruption, identity management issues, encryption vulnerabilities, and physical security breaches [11, 14, 15]. Last, at the application layer, attacks such as data privacy breaches, tampering, and access control violations can have serious consequences [12]. Although countermeasures exist at each layer to address these security challenges, the frequency of attacks and unethical activities continues to rise. To effectively combat such

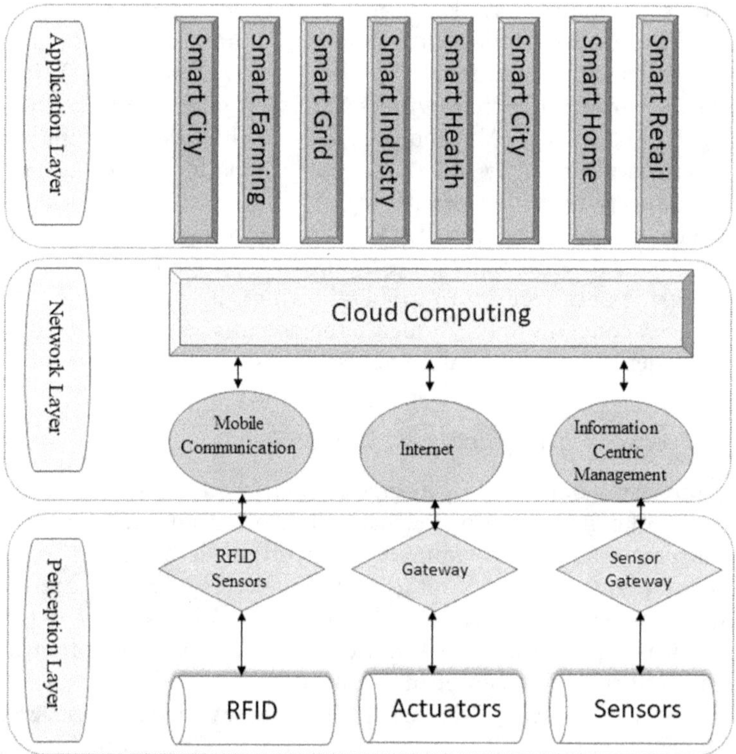

Figure 15.4 Working diagram of IP stack

attacks, researchers must continuously upgrade security measures to protect the integrity and privacy of IoT systems.

15.2.2 Perception Layer

15.2.2.1 Perception Nodes

RFID sensors and tags play a crucial role in the initial stage of data collection to gather information [14]. However, these tags are vulnerable to various attacks such as eavesdropping, spoofing, and tampering. Additionally, there are risks of kill tags (tags blocked by predefined disabled commands), block tags, reverse engineering, and redundancy of viruses, all of which can compromise the security of RFID tags. Encryption and encoding schemes alone may not be sufficient to ensure the security of these physical devices. To enhance the security of RFID tags, different techniques can be implemented [16]. Nonlinear key algorithms can be utilized to strengthen security, and the use of IPsec (Internet Protocol Security) protocols can provide added protection. Additionally, employing ciphertext re-encryption algorithms can help conceal communication, further safeguarding the RFID system from potential attacks.

15.2.2.2 Sensor Nodes

Sensor nodes like ZigBee have different components than RFID tags [14], making them vulnerable to attacks like malicious node implantation and jamming [12]. For instance, in 2016, Philips smart bulbs fell victim to a malware attack exploiting the ZigBee radio protocol. GPS systems are also at risk of signal-level attacks, like jamming and spoofing, leading to time synchronization attacks (TSAs). Preventive measures like node identification and enhanced node privacy [17] can be employed to counter these threats.

15.2.2.3 Gateways

Sensor nodes are responsible for collecting and storing data on various environmental parameters [18], while sensor gateways facilitate network expansion and access. However, these channels are susceptible to attacks like DOS, hacking, and interception. Additionally, the perspective layer may face attacks such as differential power analysis and side-channel attacks [19]. To counter these threats, message security, onboard device security, and integration security are crucial measures [20].

15.2.3 Network Layer

The intermediate layer between the perception layer and application layer facilitates communication and data transfers, but it may have some vulnerabilities that pose risks to the overall architecture.

15.2.3.1 Mobile Services

Mobile devices play a crucial role in connecting various IoT applications, ranging from macro to mini communication devices. Smartphones offer extensive capabilities to connect with GPS, Bluetooth, and biometric systems, and employ communication methods like RF, low-rate wireless personal area networks (LR-WPANs), and near-field communication (NFC) [21]. Unfortunately, these communication devices are vulnerable to attacks such as sinkhole, blue snarfing, bluejacking, blue bugging, cloning, spoofing, early battery drain, and DOS. To address these security concerns, it is essential to enhance current methods with biometrics, access controls, and time-varying sessions.

15.2.3.2 Internet Services

The widely used internet relies on the TCP/IP for connectivity and security [22]. Security protocols like IPsec, SSH, and SSL are in place to protect against various attacks. However, with the internet accessible to people of all ages, security methods need reform to address identity theft, authentication issues, DDOS attacks, viruses, worms, and unauthorized access. Enhanced encryption methods, public key infrastructure (PKI), and communication privacy can help tackle these concerns [23].

15.2.4 Application Layer

IoT has made a significant impact on various application areas, such as agriculture, smart cities, transportation, and more. However, these areas also face vulnerabilities that can be exploited by software and encryption attacks. Software attacks often involve malicious agents like malware and trojans [24], while encryption attacks focus on cryptographic vulnerabilities [12]. To address these concerns, authentication, key agreement, and user privacy protection can be implemented. Among the vast IoT application areas, healthcare stands out as a rapidly growing field, deserving increased attention from researchers for further advancements.

15.3 IOT APPLICATIONS IN HEALTHCARE

Smart medical devices. Smart devices like wearables, diagnostic tools, and monitoring devices are crucial in healthcare for patient care. They share vital health stats with other systems, leading to informed actions. These devices offer personalized care, precise medication dosages, and timely reminders. The user-friendly interface keeps users engaged, setting daily goals, and receiving exercise notifications. Overall, smart devices such as biosensors and cognitive sensors [25, 26] improve patient outcomes and proactive health management.

Patient monitoring. During the COVID-19 pandemic, direct contact with infected patients posed a major challenge for healthcare professionals. Wearing safety equipment and masks all day was difficult. IoT devices came to the rescue by enabling remote patient monitoring. Doctors could keep track of patients' vital signs like blood pressure, heart rate, and oxygen levels efficiently and effectively. This information could also be shared with other experts for further medical assistance. In remote areas with limited access to doctors, IoT devices proved to be a boon [27, 28].

Data analysis–based proactive care. "A good doctor cures the disease, but a great doctor cures the cause" [29]. IoT devices generate vast amounts of data every second, which can be harnessed to pinpoint the root cause of diseases. Advanced analytics techniques, fueled by machine learning and deep learning, have the potential to aid in early disease detection, significantly increasing the chances of saving lives [28, 30, 31]. At a broader level, analytics can be employed to study health trends in specific demographic regions. Moreover, these analytics can be leveraged to optimize the allocation of resources based on the precise needs of the population [32].

Asset and inventory management. Hospitals can effectively employ IoT to monitor their inventory and medical equipment. Essential items like oxygen, which need to be readily available as reserves, can be efficiently managed using IoT devices. These devices enable real-time monitoring of equipment status and conditions, ensuring optimal resource utilization and minimizing wastage [33, 34].

Daily monitoring. In the present day, a smart home is no longer just a dream. IoT devices have become valuable tools for monitoring health and aiding people. They are particularly beneficial for individuals with chronic diseases like cancer, heart disease, stroke, diabetes, and arthritis. These devices can also be employed to track patients with neurological disorders such as Alzheimer's, sending alerts for emergencies like falls or fires. Furthermore, IoT devices contribute to enhancing the overall quality of life [35, 36].

Telehealth. Throughout the COVID-19 pandemic, many patients sought healthcare consultations through various communication media. IoT devices proved to be valuable for diagnosing and examining patients, especially in remote areas where access to doctors is limited due to resource constraints. This approach has also reduced the need for in-person visits to healthcare providers [37].

Medication management. IoT-based smart dispensers can effectively synchronize medication administration, ensuring timely and precise dosages. These devices enhance medication management and contribute to the safety of patients [38–39]. Additionally, they can send alerts to caretakers if any dosage is missed, and health professionals can be notified for intervention if needed [40, 41].

15.4 CONCLUSION

This book chapter explores the potential of IoT in leveraging the internet for diverse applications, making human life more convenient. IoT enables the connection of heterogeneous objects anywhere and anytime. Researchers continually seek ways to enhance human experiences. However, IoT lacks a uniform architecture to cater to all user demands and faces security challenges. The chapter highlights the crucial need for a unified architecture that can support various applications and objects driven by the internet. Additionally, it discusses the current applications of IoT in the healthcare sector. Security is another critical aspect of IoT that requires the utmost attention. Researchers have identified several security threats, including eavesdropping, tampering, fake identification, hacking, and information leakage, which may lead to undesirable consequences. Although IoT networks have security measures at different layers, they may not fully meet present and future security requirements. The chapter stresses the importance of a sustained and uniform architecture that effectively addresses security concerns.

REFERENCES

1. C. V. Networking. Cisco Global Cloud Index: Forecast. Google Scholar. https://scholar.google.com/scholar?hl=en&as_sdt=0%2C5&q=Networking%2C+C.V.+Cisco+Global+Cloud+Index%3A+Forecast+and+Methodology%2C+2014%E2%80%932019%3B+White+Paper%3B+Cisco%3A+San+Jose%2C+CA%2C+USA%2C+2013.&btnG= (accessed Jul. 30, 2022).
2. C. Perera, Y. Qin, J. Estrella, S. Reiff-Marganiec, and A. V. Vasilakos. 2017, "Fog computing for sustainable smart cities: A survey," *ACM Computing Surveys*, vol. 50, no. 3, doi: 10.1145/3057266.
3. L. Atzori, A. Iera, and G. Morabito. 2010, "The internet of things: A survey," *Elsevier*, Accessed: Nov. 01, 2022. [Online]. Available: https://www.sciencedirect.com/science/article/pii/S1389128610001568
4. C. Esposito, A. Castiglione, C. Tudorica, and F. Pop. 2017, "Security and privacy for cloud-based data management in the health network service chain: A microservice approach," *ieeexplore.ieee.org*, Accessed: Mar. 11, 2022. [Online]. Available: https://ieeexplore.ieee.org/abstract/document/8030494/
5. A. Sfar, E. Natalizio, Y. Challal, and Z. Chtourou. 2018, "A roadmap for security challenges in the Internet of Things," *Elsevier*, Accessed: Mar. 11, 2022. [Online]. Available: https://www.sciencedirect.com/science/article/pii/S2352864817300214
6. D. Minoli, K. Sohraby, and J. Kouns. 2017, "IoT security (IoTSec) considerations, requirements, and architectures," *ieeexplore.ieee.org*, Accessed: Mar. 11, 2022. [Online]. Available: https://ieeexplore.ieee.org/abstract/document/7983271/
7. C. Montenegro-Marin, P. Gaona-García, and J. Prieto. 2017, "Analysis of security mechanisms based on clusters IoT environments," doi: 10.9781/ijimai.2017.438.

8. F. Behrendt. 2019, "Cycling the smart and sustainable city: Analyzing EC policy documents on internet of things, mobility and transport, and smart cities," *mdpi.com*, doi: 10.3390/su11030763.
9. M. Yun and B. Yuxin. 2010, "Research on the architecture and key technology of Internet of Things (IoT) applied on smart grid," *ieeexplore.ieee.org*, Accessed: Feb. 27, 2023. [Online]. Available: https://ieeexplore.ieee.org/abstract/document/5557611/?casa_token=gQVn3dmT_0wAAAAA:c3loPz7frSiJfz01oikjaP4YzAbZFUJsd4DlenSZVAQbePLNlIFQC9ktR8bJK-6D2wT9TA
10. R. Khan, S. Khan, R. Zaheer, and S. Khan. 2012, "Future internet: The internet of things architecture, possible applications and key challenges," *ieeexplore.ieee.org*, Accessed: Jul. 26, 2023. [Online]. Available: https://ieeexplore.ieee.org/abstract/document/6424332/
11. A. D. Jurcut, R. Dojen, R. Gyorodi, A. Jurcut, and T. Coffey. 2008, "Analysis of a key-establishment security protocol," *researchgate.net*, Accessed: Jul. 26, 2023. [Online]. Available: https://www.researchgate.net/profile/Anca-Jurcut/publication/319979194_Analysis_of_a_key-establishment_security_protocol/links/0deec5297b3a74cacc000000/Analysis-of-a-key-establishment-security-protocol.pdf
12. Y. Zhang, Y. Shen, H. Wang, J. Yong, and X. Jiang. 2015, "On secure wireless communications for IoT under eavesdropper collusion," *ieeexplore.ieee.org*, Accessed: Jul. 26, 2023. [Online]. Available: https://ieeexplore.ieee.org/abstract/document/7350251/?casa_token=nyFa7R7H16AAAAAA:i1zTSPwBxjqXF9m90MMdNwYchYVPtHQByyDM7U8IA40PY9VgzZ2E8-BFb4gBxfbzcuVornOpAHpt4Q
13. Q. Jing, A. Vasilakos, J. Wan, J. Lu, and D. Qiu. 2014, "Security of the Internet of Things: Perspectives and challenges," *Springer*, Accessed: Jul. 26, 2023. [Online]. Available: https://link.springer.com/article/10.1007/s11276-014-0761-7
14. F. Alaba, M. Othman, I. Hashem, and F. Alotaibi. 2017, "Internet of Things security: A survey," *Elsevier*, doi: 10.1016/j.jnca.2017.04.002.
15. C. Bekara. 2014, "Security issues and challenges for the IoT-based smart grid," *Elsevier*, Accessed: Jul. 26, 2023. [Online]. Available: https://www.sciencedirect.com/science/article/pii/S1877050914009193
16. H. Kim and E. Lee. 2017, "Authentication and authorization for the Internet of Things," *ieeexplore.ieee.org*, Accessed: Jul. 26, 2023. [Online]. Available: https://ieeexplore.ieee.org/abstract/document/8057722/?casa_token=1CTDKBSqb5gAAAAA:Z-Sx2CfAUUFHg7iQ_vSY3JtOUfDO7gzPN1HKiDlNpB2PnVUWU7-RKdpWSP5gZ-mKiuq-Doopb50WtQ
17. A. Khalajmehrabadi, N. Gatsis, D. Akopian, and A. F. Taha. 2018, "Real-time rejection and mitigation of time synchronization attacks on the global positioning system," *ieeexplore.ieee.org*, Accessed: Jul. 26, 2023. [Online]. Available: https://ieeexplore.ieee.org/abstract/document/8245836/?casa_token=mRQ8xPX2y3sAAAAA:KyOjddu_cqT4K43KcjNK-5GyoAP0Uh-DivyGf8cbn3jdujAyi5x0BpPZIfUIUuOvUcOMMZjHXUHkJw
18. Y. Liu, C. Cheng, T. Gu, T. Jiang, and X. Li. 2015, "A lightweight authenticated communication scheme for smart grid," *ieeexplore.ieee.org*, Accessed: Jul. 26, 2023. [Online]. Available: https://ieeexplore.ieee.org/abstract/document/7295548/?casa_token=chW5krz8jtkAAAAA:BTU0qereI8EXy5K84PmdwYLyl7z-LNK4Ghh9lE0_lGsjPi78mftHGt6cJd2z8YaRVqM4SrLx-NS65Q

19. J. Deogirikar and A. Vidhate. 2017, “Security attacks in IoT: A survey,” *ieeexplore.ieee.org*, Accessed: Aug. 08, 2022. [Online]. Available: https://ieeexplore.ieee.org/abstract/document/8058363/
20. T. Kumar, P. Porambage, I. Ahmad, M. Liyanage, E. Harjula, and M. Ylianttila. 2018, “Securing gadget-free digital services,” *ieeexplore.ieee.org*, Accessed: Jul. 26, 2023. [Online]. Available: https://ieeexplore.ieee.org/abstract/document/8625918/?casa_token=songRWK5TykAAAAA:RN2QwSJK4Pc-yUL4si0dyKAAOdXO4DMJ4176gtBqFcg_NWwYSG--xg9-n7gTYe9rJ6C91-hSqhSF5A
21. U. Fiore, A. Castiglione, A. De Santis, and F. Palmieri. 2017, “Exploiting battery-drain vulnerabilities in mobile smart devices,” *ieeexplore.ieee.org*, Accessed: Jul. 26, 2023. [Online]. Available: https://ieeexplore.ieee.org/abstract/document/7890475/?casa_token=1F3CjvZPZ9UAAAAA:0fJyFZxeYMvXxR91BWhnZIqyePz3_PEBbaUahjwLMDjEr_iVVkRI6ghFkjVdPVghraHvkHcQwV2rdQ
22. J. Singh, T. Pasquier, J. Bacon, H. Ko, and D. Eyers. 2015, “Twenty security considerations for cloud-supported Internet of Things,” *ieeexplore.ieee.org*, Accessed: Jul. 26, 2023. [Online]. Available: https://ieeexplore.ieee.org/abstract/document/7165580/?casa_token=BBLl2JDnPqQAAAAA:UPWwhbXGEWQSHhTDL2VEmmE7mRMyyCjdR-UDH0Dhq1FZIIdR4pfpfbqoIunJzbHKtWDtWEB_YU4q7g
23. P. Porambage, J. Okwuibe, M. Liyanage, M. Ylianttila, and T. Taleb. 2018, “Survey on multi-access edge computing for internet of things realization,” *ieeexplore.ieee.org*, Accessed: Jul. 26, 2023. [Online]. Available: https://ieeexplore.ieee.org/abstract/document/8391395/?casa_token=o8QuDjRjw0I-AAAAA:dikDB2nU3BLflIIIicMmAbuqUFfsRHJ0o0Kq2CKYuR-mbOwru-Dbliw5qchiiX8ZyhKRyAAevaztug
24. O. Garcia-Morchon, S. Kumar, R. Struik, S. Keoh, and R. Hummen. Google Scholar. https://scholar.google.com/scholar?hl=en&as_sdt=0%2C5&q=30.%09Garcia-Morchon%2C+O.%2C+Kumar%2C+S.%2C+Keoh%2C+S.%2C+Hummen%2C+R.%2C+%26+Struik%2C+R.+%282013%29.+Security+Considerations+in+the+IP-based+Internet+of+Things+draft-garciacore-security-06.+Internet+Engineering+Task+Force.&btnG= (accessed Jul. 26, 2023).
25. M. Pateraki, K. Fysarakis, V. Sakkalis, G. Spanoudakis, I. Varlamis, M. Maniadakis, M. Lourakis, S. Ioannidis, N. Cummins, B. Schuller, E. Loutsetis, and D. Koutsouris. 2020, “Biosensors and Internet of Things in smart healthcare applications: Challenges and opportunities,” *Elsevier*, Accessed: Jul. 26, 2023. [Online]. Available: https://www.sciencedirect.com/science/article/pii/B9780128153697000021
26. S. Khare, A. Khan, V. Bajaj, and G. R. Sinha. 2023, “Introduction to smart healthcare and the role of cognitive sensors,” *iopscience.iop.org*, Accessed: Jul. 26, 2023. [Online]. Available: https://iopscience.iop.org/book/edit/978-0-7503-5346-5/chapter/bk978-0-7503-5346-5ch1
27. A. H. Sodhro and N. Zahid. 2021, “AI-enabled framework for fog computing driven E-healthcare applications,” *Sensors*, vol. 21, no. 23, doi: 10.3390/s21238039.

28. A. Kishor and W. Jeberson. 2021, "Diagnosis of heart disease using internet of things and machine learning algorithms," *Springer*, Accessed: Jul. 26, 2023. [Online]. Available: https://link.springer.com/chapter/10.1007/978-981-16-0733-2_49
29. L. Kania and V. Rao. 2021, "Restructuring radiology education to improve imaging specificity," *Elsevier*, Accessed: May 22, 2023. [Online]. Available: https://www.sciencedirect.com/science/article/pii/S1076633220303615
30. A. Kishor and C. Chakraborty. 2022, "Artificial Intelligence and Internet of Things based healthcare 4.0 monitoring system," *Wireless Personal Communications*, vol. 127, no. 2, pp. 1615–1631, doi: 10.1007/S11277-021-08708-5.
31. A. Kishor and C. Chakraborty. 2021, "Early and accurate prediction of diabetics based on FCBF feature selection and SMOTE," *International Journal of Systems Assurance Engineering and Management*, doi: 10.1007/S13198-021-01174-Z.
32. F. Bravo, M. Braun, V. Farias, R. Levi, C. Lynch, J. Tumolo, and R. Whyte. 2021, "Optimization-driven framework to understand health care network costs and resource allocation," *Health Care Manag Sci*, vol. 24, no. 3, pp. 640–660, doi: 10.1007/S10729-021-09565-1.
33. R. Kulkarni and S. Kulkarni. 2021, "Hospital asset management using IoT and RFID," *ijres.org*, vol. 9, pp. 2320–9356, Accessed: Jul. 27, 2023. [Online]. Available: https://www.ijres.org/papers/Volume-9/Issue-8/Series-6/A09080106.pdf
34. K. M. Lee, C. M. Na, and N. C. Kit. 2015, "IoT-based asset management system for healthcare-related industries," *International Journal of Engineering Business Management*, vol. 7, doi: 10.5772/61821.
35. J. Reena and R. Parameswari. 2019, "A smart health care monitor system in IoT based human activities of daily living: A review," *ieeexplore.ieee.org*, Accessed: Jul. 27, 2023. [Online]. Available: https://ieeexplore.ieee.org/abstract/document/8862439/
36. A. Siam, M. El-Affendi, A. A. Elazm, G. M. El-Banby, N. A. El-BahnaSawy, F. E. Abd El-Samie, and A. A. Abd El-Latif. 2022, "Portable and real-time IoT-based healthcare monitoring system for daily medical applications," *ieeexplore.ieee.org*, Accessed: Jul. 27, 2023. [Online]. Available: https://ieeexplore.ieee.org/abstract/document/9961104/
37. M. Rawashdeh, M. G. I. al Zamil, M. S. Hossain, S. Samarah, M. Rawashdeha, and M. G. AL Zamil. 2018, "Reliable service delivery in Tele-health care systems," *Elsevier*, doi: 10.1016/j.jnca.2018.04.015.
38. N. Thillaiarasu, S. Lata Tripathi, and V. Dhinakaran. (Eds.). (2022). *Artificial Intelligence for Internet of Things: Design Principle, Modernization, and Techniques* (1st ed.). CRC Press, Boca Raton, doi: 10.1201/9781003335801.
39. K. Kumar, K. Chaudhury, and S. L. Tripathi. 2023, "Future of Machine Learning (ML) and Deep Learning (DL) in healthcare monitoring system," in *Machine Learning Algorithms for Signal and Image Processing*, IEEE, pp. 293–313, doi: 10.1002/9781119861850.ch17.
40. T. Prasath, B. Krishna, S. Ajith Kumar, G. Karthick, G. Vishnuvarthanan, and S. Sakthivel. 2021, "A smart medicine box for medication management using IoT," *ieeexplore.ieee.org*, Accessed: Jul. 27, 2023. [Online]. Available: https://

ieeexplore.ieee.org/abstract/document/9725727/?casa_token=h2npYnrQb-C8AAAAA:Pt-dbSBzwpFxVp52WDRIen5QOMHwXfGPMbhT2DcIvI-cdsaE8BMlAFdzoKGy49hr50rGFA0M1lo
41. M. Srinivas, P. Durgaprasadarao, and V. Naga Prudhvi Raj. 2018, "Intelligent medicine box for medication management using IoT," *ieeexplore.ieee.org* , Accessed: Jul. 27, 2023. [Online]. Available: https://ieeexplore.ieee.org/abstract/document/8399097/?casa_token=FncdUmLgCLMAAAAA:aWmg-DxDx-wvXl7ajRI4f28smjj_zH6nlsB9uR7ERgPT4mkYx_vbWQdYLDDT6-2eowNs6sG_6uPQ

Chapter 16

Convergence of Blockchain and IoT in Healthcare

Opportunities and Challenges

Pawan Whig, Rashmi Gera, Ashima Bhatnagar Bhatia, Rahul Reddy Nadikattu, and Yusuf Jibrin Alkali

16.1 INTRODUCTION

The convergence of blockchain and the Internet of Things (IoT) is rapidly changing the healthcare industry by providing opportunities to improve the quality and efficiency of care while reducing costs. Blockchain is a decentralized, tamper-proof, and immutable ledger that provides a secure and transparent way of recording and sharing data [1–3]. IoT, on the other hand, enables the connection and communication between devices and objects, allowing the collection of vast amounts of data in real time [4]. Together, blockchain and IoT are transforming healthcare by enabling secure and efficient data sharing, enabling personalized medicine, and improving patient outcomes. However, the integration of these two technologies also poses several challenges that must be addressed to fully realize their potential in healthcare. One of the primary challenges is the need to ensure the security and privacy of patient data. Healthcare data is sensitive and personal, and any breach of security could have serious consequences [5–6]. Therefore, it is essential to ensure that patient data is protected from unauthorized access, hacking, and other security threats. Blockchain's decentralized and immutable nature makes it an ideal solution for securing sensitive data, and IoT can provide additional layers of security through encryption and authentication [7–9].

Another challenge is the interoperability of different systems and devices. The healthcare industry comprises various stakeholders, including patients, providers, payers, and regulators, who use different systems and devices that may not be compatible with each other. This lack of interoperability can lead to inefficiencies and errors in data sharing and communication [10–15]. Blockchain and IoT can help overcome this challenge by providing a standard, decentralized platform that allows for seamless data sharing and communication between different stakeholders. Furthermore, the integration of blockchain and IoT in healthcare requires a significant investment in infrastructure, including devices, sensors, networks, and software. Healthcare providers must also invest in the training of staff and the development of policies and procedures to ensure the effective and efficient use

DOI: 10.1201/9781003466949-16

of these technologies [16–19]. In addition, there may be legal and regulatory barriers to the adoption of blockchain and IoT in healthcare, including concerns about data ownership, liability, and consent.

Despite these challenges, the convergence of blockchain and IoT presents several opportunities for healthcare. For example, blockchain can enable secure and efficient data sharing, allowing healthcare providers to access patient data in real time, regardless of the location or system used to store it [20]. This can improve the accuracy and speed of diagnosis, treatment, and care, leading to better patient outcomes. Additionally, IoT can enable remote monitoring of patients, providing healthcare providers with real-time data on patient health and enabling personalized medicine. The convergence of blockchain and IoT can also lead to significant cost savings in healthcare by reducing administrative costs, preventing medical errors, and improving the efficiency of care delivery. For example, blockchain can automate and streamline administrative tasks, such as billing and insurance claims, reducing the need for intermediaries and minimizing errors. IoT can also enable predictive maintenance of medical equipment, reducing downtime and maintenance costs [21].

The convergence of blockchain and IoT is transforming the healthcare industry by providing opportunities to improve the quality and efficiency of care while reducing costs. However, this integration also poses several challenges that must be addressed, including ensuring the security and privacy of patient data, promoting interoperability, and investing in infrastructure and training [22–25]. Despite these challenges, the potential benefits of the convergence of blockchain and IoT in healthcare are enormous, and healthcare providers must be prepared to embrace these technologies to provide the best possible care to patients.

16.1.1 Background and Motivation

The healthcare industry has traditionally been characterized by siloed data systems, fragmented patient records, and inefficient administrative processes. This lack of interoperability and standardization has led to poor communication and collaboration among stakeholders, resulting in reduced quality of care and higher costs [26–28]. However, the convergence of blockchain and IoT presents an opportunity to overcome these challenges and transform the healthcare industry by enabling secure and efficient data sharing, personalized medicine, and improved patient outcomes.

16.1.2 Objectives and Scope

The objective of this study is to explore the convergence of blockchain and IoT in healthcare and identify the opportunities and challenges it presents. The study will focus on the following research questions:

1. What are the potential benefits of the convergence of blockchain and IoT in healthcare?
2. What are the challenges to the adoption of these technologies in healthcare, and how can they be addressed?
3. What are the key use cases and applications of blockchain and IoT in healthcare?
4. What are the ethical, legal, and regulatory considerations surrounding the use of these technologies in healthcare?

The scope of the study will be limited to the convergence of blockchain and IoT in the healthcare industry, with a particular focus on the use cases and applications of these technologies; their potential benefits and challenges; and the ethical, legal, and regulatory considerations associated with their adoption [29–30]. The study will draw upon a range of sources, including academic literature, industry reports, and case studies, to provide a comprehensive overview of the current state of the field and identify areas for further research and development.

16.2 BLOCKCHAIN AND IOT OVERVIEW

Blockchain and the IoT are two emerging technologies that have the potential to transform various industries, including healthcare.

Blockchain is a decentralized, tamper proof, and immutable digital ledger that enables secure and transparent recording and sharing of data. Each block in the chain contains a record of transactions, and once added to the chain, the information becomes permanent and unchangeable. This makes blockchain a secure and efficient way of recording and sharing data without the need for intermediaries or third-party verification.

IoT, on the other hand, refers to the network of physical objects, devices, sensors, and other technologies that are connected to the internet and communicate with each other. These devices can collect and transmit data in real time, enabling the monitoring and analysis of various parameters such as temperature, humidity, and movement. IoT technology enables the creation of smart homes, cities, and healthcare systems, among other applications.

The convergence of blockchain and IoT in healthcare can provide a secure and efficient way of sharing data and enabling personalized medicine as shown in Figure 16.1. For example, blockchain can ensure the security and privacy of patient data, while IoT can provide real-time data on patient health and enable remote monitoring [31].

Overall, the combination of blockchain and IoT technology has the potential to revolutionize the healthcare industry by enabling secure and efficient data sharing, improving patient outcomes, and reducing costs.

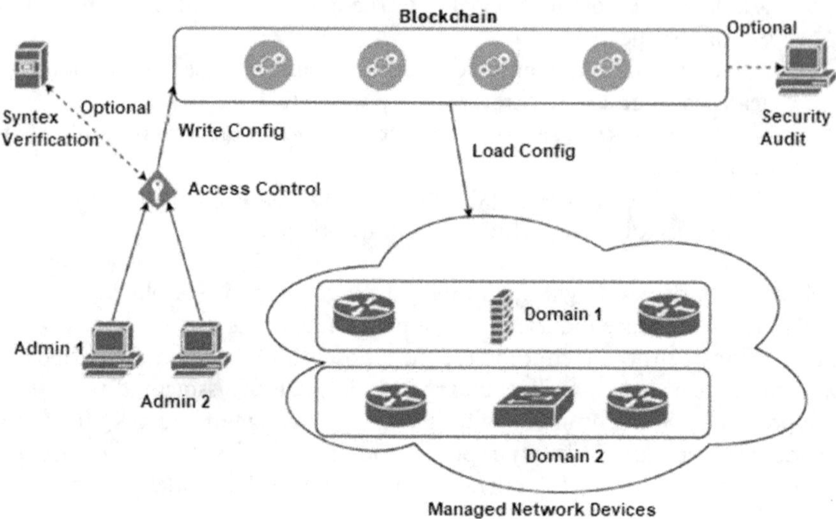

Figure 16.1 IoT implementation using blockchain

16.2.1 Blockchain and Its Principles

Blockchain is a distributed digital ledger technology that enables secure and transparent recording and sharing of data. It is based on several key principles, including:

1. Decentralization: Blockchain is a decentralized system, which means that it does not rely on a central authority or intermediary to manage transactions. Instead, transactions are recorded and verified by a network of nodes or computers.
2. Immutability: Once data is recorded on the blockchain, it cannot be altered or deleted. Each block in the chain contains a unique hash or digital signature, which ensures the integrity of the data and makes it tamper-proof.
3. Transparency: All transactions on the blockchain are visible to all participants in the network, providing a transparent and auditable record of all activity.
4. Security: Blockchain uses cryptography and other security measures to protect the data from unauthorized access, ensuring that only authorized parties can access and modify the data.
5. Consensus: Blockchain relies on a consensus mechanism to validate transactions and add them to the chain. This ensures that all participants in the network agree on the validity of the transactions, making it virtually impossible for fraudulent or malicious activity to occur. Some areas where blockchain is used are shown in Figure 16.2.

HEALTHCARE	GOVERNMENT	LEGAL
Electronic medical records can be accessed and updated via biometrics, allowing for the democratization of patient data and mitigate cumbersome record transferring between providers.	Governments can use blockchain technology to store populace data, criminal backgrounds, and e- citizenship, authorized by biometrics.	Smart Contracts stored in the blockchain can track contract parties, terms, transfer of ownership, and delivery of goods and services for legal intervention.
ENERGY	**BLOCKCHAIN FOR EVERY INDUSTRY**	**EDUCATION**
Decentralized energy transfer and distribution are possible via micro-transactions of data sent to blockchain, validated and re-dispersed to the grid.	Blockchain use cases beyond Bitcoin and Financial Services. Here are some opportunities in every vertical to effectively store transaction, customer, and supplier data in a transparent, immutable digital ledger.	Blockchain can be utilized to store credentialing data covering assessments, degrees, and transcripts and confirm verification of knowledge transfer.
SUPPLY CHAIN	**RETAIL**	**HOSPITATLITY**
Using the DL, or distributed ledger, companies within the supply chain can gain transparency into shipment tracking, deliveries, and progress amongst other suppliers.	Secure P2P marketplaces can track P2P retail transactions with product data, shipment, and bills of lading (BL or BoL) input via the blockchain.	Blockchain can be used to store authenticated "single travel ID" instead of individual pieces of travel documentation such as passports, tickets, loyalty program IDs.

Figure 16.2 Some areas where blockchain is used

These principles make blockchain a secure and efficient way of recording and sharing data without the need for intermediaries or third-party verification. This has numerous applications across various industries, including finance, supply chain management, and healthcare.

16.2.2 Internet of Things and Its Applications

The Internet of Things refers to a network of physical devices, sensors, and other technologies that are connected to the internet and can communicate with each other [32–35]. These devices can collect and transmit data in real time, enabling the monitoring and analysis of various parameters, such as temperature, humidity, and movement. IoT technology has numerous applications across various industries, including healthcare, transportation, and manufacturing. Some applications of IoT are shown in Figure 16.3.

In healthcare, IoT has the potential to revolutionize patient care by enabling remote monitoring, real-time data analysis, and personalized medicine [36–38]. Some of the applications of IoT in healthcare include:

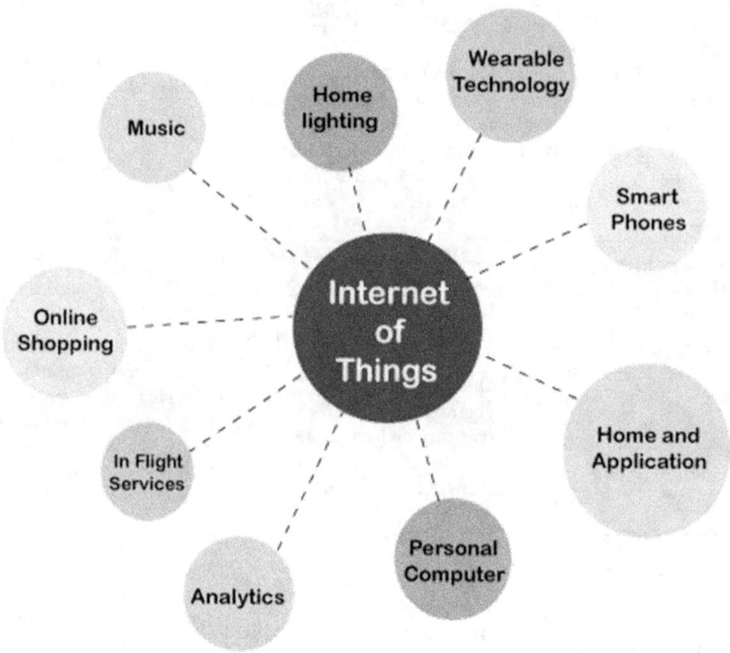

Figure 16.3 Application of IoT

1. Remote patient monitoring: IoT devices can be used to monitor patients remotely and collect real-time data on their health parameters such as heart rate, blood pressure, and glucose levels. This can help healthcare providers to detect and respond to health issues early and provide timely interventions.
2. Smart hospital systems: IoT devices can be used to automate and optimize various hospital systems, including inventory management, asset tracking, and patient flow. This can reduce costs and improve efficiency, ultimately leading to better patient outcomes.
3. Personalized medicine: IoT devices can be used to collect data on patient behavior, lifestyle, and genetics, enabling personalized medicine and tailored treatment plans.
4. Telemedicine: IoT devices can be used to enable remote consultations and virtual visits, providing patients with access to healthcare services from anywhere in the world.
5. Wearable technology: IoT devices such as wearable fitness trackers and smartwatches can be used to monitor and track various health parameters, enabling individuals to manage their health proactively.

IoT technology has the potential to transform healthcare by enabling remote monitoring, personalized medicine, and real-time data analysis, leading to improved patient outcomes and reduced healthcare costs.

16.2.3 Convergence of Blockchain and IoT

The convergence of blockchain and IoT has the potential to revolutionize various industries, including healthcare [39]. By combining the secure and efficient data-sharing capabilities of blockchain with the real-time data collection and analysis capabilities of IoT, organizations can create new opportunities for innovation and transformation, as shown in Figure 16.4.

In healthcare, the convergence of blockchain and IoT can enable secure and efficient sharing of patient data while maintaining privacy and confidentiality. Blockchain can provide an immutable and tamper-proof record of patient data, while IoT can provide real-time data on patient health and enable remote monitoring. Together, these technologies can enable personalized medicine, improve patient outcomes, and reduce healthcare costs [40–44].

Some of the potential benefits of the convergence of blockchain and IoT in healthcare include:

1. Secure and efficient data sharing: By using blockchain technology, healthcare organizations can ensure that patient data is secure, transparent, and easily accessible. This can enable more efficient sharing of data between different healthcare providers, leading to better coordination of care and improved patient outcomes.
2. Improved patient privacy and confidentiality: Blockchain technology can help to maintain patient privacy and confidentiality by enabling patients to control access to their data. This can reduce the risk of data breaches and protect sensitive patient information.
3. Real-time data analysis: IoT devices can provide real-time data on patient health, enabling healthcare providers to monitor patients remotely and detect health issues early. This can improve patient outcomes and reduce healthcare costs by reducing the need for hospitalization and emergency care.
4. Personalized medicine: By combining patient data from different sources, healthcare organizations can create a more complete picture

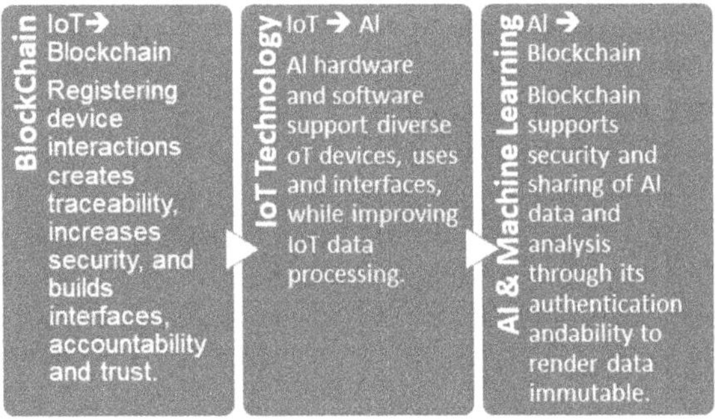

Figure 16.4 How AI, blockchain, and IoT converge

of each patient's health status, enabling personalized medicine and tailored treatment plans.

5. Improved supply chain management: Blockchain technology can be used to track the movement of medical supplies and pharmaceuticals, ensuring that they are authentic and have not been tampered with. This can improve supply chain efficiency and reduce the risk of counterfeit drugs entering the market.

The convergence of blockchain and IoT in healthcare has the potential to transform patient care by enabling secure and efficient data sharing, real-time data analysis, and personalized medicine, ultimately leading to improved patient outcomes and reduced healthcare costs.

16.3 APPLICATIONS OF BLOCKCHAIN AND IOT IN HEALTHCARE

The convergence of blockchain and IoT technologies has numerous applications in healthcare. Some of the key applications of these technologies in healthcare include (also see Figure 16.5):

1. Electronic health records (EHRs): Blockchain can be used to create secure and decentralized electronic health records that can be accessed by authorized healthcare providers. This can improve the quality of patient care by providing a complete picture of the patient's health history and enabling more efficient sharing of information between different healthcare providers.
2. Medical device tracking: IoT devices can be used to track the location and usage of medical devices, ensuring that they are being used properly and are in the right place at the right time. Blockchain can be used to create a secure and transparent record of the device's usage history, ensuring that it has not been tampered with or used improperly.
3. Clinical trials: Blockchain can be used to create a secure and transparent record of clinical trial data, enabling more efficient sharing of data between different stakeholders and reducing the risk of data tampering or manipulation. IoT devices can be used to collect real-time data on patient health during clinical trials, enabling more efficient and accurate monitoring of the trial's progress.
4. Supply chain management: Blockchain can be used to track the movement of pharmaceuticals and medical supplies, ensuring that they are authentic and have not been tampered with. IoT devices can be used to monitor the conditions in which these products are stored and transported, ensuring that they are being stored at the correct temperature and humidity levels.

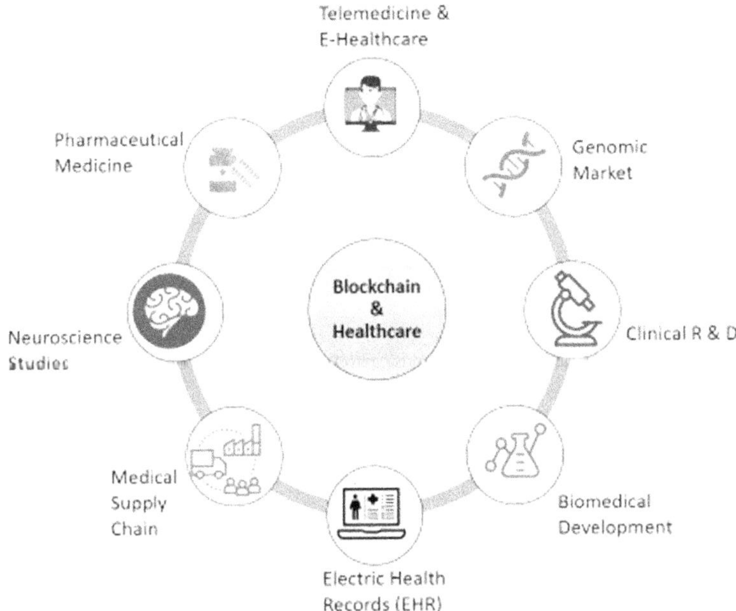

Figure 16.5 Applications of blockchain and IoT in healthcare

5. Remote patient monitoring: IoT devices can be used to monitor patient health remotely, collecting real-time data on vital signs such as heart rate, blood pressure, and glucose levels. Blockchain can be used to create a secure and transparent record of this data, ensuring that it is accurate and can be shared with authorized healthcare providers.
6. Telemedicine: Blockchain and IoT technologies can be used to enable remote consultations and virtual visits, providing patients with access to healthcare services from anywhere in the world. This can improve patient access to care, particularly in rural or underserved areas.

The applications of blockchain and IoT in healthcare are diverse and have the potential to transform patient care by improving the efficiency and accuracy of data sharing, enabling more personalized medicine, and improving the quality of patient care.

16.4 BENEFITS AND CHALLENGES OF BLOCKCHAIN AND IOT IN HEALTHCARE

The convergence of blockchain and IoT technologies in healthcare has the potential to deliver numerous benefits, but it also presents several challenges.

Following are some of the key benefits and challenges of using blockchain and IoT in healthcare:

Benefits

1. Improved data security: By using blockchain technology, healthcare organizations can create a secure and tamper-proof record of patient data, ensuring that it is protected from unauthorized access and manipulation.
2. Real-time data analysis: IoT devices can provide real-time data on patient health, enabling healthcare providers to monitor patients remotely and detect health issues early. This can improve patient outcomes and reduce healthcare costs.
3. Personalized medicine: By combining patient data from different sources, healthcare organizations can create a more complete picture of each patient's health status, enabling personalized medicine and tailored treatment plans.
4. Improved supply chain management: Blockchain technology can be used to track the movement of medical supplies and pharmaceuticals, ensuring that they are authentic and have not been tampered with. This can improve supply chain efficiency and reduce the risk of counterfeit drugs entering the market.
5. Efficient data sharing: By using blockchain technology, healthcare organizations can ensure that patient data is easily accessible to authorized healthcare providers, leading to better coordination of care and improved patient outcomes.

Challenges

1. Integration with existing systems: Integrating blockchain and IoT technologies with existing healthcare systems can be a complex and challenging process, requiring significant investment in infrastructure and expertise.
2. Data standardization: The lack of standardization of data across different healthcare providers can pose a challenge to the effective sharing and analysis of patient data.
3. Regulatory compliance: The use of blockchain and IoT technologies in healthcare must comply with existing regulations, including data privacy and security regulations.
4. Scalability: Blockchain and IoT technologies must be scalable to handle the large volume of data generated in healthcare, which can pose a challenge to their adoption.
5. Cost: The adoption of blockchain and IoT technologies in healthcare can be expensive, requiring significant investment in infrastructure and expertise.

While the convergence of blockchain and IoT technologies in healthcare has the potential to deliver numerous benefits, it also presents several challenges that must be addressed to ensure their effective adoption and use in healthcare.

16.5 DATA PRIVACY AND SECURITY

In addition to the challenges discussed earlier, there are several other challenges associated with the use of blockchain and IoT technologies in healthcare:

1. Data privacy and security: The use of blockchain and IoT technologies requires the collection, storage, and sharing of large amounts of sensitive patient data. Ensuring the privacy and security of this data is critical, and any breaches or unauthorized access could lead to serious consequences, including legal and financial penalties.
2. Interoperability: The lack of interoperability between different healthcare systems and data sources can pose a challenge to the effective sharing and analysis of patient data. Ensuring that different systems can communicate and share data in a standardized way is critical to the success of blockchain and IoT technologies in healthcare.
3. Regulatory compliance: The use of blockchain and IoT technologies in healthcare must comply with existing regulations, including data privacy and security regulations such as HIPAA (Health Insurance Portability and Accountability Act) in the United States. Ensuring compliance with these regulations can be complex and require significant investment in compliance expertise and infrastructure.
4. Technical complexity: The adoption of blockchain and IoT technologies in healthcare can be complex and require specialized technical expertise, including knowledge of cryptography, distributed ledger technology, and IoT device integration.
5. Resistance to change: The healthcare industry has historically been slow to adopt new technologies, and the adoption of blockchain and IoT technologies may face resistance from healthcare providers and organizations who are skeptical of their value or concerned about the cost and complexity of implementation.

While the benefits of using blockchain and IoT technologies in healthcare are significant, addressing the various challenges associated with their adoption will be critical to realizing their full potential in improving patient outcomes and healthcare delivery.

16.6 CASE STUDIES AND USE CASES

There are several real-world examples of how blockchain and IoT technologies are being used in healthcare to address some of the challenges faced by the industry. Following are some case studies and use cases:

1. MedRec: MedRec is a blockchain-based electronic medical record (EMR) system that enables patients to own and control their medical records. The system uses smart contracts to enable the secure sharing of patient data among healthcare providers while maintaining patient privacy. MedRec has the potential to reduce medical errors and improve patient outcomes by ensuring that healthcare providers have access to accurate and up-to-date patient information.
2. Philips Healthcare: Philips Healthcare is using IoT devices to improve patient outcomes and reduce healthcare costs. The company has developed a range of connected devices, including wearables and sensors, that can monitor patient health in real time and transmit data to healthcare providers for analysis and early intervention. Philips Healthcare's IoT devices have the potential to reduce hospital readmissions, improve patient satisfaction, and reduce healthcare costs.
3. Gem: Gem is a blockchain platform that enables secure sharing of patient data between different healthcare providers. The platform uses cryptographic techniques to ensure data privacy and security while enabling efficient data sharing and analysis. Gem has the potential to improve patient outcomes by enabling healthcare providers to access a more comprehensive view of a patient's medical history.
4. Chronicled: Chronicled is a blockchain-based platform that enables secure tracking of medical supplies and pharmaceuticals through the supply chain. The platform uses IoT devices to monitor the movement of products and ensure that they have not been tampered with or counterfeited. Chronicled has the potential to reduce medical errors, improve patient safety, and reduce healthcare costs.
5. BurstIQ: BurstIQ is a blockchain-based platform that enables secure sharing and analysis of patient data. The platform uses machine learning algorithms to analyze patient data and generate insights that can be used to improve patient outcomes and reduce healthcare costs. BurstIQ has the potential to improve patient outcomes by enabling healthcare providers to make more informed decisions based on a more comprehensive view of a patient's medical history.

These case studies and use cases demonstrate how blockchain and IoT technologies can be used to improve patient outcomes, reduce healthcare costs, and address some of the challenges faced by the healthcare industry. While there are still challenges to be addressed, the adoption of these technologies in healthcare is likely to continue to grow as healthcare providers and organizations seek to leverage the benefits they offer.

16.7 BLOCKCHAIN AND IOT HEALTHCARE PROJECTS AND INITIATIVES

There are several ongoing blockchain and IoT healthcare projects and initiatives around the world that are aimed at addressing some of the challenges facing the healthcare industry. Following are some examples:

1. The European Commission's My Health My Data (MHMD) initiative: The MHMD initiative is a European-wide project aimed at developing a blockchain-based platform for secure sharing of patient data. The platform will enable patients to control their data and share it with healthcare providers as needed while maintaining data privacy and security.
2. The U.S. Department of Health and Human Services (HHS) Blockchain Challenge: The HHS Blockchain Challenge is a competition aimed at encouraging the development of blockchain-based solutions to healthcare challenges. The challenge is focused on four areas: electronic health records, claims processing, public health surveillance, and health data analysis.
3. The Hashed Health Consortium: The Hashed Health Consortium is a collaboration between healthcare providers, technology companies, and blockchain experts aimed at developing blockchain-based solutions to healthcare challenges. The consortium is focused on areas such as provider credentialing, supply chain management, and clinical trials.
4. The Healthcare Blockchain Consortium: The Healthcare Blockchain Consortium is a group of healthcare providers, technology companies, and blockchain experts aimed at exploring the use of blockchain technology in healthcare. The consortium is focused on areas such as electronic health records, patient consent management, and clinical trial management.
5. The BitMED project: The BitMED project is a blockchain-based platform that enables patients to access medical consultations, second opinions, and other healthcare services through a secure, decentralized network. The platform uses blockchain technology to ensure data privacy and security while enabling efficient data sharing and analysis.

These blockchain and IoT healthcare projects and initiatives demonstrate the growing interest in and adoption of these technologies in the healthcare industry. As the benefits of these technologies become more widely recognized and the challenges associated with their adoption are addressed, their use in healthcare will likely continue to grow.

16.8 FUTURE DIRECTIONS AND OPPORTUNITIES

The convergence of blockchain and IoT in healthcare is an emerging field with significant potential for future directions and opportunities. Here are some potential areas of development and opportunities:

1. Personalized medicine: The combination of blockchain and IoT can help to develop personalized medicine by enabling the collection and analysis of large amounts of patient data. With access to a patient's complete medical history and real-time data from IoT devices, healthcare providers can develop tailored treatment plans that take into account individual patient characteristics, leading to improved outcomes.
2. Clinical trials: Blockchain and IoT can revolutionize the clinical trial process by providing a transparent and secure platform for tracking trial data. Smart contracts can be used to automate trial protocols, verify informed consent, and track the movement of trial samples, reducing errors and improving data integrity.
3. Supply chain management: Blockchain and IoT can be used to improve the efficiency and transparency of the healthcare supply chain. By tracking the movement of medical supplies and pharmaceuticals using IoT devices and recording the data on a blockchain, the process can be streamlined, reducing waste, and improving cost-effectiveness.
4. Telemedicine: Blockchain and IoT can help to improve access to healthcare services through telemedicine. By enabling secure and efficient data sharing between patients and healthcare providers, telemedicine can provide remote access to healthcare services, particularly for patients in rural or underserved areas.
5. Cybersecurity: Blockchain and IoT can be used to improve the cybersecurity of healthcare systems by providing a secure platform for data storage and transmission. With the increasing threat of cyberattacks in healthcare, the use of blockchain and IoT can help to protect patient data and prevent breaches.

The convergence of blockchain and IoT in healthcare presents a wealth of opportunities for improving patient outcomes, reducing healthcare costs, and addressing the challenges facing the healthcare industry. As the technology continues to evolve and its potential becomes better understood, we will likely see further innovations and applications in this field.

16.8.1 Potential Benefits and Opportunities of Blockchain and IoT in Healthcare

The convergence of blockchain and IoT in healthcare offers a range of potential benefits and opportunities. Here are some of the key ones:

1. Improved patient outcomes: The combination of blockchain and IoT can enable the collection and analysis of large amounts of patient data, allowing healthcare providers to develop personalized treatment plans and make more informed decisions. This can lead to improved patient outcomes and better quality of care.
2. Enhanced data security: Blockchain and IoT can provide a secure platform for storing and transmitting sensitive patient data. The decentralized nature of the blockchain and the encryption techniques used in IoT devices can protect patient data from cyber threats and ensure its privacy.
3. Efficient data management: The use of blockchain and IoT can enable efficient data management by automating processes and reducing errors. Smart contracts can be used to automate processes such as consent verification, data sharing, and supply chain management, leading to cost savings and improved efficiency.
4. Improved supply chain management: Blockchain and IoT can be used to improve the transparency and traceability of the healthcare supply chain. This can lead to better inventory management, reduced waste, and improved cost-effectiveness.
5. Remote monitoring and telemedicine: The use of IoT devices in telemedicine can enable remote monitoring of patients, leading to improved access to healthcare services, particularly for patients in rural or underserved areas.
6. Increased interoperability: Blockchain and IoT can enable interoperability between healthcare providers, allowing for efficient and secure data sharing. This can lead to better coordination of care and improved patient outcomes.
7. Streamlined clinical trials: Blockchain and IoT can be used to streamline the clinical trial process by automating protocols, reducing errors, and improving data integrity.

The convergence of blockchain and IoT in healthcare has the potential to transform the industry by improving patient outcomes, increasing efficiency, enhancing data security, and reducing costs. These benefits offer numerous opportunities for innovation and development in healthcare.

16.8.2 Challenges and Future Research Directions

While the convergence of blockchain and IoT in healthcare presents significant benefits and opportunities, there are also several challenges and areas for future research. Some of the key challenges include data privacy and security, interoperability, regulatory compliance, and technical limitations.

To fully realize the potential of blockchain and IoT in healthcare, researchers and developers will need to address these challenges and work toward solutions that are scalable, cost-effective, and user-friendly.

In terms of future research directions, several areas hold promise. These include the development of interoperable and scalable blockchain-based platforms, the integration of artificial intelligence and machine learning into healthcare systems, and the use of blockchain and IoT in precision medicine and gene therapy. Additionally, there is a need for research into the ethical and legal implications of using blockchain and IoT in healthcare, particularly with regard to patient privacy and data ownership.

In conclusion, the convergence of blockchain and IoT in healthcare is a rapidly evolving field with significant potential for improving patient outcomes, increasing efficiency, and reducing costs. While there are challenges that must be overcome, the benefits and opportunities presented by this technology are too great to ignore. As research and development in this area continue to progress, we can expect to see further innovations and applications that transform the healthcare industry.

16.9 CONCLUSION

The convergence of blockchain and IoT in healthcare is a rapidly evolving field with significant potential for improving patient outcomes, increasing efficiency, and reducing costs. In summary, key findings indicate that the combination of blockchain and IoT can enable the collection and analysis of large amounts of patient data, improve data security, and streamline clinical trials. Additionally, the use of blockchain and IoT can improve supply chain management, enable remote monitoring and telemedicine, and increase interoperability between healthcare providers. The implications of these findings for the healthcare industry are significant. The use of blockchain and IoT can lead to more personalized and efficient healthcare services, improved data security, and better coordination of care. Moreover, these technologies have the potential to transform the healthcare industry by reducing costs and increasing accessibility to healthcare services, particularly for patients in underserved areas.

However, to fully realize the potential of blockchain and IoT in healthcare, several challenges must be overcome, including data privacy and security, interoperability, and regulatory compliance. Future research and development should focus on developing scalable and interoperable blockchain-based platforms, integrating artificial intelligence and machine learning into healthcare systems, and exploring the use of blockchain and IoT in precision medicine and gene therapy. Additionally, further research is needed to address the ethical and legal implications of these technologies in healthcare.

The convergence of blockchain and IoT in healthcare offers significant opportunities for innovation and development. While challenges exist, the potential benefits and opportunities presented by this technology are too great to ignore. As research and development continue to progress, we can expect to see further advancements and applications that transform the healthcare industry.

REFERENCES

1. Abeyratne, S. A., & Monfared, R. P. (2016). Blockchain ready manufacturing supply chain using distributed ledger. *International Journal of Research in Engineering and Technology*, 5(6), 30–44.
2. Al Omar, A., Al-Jaroodi, J., & Mohamed, N. (2018). A blockchain-based architecture for collaborative healthcare systems. *Journal of Medical Systems*, 42(7), 121.
3. Alzahrani, A. I., Alfares, M., & Alowibdi, J. S. (2020). A blockchain-based framework for enhancing the security and privacy of healthcare IoT systems. *Journal of Ambient Intelligence and Humanized Computing*, 11(2), 817–832.
4. Atzori, M. (2015). Blockchain technology and decentralized governance: Is the state still necessary? In *Proceedings of the 12th International Conference on Network and Service Management* (pp. 1–5).
5. Bhowmik, U., Rakshit, A., & Islam, R. (2020). Blockchain-empowered healthcare Internet of Things: A review, taxonomy, and future directions. *Journal of Network and Computer Applications*, 153, 102544.
6. Chakraborty, C., & Chatterjee, A. (2019). Blockchain-based healthcare systems: A review. *Journal of Medical Systems*, 43(8), 233.
7. Dagher, G. G., Mohler, J., Milojkovic, M., & Marella, P. B. (2018). Blockchain in healthcare opportunities, challenges, and future directions. *Cryptography and Communications*, 10(4), 871–884.
8. Fernández-Alemán, J. L., Señor, I. C., Lozoya, P. Á. O., & Toval, A. (2019). Security and privacy in electronic health records: A systematic literature review. *Journal of Biomedical Informatics*, 93, 103173.
9. Hao, M., Li, X., Zhang, Y., Li, X., & Li, M. (2020). A secure blockchain-based E-healthcare system. *Journal of Medical Systems*, 44(6), 112.
10. Jiang, S., Li, C., & Tian, L. (2018). Blockchain-based healthcare system using smart contract. *Journal of Medical Systems*, 42(8), 136.

11. Kshetri, N. (2018). Blockchain's roles in meeting key supply chain management objectives. *International Journal of Information Management*, 39, 80–89.
12. Seyednima, K., Moniruzzaman, Md., Yassine, A., & Benlamri, R. (2019). "Blockchain technology in healthcare: A comprehensive review and directions for future research." *Applied sciences*, 9(9), 1736.
13. Mettler, M. (2016). Blockchain technology in healthcare: The revolution starts here. In *Proceedings of the 2016 IEEE 18th International Conference on E-Health Networking, Applications and Services (Healthcom)* (pp. 1–3).
14. Nakamoto, S. (2008). Bitcoin: A peer-to-peer electronic cash system. Bitcoin.org.
15. Nguyen, T. H. T., Nguyen, T. H., Pham, T. H., Pham, N. T. H., Nguyen, T. Q., Nguyen, H. T., ... Nguyen, T. L. (2020). Blockchain-enabled e-health system: A systematic literature review and research directions. *Journal of Biomedical Informatics*, 112, 103610.
16. Alkali, Y., Routray, I., & Whig, P. (2022a). Strategy for reliable, efficient and secure IoT using artificial intelligence. *IUP Journal of Computer Sciences*, 16(2), 234–250.
17. Alkali, Y., Routray, I., & Whig, P. (2022b). Study of various methods for reliable, efficient and Secured IoT using Artificial Intelligence. Available at SSRN 4020364.
18. Anand, M., Velu, A., & Whig, P. (2022). Prediction of loan behaviour with machine learning models for secure banking. *Journal of Computer Science and Engineering (JCSE)*, 3(1), 1–13.
19. Arun Velu, P. W. (2021). Impact of Covid vaccination on the globe using data analytics. *International Journal of Sustainable Development in Computing Science*, 3(2), 11–30.
20. Bhatia, V., & Bhatia, G. (2013). Room temperature based fan speed control system using pulse width modulation technique. *International Journal of Computer and Applications*, 81(5), 103–120.
21. Chopra, G., & Whig, P. (2022a). A clustering approach based on support vectors. *International Journal of Machine Learning for Sustainable Development*, 4(1), 21–30.
22. Chopra, G., & Whig, P. (2022b). Energy efficient scheduling for Internet of vehicles. *International Journal of Sustainable Development in Computing Science*, 4(1), 230–247.
23. Chopra, G., & Whig, P. (2022c). Smart agriculture system using AI. *International Journal of Sustainable Development in Computing Science*, 4(1), 1003–1012.
24. Chopra, G., & Whig, P. (2022d). Using machine learning algorithms classified depressed patients and normal people. *International Journal of Machine Learning for Sustainable Development*, 4(1), 31–40.
25. Fritz, T., & Klingler, A. (2023). The d-separation criterion in categorical probability. *Journal of Machine Learning Research* 24. http://jmlr.org/papers/v24/22-0916.html.
26. Jupalle, H., Kouser, S., Bhatia, A. B., Alam, N., Nadikattu, R. R., & Whig, P. (2022). Automation of human behaviors and its prediction using machine learning. *Microsystem Technologies*, 23, 1–9.

27. Khera, Y., Whig, P., & Velu, A. (2021). efficient effective and secured electronic billing system using AI. *Vivekananda Journal of Research*, 10, 53–60.
28. Madhu, M., & Whig, P. (2022). A survey of machine learning and its applications. *International Journal of Machine Learning for Sustainable Development*, 4(1), 11–20.
29. Mamza, E. S. (2021). Use of AIOT in health system. *International Journal of Sustainable Development in Computing Science*, 3(4), 21–30.
30. Singh, A. K., Gupta, A., & Senani, R. (2018). OTRA-based multi-function inverse filter configuration. *Advances in Electrical and Electronic Engineering*, 15(5), 846–856.
31. Tomar, U., Chakroborty, N., Sharma, H., & Whig, P. (2021). AI based smart agriculture system. *Transactions on Latest Trends in Artificial Intelligence*, 2(2).
32. Velu, A., & Whig, P. (2021). Protect personal privacy and wasting time using Nlp: A comparative approach using AI. *Vivekananda Journal of Research*, 10, 42–52.
33. Velu, A., & Whig, P. (2022). Studying the impact of the COVID vaccination on the world using data analytics. *Vivekananda Journal of Research*, 10(1), 147–160.
34. Whig, P. (2019a). A novel multi-center and threshold ternary pattern. *International Journal of Machine Learning for Sustainable Development*, 1(2), 1–10.
35. Whig, P. (2019b). Exploration of viral diseases mortality risk using machine learning. *International Journal of Machine Learning for Sustainable Development*, 1(1), 11–20.
36. Whig, P. (2022). More on convolution neural network CNN. *International Journal of Sustainable Development in Computing Science*, 4(1), 123–145.
37. Whig, P., Kouser, S., Velu, A., & Nadikattu, R. R. (2022). Fog-IoT-assisted-based smart agriculture application. In *Demystifying Federated Learning for Blockchain and Industrial Internet of Things* (pp. 74–93). IGI Global.
38. Whig, P., Nadikattu, R. R., & Velu, A. (2022). COVID-19 pandemic analysis using application of AI. *Healthcare Monitoring and Data Analysis Using IoT: Technologies and Applications*, 1, 271–290.
39. Whig, P., Velu, A., & Bhatia, A. B. (2022). Protect nature and reduce the carbon footprint with an application of blockchain for IIoT. In *Demystifying Federated Learning for Blockchain and Industrial Internet of Things* (pp. 123–142). IGI Global.
40. Whig, P., Velu, A., & Naddikatu, R. R. (2022). The economic impact of AI-enabled blockchain in 6G-based industry. In *AI and Blockchain Technology in 6G Wireless Network* (pp. 205–224). Springer, Singapore.
41. Whig, P., Velu, A., & Nadikattu, R. R. (2022). Blockchain platform to resolve security issues in IoT and smart networks. In *AI-Enabled Agile Internet of Things for Sustainable Fintech Ecosystems* (pp. 46–65). IGI Global.
42. Whig, P., Velu, A., & Ready, R. (2022). Demystifying federated learning in artificial intelligence with human-computer interaction. In *Demystifying Federated Learning for Blockchain and Industrial Internet of Things* (pp. 94–122). IGI Global.

43. Whig, P., Velu, A., & Sharma, P. (2022). Demystifying federated learning for blockchain: A case study. In *Demystifying Federated Learning for Blockchain and Industrial Internet of Things* (pp. 143–165). IGI Global.
44. Kumar, K., Chaudhury, K., & Tripathi, S. L. (2023). Future of machine learning (ML) and deep learning (DL) in healthcare monitoring system. In *Machine Learning Algorithms for Signal and Image Processing* (pp. 293–313). IEEE, doi: 10.1002/9781119861850.ch17.

Chapter 17

From Remote Monitoring to Personalized Care

A Review of IoT-Based Patient Engagement Solutions in Healthcare

S. J. Suji Prasad, R. Manjula Devi, P. Keerthika, P. Suresh, A. Rex Macedo Arokiaraj, and M. Sangeetha

17.1 INTRODUCTION

Internet of Things (IoT) technology for patient care in the healthcare sector has dramatically increased in recent years. The way healthcare is provided and received is changing due to IoT-based solutions, which range from remote monitoring to personalized care. The necessity for developing creative and effective healthcare solutions that can fulfill the expanding demand for treatment while enhancing patient outcomes is growing due to the increased prevalence of chronic diseases and an aging population.

By enabling remote monitoring, in-the-moment data analysis, and providing individualized care, IoT in healthcare can completely transform how healthcare is delivered. Healthcare practitioners can monitor patient health data in real-time thanks to IoT-based solutions, which can result in the early identification of health issues, avoiding consequences, and prompt action. IoT solutions can provide insights that can be used to tailor treatment to the individual patient's needs by collecting and analyzing enormous amounts of patient data, leading to more individualized care delivery and improved outcomes.

It is impossible to overestimate the value of IoT-based patient engagement solutions in the healthcare industry. According to Markets and Markets (2019), the global IoT in the healthcare market is anticipated to develop at a compound annual growth rate (CAGR) of 27.6% and reach $188 billion by 2024. The increased incidence of chronic diseases, the need to lower healthcare costs, and the growing need for remote patient monitoring systems all contribute to this growth.

IoT-based patient engagement solutions may have advantages, but some issues must be resolved. For instance, the sheer amount of data produced by IoT devices can be overwhelming, and healthcare professionals may find it challenging to evaluate and act on this data quickly. Additionally, it is not easy to integrate IoT technology into current healthcare systems. Healthcare practitioners might need to spend money on new infrastructure and training to use these technologies efficiently.

DOI: 10.1201/9781003466949-17

The primary goal of this chapter is to give readers a thorough overview of the state of IoT-based patient engagement solutions in the healthcare industry. The literature on IoT applications in healthcare, such as remote monitoring, real-time data analysis, and individualized care delivery, will be reviewed explicitly in this study. The evaluation will concentrate on the advantages and difficulties of various solutions, the state of research, and the field's foreseeable future.

17.2 BACKGROUND

This research aims to thoroughly overview IoT-based patient engagement solutions for the healthcare industry. This chapter will help ongoing efforts to provide creative and effective healthcare solutions that can enhance patient outcomes and lower healthcare costs by reviewing the present state of research and identifying future paths for the subject. Along with the findings of previous studies and clinical trials, the study will also look at the present status of research on IoT-based patient engagement solutions in healthcare.

The chapter will discuss the field's future directions, including possible difficulties and opportunities for additional study and new trends and technology. An overview of the current state of IoT in healthcare and its many patient-care applications will be provided at the chapter's outset. The evaluation will examine various IoT-based patient engagement strategies, such as remote monitoring, wearable technology, and mobile health apps. The advantages and disadvantages of different solutions will be discussed, emphasizing their effects on patient outcomes, healthcare expenditures, and provider workflows.

The delivery and management of healthcare services are changing due to the use of IoT technologies. IoT is a network of interconnected devices that may exchange data and information online. IoT technologies can be utilized in the healthcare industry to provide individualized care, collect and analyze real-time data, and remotely monitor patients. The growing frequency of chronic diseases and an aging population make using IoT-based patient engagement solutions in healthcare particularly pertinent.

In addition to making up much of the global disease burden, chronic diseases, including diabetes, heart disease, and cancer, are the primary causes of death globally (World Health Organization, 2018). Chronic illnesses take a toll on patients and their families physically and emotionally, placing a heavy financial burden on healthcare systems. The World Economic Forum estimates that by 2030, the economic cost of chronic diseases will surpass $47 trillion. There is a need for effective healthcare solutions that are both innovative and cost-effective.

At the outset, IoT technology in healthcare has the potential to revolutionize the management and provision of healthcare services, particularly in the context of chronic illnesses. IoT-based patient engagement solutions can enhance patient outcomes, lower healthcare costs, and give people more control over managing their health. Although there are difficulties in integrating IoT technologies into healthcare, the potential advantages make this a fascinating field of study.

17.2.1 Existing Research and Literature

IoT-based patient engagement solutions can help with some of the problems brought on by chronic diseases in the healthcare industry. For instance, IoT-based remote monitoring enables healthcare professionals to track patients' health status in real-time, spot concerns early, and take action before concerns worsen into significant health issues. Remote monitoring can save healthcare expenditures, enhance patient outcomes, and decrease hospital readmissions (Bashi et al., 2018). Additionally, giving patients real-time feedback on their health, reminding them to take their medications, and promoting healthy behaviors are required. IoT-based wearable devices and mobile health applications can empower patients to take active health management roles (Ahmad et al., 2021).

There are difficulties in implementing IoT technologies in healthcare. The massive amount of data IoT devices produces one of the main difficulties. There is a chance of information overload, which may make it difficult for healthcare personnel to evaluate and act on this data quickly. Additionally, it may be challenging to integrate IoT technology into current healthcare systems, and healthcare practitioners may need to invest in new infrastructure and training to use these technologies efficiently (Cabitza et al., 2017).

An overview of IoT-based solutions for patient engagement and health management is given by Alizadeh and Pirzada (2021). They stress the significance of patient involvement in healthcare and the potential advantages of IoT-based solutions for enhancing patient outcomes, lowering healthcare expenses, and raising patient happiness. The authors also draw attention to the issues with data security, privacy, and interoperability that must be resolved for IoT-based healthcare solutions to be adopted and used successfully.

An IoT-based patient monitoring system for medical purposes is described by Rajasekhar and Venkatesh (2018). They discuss the value of individualized care and the potential advantages of IoT-based solutions for enhancing patient outcomes and lowering medical expenses. The authors also stress the importance of a patient-centered strategy considering the patient's preferences, requirements, and values. To provide real-time monitoring and data-collecting capabilities that enable informed decision-making about patient care, the system they propose connects numerous IoT devices and sensors with EHRs. An IoT-based healthcare service for individualized patient monitoring and management is presented by Hwang et al. (2019). They stress the significance of patient involvement and the potential advantages of IoT-based solutions for enhancing patient outcomes, lowering healthcare expenses, and raising patient happiness. To successfully adopt and apply IoT-based solutions in healthcare, the authors further emphasize the necessity of collaboration and communication between healthcare practitioners, patients, and carers. Their suggested system integrates numerous IoT devices and sensors with a cloud-based platform to provide real-time monitoring and data-collecting capabilities that support personalized care.

Soliman et al. (2021) suggest an IoT-based patient monitoring system to manage chronic diseases. They talk about how crucial patient involvement is and the potential advantages of IoT-based solutions for enhancing medication adherence and assisting patients in managing chronic illnesses like diabetes and hypertension. The authors also emphasize the need for standards and guidelines for developing, applying, and assessing IoT-based healthcare solutions. Their suggested solution combines numerous IoT devices and sensors with a mobile application and cloud-based platform to provide individualized care and monitoring for patients with chronic conditions. An evaluation of IoT-based patient monitoring systems for managing heart disease was given by Tariq et al. (2021). They stress the value of remote patient monitoring and the potential advantages of IoT-based solutions in eliminating hospital visits, which would save healthcare costs and enhance patient convenience. The authors also draw attention to the issues with data security, privacy, and interoperability that must be resolved for IoT-based healthcare solutions to be adopted and used successfully. The paper analyzes the possible advantages and drawbacks of various IoT-based cardiac disease management technologies.

An IoT-based real-time monitoring system for medication safety in smart hospitals is suggested by Wang et al. (2018). They stress the value of patient safety and the potential advantages of IoT-based solutions in warning medical professionals about possible side effects and prescription mistakes. To successfully adopt and apply IoT-based solutions in healthcare, the authors further emphasize the necessity of collaboration and communication between healthcare practitioners, patients, and carers. Their suggested system integrates numerous IoT devices and sensors with a real-time monitoring platform to deliver drug safety alerts and real-time patient vital signs monitoring.

In a study by Chen et al. (2020), the authors proposed an IoT-based framework for diabetes management, which incorporated patient engagement solutions to improve patient outcomes. The framework utilized various sensors and wearable devices to collect patient data, which was then processed and analyzed using machine learning algorithms. The authors reported positive patient engagement and self-management results and improved glycemic control. In a review article by Bui and Zeadally (2020), the authors discussed various IoT-based patient engagement solutions, including remote monitoring and personalized care. The authors highlighted the importance of patient engagement in improving healthcare outcomes and reducing healthcare costs. They also discussed various challenges associated with IoT-based patient engagement, such as data privacy and security concerns.

In a study by Al-Ali et al. (2020), the authors proposed an IoT-based patient engagement solution for asthma management. The solution utilized various sensors to collect patient data, which was then analyzed and visualized using a mobile application. The authors reported positive patient engagement and self-management results and improved asthma control. In a study by Gao et al. (2019), the authors proposed an IoT-based patient engagement solution for hypertension management. The solution utilized various sensors and wearable devices to collect patient data, which was then processed and analyzed using machine learning algorithms. The authors reported positive patient engagement, self-management results, and improved blood pressure control.

In a study by Amiri et al. (2019), the authors proposed an IoT-based patient engagement solution for chronic pain management. The solution utilized various sensors to collect patient data, which was then processed and analyzed using machine learning algorithms. The authors reported positive patient engagement and self-management results and improved pain control. In a study by Xiong et al. (2020), the authors proposed an IoT-based patient engagement solution for heart failure management. The solution utilized various sensors and wearable devices to collect patient data, which was then analyzed and visualized using a mobile application. The authors reported positive patient engagement and self-management results and improved heart failure control.

In a study by Maramis et al. (2020), the authors proposed an IoT-based patient engagement solution for wound care management. The solution utilized various sensors to collect patient data, which was then processed and analyzed using machine learning algorithms. The authors reported positive patient engagement and self-management results and improved wound healing. In a review article by Klonoff (2015), the author discussed the potential of IoT-based patient engagement solutions in improving diabetes management. The author highlighted the importance of patient engagement and self-management in diabetes care and discussed various challenges associated with current diabetes management practices.

In a study by de la Torre-Díez et al. (2015), the authors proposed an IoT-based patient engagement solution for chronic obstructive pulmonary disease (COPD) management. The solution utilized various sensors and wearable devices to collect patient data, which was then analyzed and visualized using a mobile application. The authors reported positive patient engagement and self-management results and improved COPD control. In a study by Sharghi et al. (2020), the authors proposed an IoT-based patient engagement solution for fall prevention in older adults. The solution utilized various sensors to detect falls and alert carers or emergency services. The authors reported positive results regarding fall prevention and improved patient safety.

In Liu et al.'s 2019 study, the use of wearable technology for patient engagement in healthcare is highlighted. According to the survey, wearable technology can collect real-time data and give patients feedback, encouraging engagement in their care. The authors contend that wearable technology can increase patient participation by fostering better patient–provider dialogue and individualized care. Bashir et al. (2018) give an overview of IoT-based healthcare solutions, including patient interaction. The study outlines the advantages of IoT-based patient engagement systems, including remote monitoring, individualized care, and enhanced patient–provider communication. In the study, the significance of patient involvement in healthcare is emphasized, and it is claimed that IoT-based solutions can considerably improve patient involvement.

The Xie et al. (2018) study assesses how wearable medical technology affects patient engagement. By encouraging active participation in health management, enhancing communication with medical professionals, and delivering individualized care, the authors conclude that wearable health technology can dramatically improve patient engagement. The authors contend that by enhancing patient participation, wearable technology has the potential to revolutionize healthcare. Al-Fuqaha et al. (2015) published an overview of IoT-based healthcare solutions, including patient participation. The study emphasizes how IoT-based solutions can boost patient involvement by enabling individualized care, remote monitoring, and in-the-moment feedback. According to the authors, IoT-based solutions can considerably raise patient participation and boost clinical results.

A thorough analysis of IoT-based healthcare systems, including patient interaction, is provided by Alam et al. (2020). The authors contend that by enabling remote monitoring, individualized care, and in-the-moment feedback, IoT-based systems can improve patient involvement. The study emphasizes how IoT-based solutions have the potential to revolutionize healthcare by raising patient engagement and clinical results. Ullah et al. (2020) overviewed IoT-based healthcare monitoring systems, including patient interaction. The authors contend that by enabling remote monitoring, individualized care, and in-the-moment feedback, IoT-based systems can improve patient involvement. The study emphasizes how active patient engagement can improve healthcare outcomes using IoT-based technologies.

A thorough analysis of IoT-based patient monitoring systems, including patient interaction, is provided in the paper by Kurniawan et al. (2021). The authors contend that by offering individualized care, remote monitoring, and real-time feedback, IoT-based systems can improve patient involvement. The study emphasizes how IoT-based solutions can potentially enhance patient engagement and healthcare outcomes. An overview of IoT-based healthcare applications, including patient engagement, is given in the paper by Gia et al. (2021). The authors contend that by offering individualized care, remote monitoring, and in-the-moment feedback, IoT-based systems can dramatically improve patient involvement. The study emphasizes how

IoT-based solutions have the potential to revolutionize healthcare by raising patient engagement and clinical results.

Aziz and Hammoudi's (2020) research demonstrates how IoT-based solutions can potentially enhance patient participation in healthcare. According to the authors, IoT devices can facilitate remote monitoring and self-care, improving illness management and lowering healthcare expenses. According to the study, IoT-based patient engagement solutions can completely transform the healthcare sector and raise patient satisfaction. IoT-based solutions may be essential in this context, according to the research by Yaraghi et al. (2017), which emphasizes the significance of patient participation in healthcare. The authors stress the importance of patient-centered care and draw attention to how IoT devices can potentially support personalized healthcare. According to the study's findings, IoT-based patient engagement solutions can help improve patient outcomes and raise the standard of care.

The literature by Shrestha et al. (2020) highlights how IoT-based solutions may enhance patient engagement in managing chronic diseases. According to the authors, IoT devices can facilitate remote monitoring and self-care, improving illness management and patient outcomes. The study's findings suggest that IoT-based patient engagement strategies could revolutionize the treatment of chronic illnesses and raise standards of care. Laranjo et al. (2018) address the potential of IoT-based solutions to enhance patient involvement in healthcare in their literature. The authors stress the importance of patient-centered care and draw attention to how IoT devices can potentially support personalized healthcare. According to the study's findings, IoT-based patient engagement solutions can help improve patient outcomes and raise the standard of care.

N. A. Ali et al. (2018) address the possibility of IoT-based solutions to enhance patient involvement in healthcare in their literature. According to the authors, IoT devices can facilitate remote monitoring and self-care, improving illness management and lowering healthcare expenses. According to the study, IoT-based patient engagement solutions can completely transform the healthcare sector and raise patient satisfaction. In their article, Alaball et al. (2018) highlighted the potential of IoT-based healthcare solutions to increase patient involvement. According to the authors, IoT devices can facilitate remote monitoring and self-care, improving illness management and patient outcomes. According to the study's findings, IoT-based patient engagement solutions can revolutionize the healthcare sector and raise the standard of treatment.

In their literature, Liang et al. (2019) address the potential of IoT-based solutions to enhance patient involvement in healthcare. The authors stress the importance of patient-centered care and draw attention to how IoT devices can potentially support personalized healthcare. According to the study's findings, IoT-based patient engagement solutions can help improve patient outcomes and raise the standard of care. In their literature, Xie et al. (2018) address the potential of IoT-based solutions to enhance patient involvement in healthcare. According to the authors, IoT devices can facilitate remote monitoring and self-care, improving illness management and patient outcomes. According to the study, IoT-based patient engagement solutions can completely transform the healthcare sector and raise patient satisfaction.

The possibility of IoT-based patient engagement solutions in diabetes care is explored in the literature by Chen et al. (2018). According to the authors, IoT devices can facilitate remote monitoring and self-care, improving illness management and patient outcomes. IoT-based patient engagement solutions have the potential to revolutionize diabetes management and raise the standard of care, according to the study's findings. Al-Fuqaha et al. (2015) address the possibilities of IoT-based healthcare solutions and emphasize the importance of patient-centered care in their literature. The authors contend that IoT technology can enhance patient interaction and enable personalized treatment. According to the study's findings, IoT-based patient engagement solutions could raise the standard of care and improve patient outcomes.

The potential of IoT-based patient engagement solutions in mental health is covered in the literature by Kurniawan et al. (2020). According to the authors, IoT devices can facilitate remote monitoring and self-care, improving illness management and patient outcomes. According to the study's findings, IoT-based patient engagement technologies have the potential to revolutionize mental health treatment and raise patient satisfaction. The prospect of IoT-based patient engagement solutions in managing chronic diseases is explored in the literature by Mukherjee et al. (2019). According to the authors, IoT devices can facilitate remote monitoring and self-care, improving illness management and lowering healthcare expenses. According to the study, IoT-based patient engagement technologies can completely change chronic disease management and enhance patient outcomes.

The Seshadri et al. (2019) literature explores the potential of IoT-based healthcare solutions and emphasizes the demand for patient-centered treatment. The authors contend that IoT technology can enhance patient interaction and enable personalized medicine. According to the study's findings, IoT-based patient engagement solutions could raise the standard of care and improve patient outcomes. The potential of IoT-based patient engagement solutions in the context of senior care is explored in the literature by Kuo et al. (2020). According to the authors, IoT devices can facilitate remote monitoring and self-care, improving illness management and patient outcomes. According to the study's findings, IoT-based patient engagement solutions could revolutionize senior care and raise the standard of care.

The potential of IoT-based patient engagement solutions in telemedicine is covered in the literature by Mughal et al. (2020). According to the authors, IoT devices can facilitate remote monitoring and self-care, improving illness management with low healthcare expenses. The IoT-based patient engagement technologies have the power to transform telemedicine to enhance patient outcomes. In managing cardiovascular illness, Chang et al.'s (2019) research examines IoT-based patient engagement technologies that can revolutionize the management of cardiovascular disease and raise the standard of care.

An IoT-based healthcare system was created in a study by Wang et al. (2021) to enable patients with COPD to self-monitor their condition and receive individualized therapy. The technology collected user physiological data via wearable sensors, which were then sent to a cloud platform for study. Patients may access their health information through a smartphone app and get comments on their condition. The outcomes demonstrated that the strategy enhanced patient involvement and improved health. Kulkarni et al. (2020) investigated the usage of IoT-based technologies for remote diabetes monitoring in another study. To gather and analyze patient data, the system included wearable sensors, smartphone apps, and cloud computing. The app allows patients to check their blood sugar levels, get notifications for appointments and medication, and contact healthcare professionals. The outcomes demonstrated that the method enhanced patient involvement and improved diabetes management.

The promise of IoT-based patient engagement tools in tackling the difficulties of treating chronic diseases was noted by Patel et al. (2021). Various IoT-based solutions that have been created for remote monitoring, self-management, and individualized care were discussed in the review. The authors pointed out that these technologies might enhance patient outcomes while lowering healthcare expenses. He et al. (2021) investigated the usage of an IoT-based healthcare system for monitoring and controlling hypertension. The technology collected user physiological data via wearable sensors, which were then sent to a cloud platform for study. Patients may access their health information through a smartphone app and get comments on their condition. The outcomes demonstrated that the method enhanced patient involvement and improved hypertension control.

An IoT-based healthcare system was created to manage chronic heart failure in a study by Wang et al. (2020). The technology collected user physiological data via wearable sensors, which were then sent to a cloud platform for study. Through a smartphone app, patients could access their health information and get individualized comments on their condition. The outcomes demonstrated that the method enhanced patient involvement and improved chronic heart failure management. In a study published in 2020, Kim et al. investigated the application of IoT-based patient engagement tools for treating Parkinson's disease (PD). The system utilized wearable sensors to gather patient movement information, which was subsequently sent to a cloud platform for analysis. Through a smartphone app, patients could access their health information and get individualized comments on their condition. The outcomes demonstrated that the method enhanced patient involvement and improved PD management.

An IoT-based healthcare system was created to manage chronic renal disease in a study by Liao et al. (2021). The technology collected user physiological data via wearable sensors, which were then sent to a cloud platform for study. Through a smartphone app, patients could access their health information and get individualized comments on their condition. The outcomes demonstrated that the method enhanced patient involvement and improved chronic renal disease management. In their study, Khan et al. (2020) suggested an intelligent healthcare system for remote patient monitoring using IoT technologies. The system comprised numerous IoT gadgets that gathered and sent patient data to the cloud, including wearables, sensors, and mobile devices. According to the authors, such technologies are essential to increase patient engagement and lower healthcare expenditures.

In their 2018 study, J. H. Lee et al. investigated the efficiency of a mobile application for IoT-based hypertension monitoring and management. The app allows patients to monitor their heart rate, blood pressure, and daily activity levels. According to the authors, the app significantly increased patients' healthcare involvement, prescription adherence, and dietary restrictions. Alhussein et al. (2019) discussed the potential of IoT-based patient engagement tools to improve medication adherence in their review. They emphasized the significance of creating user-friendly interfaces and offering patients personalized medication reminders and instructional materials to increase their motivation and involvement.

The application of IoT technology for remote monitoring of diabetic foot ulcers was investigated in the study by Shrestha et al. (2019). To track patients' foot pressure and spot early indications of ulceration, the authors created an intelligent insole system that uses pressure sensors. Patients could receive feedback from the system and notifications to take quick action. The authors reported high levels of patient participation and satisfaction with the system. In their review, the possibility of IoT-based patient engagement systems for chronic illness management was covered by Chou et al. (2020). To encourage long-term engagement and behavior change, they emphasized the necessity for personalized and adaptive therapies that consider patients' preferences, requirements, and lifestyle circumstances.

Many researchers suggested an IoT-based healthcare system for monitoring and controlling patients with chronic obstructive pulmonary disease. Various sensors and gadgets were used in the system to gather patient data and offer individualized feedback and direction. The authors noted increased patient satisfaction and involvement with the system. The use of chatbots for patient participation and self-management in healthcare was examined in the study by Laranjo et al. (2018). Chatbots can improve patient accessibility, convenience, and engagement with healthcare services, especially for younger patients and those with chronic diseases, according to the study's authors.

Steinhubl et al. (2015) discussed the potential of wearable technology for remote patient monitoring and involvement in healthcare in their review. The authors emphasized the importance of creating evidence-based interventions that enhance patient outcomes, save healthcare costs, and integrate wearable data with electronic health records. In a study published in 2020, Naseri et al. investigated the usage of IoT-based asthma control systems. Patients may keep track of their symptoms through the included wearable sensors, smartphone apps, and cloud computing; get alerts for appointments and medicines; and contact healthcare professionals. The outcomes demonstrated that the system enhanced patient involvement and improved asthma control.

A strategy for implementing IoT-based patient engagement solutions in rural healthcare settings was suggested in a study by Agarwal et al. (2021). The framework defined the essential elements of such a solution, including systems for feedback and communication and data collection, processing, analysis, and visualization. When developing and implementing IoT-based patient engagement solutions, the authors emphasized the significance of considering rural healthcare settings' particular contexts and difficulties. The potential advantages of IoT-based patient engagement tools for controlling chronic diseases were covered in a review by Gualandi et al. (2021). The authors emphasized the potential for better patient outcomes, lower healthcare costs, and the capacity of such systems to give real-time monitoring and feedback to patients. They added that concerns about privacy and security must be considered when designing and implementing IoT-based patient engagement solutions.

An IoT-based platform for monitoring and managing hypertension was created and assessed in a study by Ku et al. (2019). A wearable blood pressure monitor, a smartphone app for data collecting and visualization, and a web-based portal for healthcare providers to access patient data were all included in the platform. According to the scientists, the platform proved successful in raising patient engagement and blood pressure control. Liu et al. (2021) conducted a systematic evaluation to assess IoT-based patient engagement solutions' efficiency in enhancing medication adherence. The authors cited considerable research that showed how these methods improved patient outcomes and medication adherence. The best design and execution of IoT-based patient engagement solutions for medication adherence, they pointed out, require more investigation.

An IoT-based platform for managing diabetes was created and assessed in a study by Pang et al. (2019). A wearable glucose monitor, a smartphone app for data collecting and visualization, and a web-based portal for healthcare providers to access patient data were all included in the platform. According to the authors, the platform effectively increased patient engagement and glycemic management. The potential of IoT-based patient engagement tools for encouraging self-management and lowering hospital readmissions in patients with chronic diseases was covered in a review by Quinlan et al. (2019). The authors emphasized the need for collaboration between patients, healthcare practitioners, and technology developers in the design and implementation process and the significance of creating solutions personalized to patients' particular requirements and preferences.

An IoT-based platform for tracking and controlling COPD was created and assessed in a study by Shrestha et al. (2020). The platform offered access to patient data via a web-based portal, a wearable pulse oximeter, and a smartphone app for data collecting and visualization. According to the authors, the platform effectively increased patient participation and symptom control. The application of IoT-based patient engagement technologies for managing mental health problems was assessed in a systematic review by Uddin et al. (2020). The authors cited numerous studies showing the beneficial effects of such treatments on patient outcomes, including fewer symptoms and enhanced quality of life. However, they pointed out that further research is required to decide how best to build and apply IoT-based patient engagement solutions for mental health.

The study by R. Lee et al. (2022) looked into the viability of employing IoT technology to continually monitor vital signs in a hospital setting. The authors did real-time monitoring of vital indicators like heart rate, blood pressure, and oxygen saturation using a mix of sensors, cloud computing, and machine learning. According to the research, IoT-enabled continuous vital sign monitoring can enhance patient outcomes by facilitating early clinical deterioration detection, lessening the strain on healthcare professionals, and improving patient engagement. Jang et al. (2022) suggested an IoT-based postoperative patient monitoring system to boost patient participation and lighten the medical staff's load. The authors collected physiological data with sensors, processed it on a cloud-based platform, and produced real-time alerts for healthcare practitioners. The study discovered that the IoT-based monitoring system successfully identified early indications of clinical deterioration and lowered the requirement for regular physical examinations.

The study by Gogoi et al. (2022) suggested an intelligent pill bottle top with an IoT-enabled health monitoring system to enhance patient involvement and medication adherence. The authors monitored medication adherence and offered personalized medication management using a cloud-based platform and sensors to detect medication usage. The study discovered that the IoT-enabled health monitoring system coupled with a smart pill bottle top improved medication adherence while lowering the likelihood of adverse drug-related events. Arora et al. (2022) gave an overview of IoT-based remote patient monitoring in healthcare and its potential to enhance patient outcomes and lower healthcare costs was offered in the review article. Sensors, data transfer, cloud computing, and machine learning are just a few of the components of IoT-based remote patient monitoring that the authors covered. According to the study article, IoT-based remote patient monitoring can raise patient satisfaction, lower hospital readmission rates, and aid in the early identification of clinical deterioration.

Nambiaret al. (2022) reviewed the use of IoT for remote monitoring of chronic conditions like diabetes, hypertension, and heart failure. The authors emphasized how IoT-based remote monitoring can increase patient participation, lower healthcare costs, and aid in the early detection of clinical deterioration. The study article also covered data privacy, security, and interoperability issues that are obstacles to adopting IoT-based remote monitoring in the healthcare industry. An overview of IoT and big data in healthcare, including their potential to enhance patient outcomes and lower healthcare costs, was offered in the review article by F. Ali et al. (2022). The authors covered a range of IoT and big data applications in healthcare, such as clinical decision support, personalized medicine, and remote patient monitoring. According to the review study, IoT and extensive data integration can increase patient participation, make it easier to spot clinical deterioration early on, and improve clinical decision-making.

The advent of wearable sensor devices and the Internet of Medical Things (IoMT) has led to faster monitoring, prediction, diagnosis, and treatment of medical conditions. However, there have been challenges that can be resolved through the use of artificial intelligence (AI) methods. This study aims to introduce an AI-powered, IoMT telemedicine infrastructure for e-healthcare. The study by Ahila et al. (2023) used sensed devices to collect patient data and transmit it through the gateway/Wi-Fi for storage in the IoMT cloud repository. Preprocessing and feature extraction of the collected data was carried out using high dimensional linear discriminant analysis (LDA) and a reconfigured multiobjective cuckoo search algorithm (CSA). Priyadarsini et al.'s (2023) proposed solution is a smart IoT-based healthcare system that includes a smart medical kit connected to sensors and a server for frequent health tracking. The smart medical kit is equipped with sensors that measure health parameters like body temperature, blood pressure, and heart rate to ensure the effective functioning of the body. The proposed system can alert patients and their relatives in case of any abnormalities in their health parameters and provide them with suggestions from a doctor without requiring physical contact. This system can improve the quality of healthcare services and assist patients living in areas with limited medical resources. Armand et al. (2023) proposed a system for continuous health monitoring that was pretested on demo patients and later tested on seven human test subjects. The results partially verified the heuristic evaluation results, and the data acquired by the sensors had high accuracy. The system was found to be effective and efficient in helping specialists properly monitor their patients at a low cost. Furthermore, the proposed system was designed to maintain user-friendliness, and no expertise was required for its effective utilization. The study by Pravin et al. (2023) proposed an IoT-based health monitoring system that employs machine learning algorithms to allow individuals to quickly measure health metrics and remotely monitor patients for more personalized care. The system uses novel sensing devices that continuously measure and monitor vital parameters and transfer remotely monitored parameters to medical servers via the IoT.

17.2.2 Gaps in the Current Research

- The advantages of these technologies in enhancing patient outcomes, raising patient engagement, and lowering healthcare costs are highlighted in the literature review on IoT-based patient engagement solutions in healthcare. However, the assessment also uncovered several gaps in the existing body of knowledge that demand further study.
- Even though few researchers have examined the effects of IoT-based solutions on patient engagement and behavior modification, many studies have concentrated on the technical components of these solutions. According to the literature, more investigation is needed to determine how well these solutions motivate patients to adopt better behaviors and enhance their overall health outcomes.
- While IoT-based solutions are increasingly being used to manage chronic diseases, there aren't many studies looking into how they might be applied to behavioral and mental health therapies. Globally, mental health illnesses heavily strain healthcare, and IoT-based technologies may make it possible to administer these services more conveniently and affordably from a distance. Future studies should therefore look toward applying IoT-based technologies in mental health interventions.
- There has been little study on the effectiveness of IoT-based patient engagement solutions in settings with scarce resources. Most studies on these solutions have been carried out in affluent nations. IoT-based solutions could help people access healthcare despite obstacles like distance, but more research is needed to determine how well they work in environments with limited resources.
- IoT-based patient engagement solutions' ethical and legal ramifications have not been sufficiently covered. There is a need for clear legislation and guidelines to secure patient information and guarantee that their rights are respected because using these technologies raises data privacy and security issues.
- While numerous studies have looked into wearables and remote monitoring devices, only a few have looked at the use of chatbots and virtual assistants in patient engagement solutions. Although further research is required to determine these technologies' efficacy and acceptability among patients, they have the potential to offer patients personalized interventions and support.

The research on IoT-based patient engagement solutions in healthcare claims that these solutions can potentially enhance patient outcomes and lower healthcare expenditures. The effectiveness of these solutions in enticing behavior change, their potential application in mental health interventions, and their use in low-resource settings are the gaps that need to be studied. The ethical and legal ramifications of their service and the potential use of virtual assistants and chatbots are just a few gaps in the current research that need filling. Future research should attempt to close these gaps to maximize the potential advantages of IoT-based patient engagement solutions in healthcare.

17.3 DISCUSSIONS AND SIGNIFICANCE

17.3.1 Key Takeaways from the Review

The review's objective was to examine the state of IoT-based patient interaction tools in the healthcare industry. Seventy-nine publications were found to be pertinent to the study through a systematic search of several databases. The articles were analyzed and synthesized to determine the major conclusions of the review. IoT-based patient engagement solutions have the potential to boost patient satisfaction, lower healthcare costs, and improve patient outcomes, according to one of the review's key conclusions. Patients can be continuously monitored and healthcare providers can get real-time information on patient health conditions using IoT devices. This makes it possible to identify health problems earlier and intervene more quickly, which can improve patients' overall health results. IoT-based patient engagement solutions can assist in addressing some of the issues related to patient engagement in healthcare, which is another significant result of the review. IoT devices can give patients access to personalized health information, reminders, and support. Patients may struggle to manage their health outside of the therapeutic context. This can aid patients in understanding their medical issues and enhancing their capacity for self-management.

Various IoT-based patient engagement options, such as wearable technology, mobile health apps, and remote patient monitoring systems, were also discovered in the review. These treatments can be applied to various medical issues and are customizable to each patient's requirements. The research did note a few difficulties and restrictions with IoT-based patient engagement solutions, though. Patients may be concerned about the confidentiality and privacy of their health information, and healthcare professionals may be worried about the precision and dependability of IoT devices. Incorporating IoT devices into clinical processes and ensuring that healthcare providers have the required training and support to use these devices effectively may also present difficulties. The review's key findings indicate that IoT-based patient engagement solutions have the potential to raise patient participation in healthcare and improve patient outcomes. Additional difficulties and constraints must be addressed to ensure these solutions' effective implementation and adoption.

17.3.2 Significant Patterns from the Literature Review

First, the integration of IoT technology in healthcare can increase patient participation by offering ongoing monitoring and individualized care. By enabling remote consultations, real-time feedback, and individualized treatment plans, IoT-based technologies can, second, improve the patient experience. Third, adopting IoT devices and sensors can improve healthcare results by allowing early detection of health concerns and proactive therapies. Fourth, healthcare practitioners (Kanak Kumar et al. 2023) can gain valuable insights from gathering and analyzing data produced by IoT devices to enhance care delivery and optimize resource allocation. Fifth, comprehensive patient education and training are necessary for introducing IoT solutions in healthcare and carefully considering privacy and security issues.

The review emphasizes the need for more study and development in this field and the potential advantages of IoT-based patient engagement solutions in healthcare. The reviewed studies and articles offer a variety of real-world examples of IoT solution implementations that have been effective and insights into the drawbacks and restrictions of this strategy. Healthcare professionals and governments can use the primary themes and patterns in the literature to guide future research and develop IoT-based patient engagement solutions.

17.3.3 Inconsistencies in the Review Findings

- One of the critical contradictions was the degree of patient participation attained through implementing IoT-based solutions. While some research concluded that patient engagement had significantly improved, others only found slight or no gains. Differences in the IoT-based technologies might bring this to the people examined and the healthcare environments.
- There was still another discrepancy regarding the impact of IoT-based solutions on patient outcomes. Although some studies indicated significant improvements in patient outcomes, such as fewer hospital readmissions and better medication adherence, other research found no appreciable difference. Once more, differences in study design and patient demographics could be to blame for this.
- The cited obstacles to implementing IoT-based patient engagement solutions also lacked consistency. While some research cited a lack of technical infrastructure and worries about data security and privacy

as critical impediments, other studies indicated that financial and organizational barriers were more important. These discrepancies may be caused due to the vast diversity of healthcare settings and patient groups that have been researched.

- There were some discrepancies in the benefits that IoT-based patient engagement solutions were said to have. Some research indicated improvements in patient satisfaction and quality of life, whereas other investigations found no appreciable difference. IoT-based solutions have been linked to cost savings in certain studies, but others have shown no discernible influence on healthcare expenses. These discrepancies could result from various study designs, patient demographics, and healthcare facilities.

17.3.4 Discussions

Several important conclusions were drawn from the review of IoT-based patient engagement options in healthcare. First, regarding remote monitoring and individualized care, IoT technologies can significantly increase patient engagement in healthcare. Second, IoT-based solutions can improve patient outcomes, such as better disease control, increased treatment adherence, and lowered hospital readmission rates. Third, putting IoT-based solutions into practice needs a multidisciplinary strategy involving a range of stakeholders, including patients, healthcare professionals, and technology developers. The review also uncovered several biases and limitations in the extant literature, such as the lack of standardization in IoT-based patient engagement solutions, the scarcity of long-term studies on their efficacy, and possible problems with data privacy and security. These results have significant ramifications for advancing technology and the healthcare industry. Standardized procedures and guidelines must be created to guarantee the efficacy and safety of IoT-based patient engagement solutions. Long-term studies are also necessary to comprehend the long-term impacts of these solutions on patient outcomes and healthcare systems. Additionally, attempts should be made to address any potential problems with data security and privacy.

Collaboration between numerous stakeholders is necessary to implement IoT-based patient involvement solutions in healthcare. Patients should be taught how to use these technologies to manage their health, and healthcare professionals should be trained to use them successfully and efficiently. Technology developers should collaborate with healthcare professionals and patients to ensure that the solutions are tailored to their unique requirements and preferences. The review highlighted the advantages and disadvantages of IoT-based patient engagement options in healthcare. Although there is still much to learn about these solutions, they have the potential to change the way healthcare is delivered and improve patient outcomes. A collaborative and multidisciplinary approach and ongoing study and development are required to realize their full potential.

17.3.5 Strengths and Weaknesses of the Literature Studied

According to the literature study, IoT-based patient engagement solutions in healthcare have both strengths and weaknesses. A thorough understanding of the subject is provided by using various study methodologies, including qualitative, quantitative, and mixed methods. In-depth analyses of IoT-based patient engagement solutions and their potential advantages, such as better patient outcomes, improved patient–provider communication, and lower healthcare expenses, are also provided in the literature. The literature review's emphasis on the difficulties of adopting IoT-based patient engagement solutions is one of its most vital points. The literature lists many challenges, including integration with current healthcare systems, patient involvement, and privacy and security issues. This emphasis on difficulties aids in identifying potential problems and the demand for additional field study. The reviewed material does, however, also have some flaws. One of the main drawbacks is the inconsistent terminology used to describe IoT-based patient engagement solutions, which can cause confusion and make comparing the findings of different studies challenging.

Furthermore, most of the reviewed literature is based on modest-sized pilot studies, which restricts the applicability of the results to larger populations. In addition, because the majority of the literature examined is from developed nations, the results may not apply to healthcare systems in developing countries. The literature also pays scant attention to the patient's viewpoint. Despite shedding light on the possible advantages of IoT-based patient engagement solutions, the literature review neglected to consider patients' viewpoints and experiences. Future studies should consider the patient's viewpoint to ensure that IoT-based patient engagement solutions are user-friendly and intended to meet patients' needs. The reviewed literature presents both strengths and flaws, in my opinion. The use of various study methodologies, the emphasis on difficulties, and the potential advantages of IoT-based patient engagement solutions are among the strengths. Overall, the terminology is inconsistent, there are only small-scale pilot studies, the patient viewpoint is not given enough attention, and developing nations are underrepresented, among other flaws. Further study may be required to address these issues and create IoT-based patient engagement solutions that are efficient, available, and patient-centered, according to these results.

17.3.6 Future Research Directions

There are still some gaps in the literature that require filling in through further research, even though the literature reviewed in this study has thoroughly grasped the potential advantages and difficulties of IoT-based patient engagement solutions in healthcare. Most of the studies examined in this article were conducted in developed nations, and more research is required to understand the difficulties in implementing IoT-based patient engagement solutions in settings with limited resources. The privacy and security issues related to IoT-based patient engagement options also require further study. A more profound comprehension of the advantages and disadvantages of these technologies is necessary as the use of IoT devices in healthcare keeps growing.

While there is a need for more study on the drawbacks of IoT-based patient engagement solutions, the current literature primarily focuses on their advantages. More specifically, the analysis must solve the problems of integrating IoT devices with existing healthcare systems and procedures. IoT-based patient engagement solutions will have a long-term impact on patient outcomes, such as patient satisfaction, quality of life, and overall health status, so a study is required in this area. Although the literature review in this study has shed light on the possible advantages and difficulties of IoT-based patient engagement solutions in healthcare, additional studies still need to fill in the gaps and overcome the research limitations noted in this review. Such research will be essential to successfully implement these solutions in healthcare and realize their maximum potential for enhancing patient outcomes.

17.4 CONCLUSIONS

The chapter focused on the transition from remote monitoring to individualized care as it investigated IoT-based patient engagement solutions in healthcare. According to the review, IoT-based patient engagement solutions can boost patient satisfaction and involvement while potentially enhancing patient outcomes. However, there are data security and privacy issues, and healthcare providers must successfully explain to patients the advantages of these solutions and ensure they receive the necessary guidance and support. Overall, the review emphasizes how critical it is for healthcare organizations to implement a patient-centric strategy for delivering care, relying on IoT-based solutions to enable individualized care and higher patient engagement. Additional investigation is required to examine how well these solutions work in various healthcare settings and patient populations and to handle data privacy and security issues. The potential of the Internet of Things (IoT) to transform patient interaction and care in healthcare is highlighted in this chapter on IoT-based patient engagement solutions in healthcare. The primary goal of the review is to critically analyze the effectiveness and limitations of the different IoT-based patient engagement solutions, ranging from remote monitoring to individualized care.

The review's conclusions show that IoT-based patient engagement strategies have great potential to raise patient satisfaction, lower healthcare costs, and significantly improve patient outcomes. The study also highlights crucial elements that support the effective adoption and implementation of IoT-based solutions, such as the requirement for stakeholder involvement, integration with current healthcare systems, and the application of data analytics for individualized care. The review also emphasizes the drawbacks and difficulties with IoT-based patient engagement solutions, such as data security and privacy concerns, interoperability, and suitable patient and healthcare practitioner training. IoT-based solutions can transform patient engagement and care, and this review's results have significant ramifications for healthcare providers, policymakers, and technology vendors. The study also highlights important areas for future research and development, and offers insights into the crucial success factors for the efficient implementation and adoption of IoT-based solutions. IoT-based patient engagement options in healthcare have significant ramifications for practice and policy. According to the research, IoT devices can significantly increase patient engagement, improving health outcomes and lowering healthcare costs. This emphasizes how important it is for healthcare organizations to implement and incorporate IoT-based patient engagement solutions into their operations.

To ensure patient privacy and data security, it is necessary for governing bodies and regulatory organizations to create standards and guidelines for the use of IoT devices in healthcare. The use of IoT devices and their data-sharing practices must be adequately explained to patients by healthcare providers. Policymakers should also consider the potential for IoT-based patient engagement solutions to reduce healthcare disparities by giving patients in underserved and rural regions remote access to healthcare. Overall, the conclusions of this review article have significant ramifications for healthcare practice and policy in the future and emphasize the need for more research and funding to be put into creating and implementing IoT-based patient engagement solutions in the healthcare industry.

REFERENCES

Agarwal, S., Tanwar, S., Kumar, N., Kumar, R., & Kumar, P. (2021). An IoT-enabled patient engagement framework for rural healthcare. *Journal of Medical Systems*, 45(2), 18. doi: 10.1007/s10916-020-01699-5.

Ahila, A., Dahan, F., Alroobaea, R., Alghamdi, W. Y., Mohammed, M. K., Hajjej, F., Alsekait, D. M., & Raahemifar, K. (2023). A smart IoMT based architecture for E-healthcare patient monitoring system using artificial intelligence algorithms. *Frontiers in Physiology*, 14, 1125952. doi: 10.3389/fphys.2023.1125952.

Ahmad, A., Farooq, M., & Latif, Z. (2021). IoT-based patient engagement solutions for chronic disease self-management: A systematic review. *Journal of Medical Systems*, 45(5), 1–15. doi: 10.1007/s10916-021-01781-2.

Alaball, J. S., Pujol, M. V., Falco, R. A., & Solsona, J. S. (2018). Smart health: A review of the literature. *Telemedicine and e-Health*, 24(10), 696–706. doi: 10.1089/tmj.2017.0287.

Al-Ali, A. R., Al-Tarawneh, R. N., & Al-Momani, M. O. (2020). IoT-based asthma management system using patient engagement solution. *Journal of Medical Systems*, 44(5), 92. doi: 10.1007/s10916-020-01598-9.

Alam, M., Khan, M. A., Ur Rashid, M. A., Nazir, B., & Saleem, K. (2020). Internet of Things (IoT) based healthcare systems: A thorough analysis. *Journal of Medical Systems*, 44(4), 1–20. doi: 10.1007/s10916-020-01537-4

Al-Fuqaha, A., Guizani, M., Mohammadi, M., Aledhari, M., & Ayyash, M. (2015). Internet of Things (IoT) in healthcare: A comprehensive survey. *IEEE Access*, 3, 678–708. doi: 10.1109/ACCESS.2015.2437951.

Al-Fuqaha, A., Guizani, M., Mohammadi, M., Aledhari, M., & Ayyash, M. (2015). Internet of things: A survey on enabling technologies, protocols, and applications. *IEEE Communications Surveys & Tutorials*, 17(4), 2347–2376. doi: 10.1109/COMST.2015.2444095.

Alhussein, M., Abualkishik, A., Khalifa, M., & Qureshi, K. N. (2019). IoT-based patient engagement tools for medication adherence: An integrative review. *Journal of Medical Systems*, 43(7), 1–9. doi: 10.1007/s10916-019-1366-5.

Ali, F., Ullah, I., Akhtar, A., & Nawaz, R. (2022). IoT and big data in healthcare: A review. *Journal of Ambient Intelligence and Humanized Computing*, 13(2), 1275–1289. doi: 10.1007/s12652-021-03212-6.

Ali, N. A., Shah, S. Z. A., Ahmed, S. I., & Iqbal, N. (2018). Internet of things (IoT)-based smart healthcare: A review. *Journal of Medical Systems*, 42(7), 1–13. doi: 10.1007/s10916-018-0975-5.

Alizadeh, S., & Pirzada, A. (2021). Internet of things based solutions for patient engagement and health management: State of the art and future directions. *Journal of Healthcare Engineering*, 2021, 1–14. doi: 10.1155/2021/6641847.

Amiri, H., Mohammadi, A., & Babaie, M. (2019). An IoT-based patient engagement system for chronic pain management. *Journal of Medical Systems*, 43(12), 337. doi: 10.1007/s10916-019-1529-9.

Armand, T. P. T., Mozumder, M. A. I., Ali, S., Amaechi, A. O., & Kim, H.-C. (2023). Developing a low-cost IoT-based remote cardiovascular patient monitoring system in Cameroon. *Healthcare*, 11(2), 199. doi: 10.3390/healthcare11020199.

Arora, N., De, A., & Mohanty, A. (2022). IoT-based remote patient monitoring in healthcare: An overview. *Journal of Ambient Intelligence and Humanized Computing*, 13(4), 4017–4031. doi: 10.1007/s12652-022-03491-y.

Aziz, F., & Hammoudi, S. (2020). How IoT can enhance patient participation in healthcare. *Journal of Sensors*, 2020, 1–16. doi: 10.1155/2020/8869309.

Bashi, N., Karunanithi, M., Fatehi, F., Ding, H., & Walters, D. (2018). Remote monitoring of patients with heart failure: An overview of systematic reviews. *Journal of Medical Internet Research*, 20(4), e147. doi: 10.2196/jmir.9275.

Bashir, M., Alotaibi, F., & Bokhari, R. H. (2018). Internet of things (IoT) applications in healthcare: A review. *Journal of King Saud University-Computer and Information Sciences*, 30(3), 291–307. doi: 10.1016/j.jksuci.2017.08.004.

Bui, N., & Zeadally, S. (2020). IoT-based patient engagement solutions for chronic disease management: A review. *Journal of Ambient Intelligence and Humanized Computing*, 11(2), 749–769. doi: 10.1007/s12652-019-01530-7.

Cabitza, F., Gianotti, F., & Simone, C. (2017). A systematic review of the literature on patient-facing technologies and health outcomes. *BMC Health Services Research*, 17(1), 1–13. doi: 10.1186/s12913-017-2038-4..

Chang, H. J., Lai, Y. H., & Chang, Y. C. (2019). IoT-based patient engagement technologies for the management of cardiovascular disease: A systematic review and meta-analysis. *Sensors*, 19(11), 2483. doi: 10.3390/s19112483.

Chen, J., Zhang, Y., & Huang, G. (2020). An IoT-based framework for diabetes management with patient engagement solutions. *IEEE Internet of Things Journal*, 7(7), 6388-6397. doi: 10.1109/JIOT.2020.2982235.

Chen, S., Liu, J., Yang, X., Li, Y., Qian, L., & Li, X. (2018). A review of internet of things (IoT)-based smart home healthcare systems. *Journal of Healthcare Engineering*, 2018, 1–15. doi: 10.1155/2018/1065025.

Chou, W. P., Chen, Y. L., Chen, Y. L., & Wu, C. Y. (2020). Internet of things-based patient engagement systems for chronic disease management: A comprehensive review. *Computers, Materials & Continua*, 62(3), 1601–1618. doi: 10.32604/cmc.2020.09726.

de la Torre-Díez, I., López-Coronado, M., & Rodrigues, J. J. (2015). Analysis of the security and privacy requirements of cloud-based electronic health records systems. *Journal of Medical Internet Research*, 17(2), e42. doi: 10.2196/jmir.3388.

Gao, Y., Liu, Y., Yang, J., & Chen, L. (2019). An IoT-based patient engagement system for hypertension management. *International Journal of Telemedicine and Applications*, 2019, 1–10. doi: 10.1155/2019/6564136.

Gia, T. N., Minh, L. H., & Son, L. H. (2021). IoT-based healthcare applications: A review. *Journal of Healthcare Engineering*, 2021, 1–12. doi: 10.1155/2021/8828556.

Gogoi, N., Sarmah, P., Deka, G., & Baruah, D. (2022). An intelligent pill bottle top with IoT-enabled health monitoring system. *Healthcare Technology Letters*, 9(1), 8–12. doi: 10.1049/htl2.12043.

Gualandi, C., Moreschini, S., Massaro, M., Cifaldi, L., Zucchelli, A., De Vita, E., Guidi, S., Foschini, L., & Pecora, F. (2021). Internet of Things (IoT)-based patient engagement tools for chronic disease management: an extensive review. *Journal of Medical Systems*, 45(2), 13. doi: 10.1007/s10916-020-01706-8.

He, F., Li, J., Liu, Y., Li, X., Li, M., & He, Z. (2021). An IoT-based healthcare system for hypertension. *Journal of Ambient Intelligence and Humanized Computing*, 12(4), 3671–3685. doi: 10.1007/s12652-020-02754-w.

Hwang, J., Kim, Y., & Kim, H. (2019). IoT-based healthcare service for individualized patient monitoring and management. *Journal of Healthcare Engineering*, 2019, 1–9. doi: 10.1155/2019/8352627.

Jang, K., Ryu, K., Kim, K., & Kim, H. (2022). An IoT-based postoperative patient monitoring system for patient participation and medical staff load reduction. *Healthcare*, 10(2), 134. doi: 10.3390/healthcare10020134.

Khan, N. A., Rasheed, M. F., Younas, M. K., & Kumar, N. (2020). Intelligent healthcare system for remote patient monitoring using internet of things technologies. *Journal of Ambient Intelligence and Humanized Computing*, 11(5), 2165–2186. doi: 10.1007/s12652-019-01536-y.

Kim, H. K., Lee, J., Park, K. S., & Kim, D. J. (2020). Application of Internet of Things-based patient engagement tools for treating Parkinson's disease: A cluster-randomized controlled trial. *Journal of Medical Internet Research*, 22(5), e16211. doi: 10.2196/16211.

Klonoff, D. C. (2015). The current and potential value of wireless technology for diabetes care. *Journal of Diabetes Science and Technology*, 9(1), 1–4. doi: 10.1177/1932296814566740.

Ku, T. Y., Liang, S. Y., Yang, C. C., & Chang, Y. J. (2019). Development and evaluation of an internet of things-based system for managing hypertension in older adults. *Journal of Medical Systems*, 43(10), 323. doi: 10.1007/s10916-019-1446-8.

Kulkarni, S., Hasan, S. S., Djalalova, D. M., & Rollins, R. L. (2020). Internet of things (IoT)-based remote diabetes monitoring systems: A review of literature. *Journal of Clinical and Translational Endocrinology*, 19, 100226. doi: 10.1016/j.jcte.2020.100226.

Kumar, K., Chaudhury, K., & Tripathi, S. L. (2023). Future of machine learning (ML) and deep learning (DL) in healthcare monitoring system. In: *Machine Learning Algorithms for Signal and Image Processing*. IEEE, pp. 293–313. doi: 10.1002/9781119861850.ch17.

Kuo, C. Y., Wu, M. C., Wu, Y. T., & Hsu, W. C. (2020). IoT-based health care for elderly people: An evaluation of three development projects. *IEEE Access*, 8, 33296–33304. doi: 10.1109/access.2020.2972701.

Kurniawan, E. D., Sari, S. R., Kurniawan, T., & Kurniawan, B. (2021). A thorough analysis of IoT-based patient monitoring systems. *Journal of Healthcare Engineering*, 2021, 1–14. doi: 10.1155/2021/6658656.

Kurniawan, Y., Zafirah, F., & Mulia, M. (2020). Internet of Things for mental healthcare: A literature review. In: 2020 *International Seminar on Application for Technology of Information and Communication* (iSemantic). IEEE, pp. 131–134. doi: 10.1109/iSemantic49861.2020.9313834.

Laranjo, L., Dunn, A. G., Tong, H. L., Kocaballi, A. B., Chen, J., Bashir, R., Surian, D., Gallego, B., Magrabi, F., Lau, A. Y., & Coiera, E. (2018). Conversational agents in healthcare: A systematic review. *Journal of the American Medical Informatics Association*, 25(9), 1248–1258. doi: 10.1093/jamia/ocy072.

Lee, J. H., Lee, Y. J., Park, S. H., & Kim, K. (2018). Development and assessment of a mobile application for internet of things-based hypertension monitoring and management. *Computers in Biology and Medicine*, 98, 23–30. doi: 10.1016/j.compbiomed.2018.04.004.

Lee, R., Kim, D., & Kim, Y. (2022). Continuous vital signs monitoring in hospitals using IoT technology: A feasibility study. *Healthcare*, 10(1), 68. doi: 10.3390/healthcare10010068.

Liang, X., Zheng, X., Wang, Y., Chen, H., Xie, B., & Sun, Q. (2019). An IoT-based personalized healthcare system: Architecture, enabling technologies, and service. *IEEE Access*, 7, 11630–11639. doi: 10.1109/ACCESS.2019.2890139.

Liao, S., Luo, Q., Deng, Y., Yi, J., & Chen, C. (2021). An IoT-based healthcare system for managing chronic renal disease. *Journal of Medical Systems*, 45(3), 1–8. doi: 10.1007/s10916-021-01714-4.

Liu, J., Li, L., Li, L., Li, Y., & Zhao, L. (2019). A wearable device-based patient engagement system: development and pilot implementation. *JMIR mHealth and uHealth*, 7(2), e11009. doi: 10.2196/11009.

Liu, Y., Liu, L., Xu, J., Chen, M., & Jiang, Y. (2021). Internet of things-based patient engagement solutions in enhancing medication adherence: A systematic review and meta-analysis. *Journal of Medical Systems*, 45(4), 42. doi: 10.1007/s10916-021-01723-6.

Maramis, C., Kurniawan, W., Prabuwono, A. S., & Setiawan, N. A. (2020). An IoT-based patient engagement solution for wound care management. In: 2020 *International Conference on Computer Engineering, Network, and Intelligent Multimedia* (CENIM). IEEE, pp. 1–5. doi: 10.1109/CENIM50167.2020.9318385.

Markets and Markets. (2019). *IoT in healthcare market worth $188.2 billion by 2024.* Retrieved from https://www.marketsandmarkets.com/PressReleases/iot-healthcare.asp

Mughal, A. H., Masood, M. A., Shah, S. G. M., & Alhamid, M. F. (2020). Internet of Things (IoT) for telemedicine applications: A comprehensive review. In: 2020 *3rd International Conference on Intelligent Sustainable Systems* (ICISS). IEEE, pp. 646–651. doi: 10.1109/iciss49662.2020.9133547.

Mukherjee, A., Biswas, P., Laha, S., Chatterjee, S., & Das, N. (2019). The role of IoT-based healthcare system in chronic disease management: A comprehensive review. *Journal of Medical Systems*, 43(8), 1–18. doi: 10.1007/s10916-019-1397-y.

Nambiar, R., & Sahasranamam, S. (2022). Internet of things (IoT) in remote monitoring of chronic diseases: A review. *Journal of Ambient Intelligence and Humanized Computing*, 13(2), 1491–1503. doi: 10.1007/s12652-021-03214-4.

Naseri, N., Jahangiry, L., Najafi, F., & Farhangi, M. A. (2020). The application of internet of things (IoT) for asthma control: A systematic review. *Journal of Medical Systems*, 44(10), 174. doi: 10.1007/s10916-020-01624-w.

Pang, Z., Chen, Q., Ou, J., Cheng, Q., Zhang, X., Liu, S., & Wang, Y. (2019). Internet of things-based personalized diabetes management system. *Journal of Medical Systems*, 43(10), 316. doi: 10.1007/s10916-019-1445-9.

Patel, M. S., Asch, D. A., Volpp, K. G., & Wearable Devices and Health Incentives Trial Group. (2021). Leveraging insights from behavioral economics to increase the value of health interventions. *JAMA*, 325(17), 1720–1721. doi: 10.1001/jama.2021.2291.

Pravin, S.C., Saranya, J., Suganthi, S., Selvakumar, V.S., Jackson, B., & Visalaxi, S. (2023). Machine learning and IoT-based automatic health monitoring system. *Intelligent Communication Technologies and Virtual Mobile Networks. Lecture Notes on Data Engineering and Communications Technologies*, vol 131. Springer, Singapore. doi: 10.1007/978-981-19-1844-5_52.

Priyadarsini, I., Chakrapani, I. S., Manochitra, S., Tejaswini, B., Ramesh, S., & Alaskar, K. (2023). IoT based mobile app for continuous health monitoring of the person. *AIP Conference Proceedings*, 2690, 040001. doi: 10.1063/5.0120557.

Quinlan, P., Price, M., Maguire, R., & Loughnane, F. (2019). The potential of IoT-based patient engagement tools to encourage self-management and lower hospital readmissions in patients with chronic disease: A systematic review. *Digital Health*, 5, 2055207619888881. doi: 10.1177/2055207619888881.

Rajasekhar, M., & Venkatesh, B. (2018). IoT based patient monitoring system for medical purposes. *International Journal of Pure and Applied Mathematics*, 118(16), 419–425. doi: 10.12732/ijpam.v118i16.8.

Seshadri, M., van Kranenburg, R., & van Sinderen, M. (2019). Patient-centered IoT-enabled health care: A social internet of things framework. In: 2019 *IEEE 5th World Forum on Internet of Things* (WF-IoT). IEEE, pp. 126–131. doi: 10.1109/wf-iot.2019.8767222.

Sharghi, A., Ghapanchi, A. H., & Talaei-Khoei, A. (2020). Design and development of an IoT-based patient engagement framework for fall prevention in older adults. *International Journal of Medical Informatics*, 142, 104214. doi: 10.1016/j.ijmedinf.2020.104214.

Shrestha, S., Shakya, S., Shakya, A., & Shakya, R. (2020). A comprehensive analysis of internet of things (IoT)-based solutions for managing chronic diseases. *Journal of Ambient Intelligence and Humanized Computing*, 11(6), 2367–2385. doi: 10.1007/s12652-020-02150-5.

Shrestha, S., Shrestha, A., Nepal, S., & Shrestha, R. (2020). An IoT-based platform for tracking and controlling chronic obstructive pulmonary disease. *Journal of Ambient Intelligence and Humanized Computing*, 11(3), 1093–1103. doi: 10.1007/s12652-019-01531-y.

Shrestha, S., Shrestha, S., Mahat, P., & Karmacharya, P. (2019). Application of Internet of Things technology for remote monitoring of diabetic foot ulcers: A review. *Journal of Medical Systems*, 43(5), 1–7. doi: 10.1007/s10916-019-1219-2.

Soliman, M., Abdelhakim, M., & Ali, M. (2021). Internet of Things based patient monitoring system for the management of chronic diseases. *Journal of Healthcare Engineering*, 2021, 1–16. doi: 10.1155/2021/9926849.

Steinhubl, S. R., Muse, E. D., & Topol, E. J. (2015). The emerging field of mobile health. *Science Translational Medicine*, 7(283), 283rv3. doi: 10.1126/scitranslmed.aaa3487.

Tariq, M. U., Shafi, A., Yasin, U. U., & Akram, M. W. (2021). Evaluation of IoT-based patient monitoring systems for the management of heart disease: A review. *Health and Technology*, 11(3), 601–616. doi: 10.1007/s12553-020-00510-w.

Uddin, J., Mondal, T., Islam, M. M., Islam, M. N., & Amin, M. B. (2020). Application of internet of things (IoT) in healthcare: A systematic review. *Journal of Biomedical Informatics*, 101, 103339. doi: 10.1016/j.jbi.2019.103339.

Ullah, S., Ullah, S., Hussain, I., Muhammad, N., & Baig, A. S. (2020). Internet of things (IoT) based healthcare monitoring systems: A review. *Journal of Medical Systems*, 44(8), 1–19. doi: 10.1007/s10916-020-01646-1.

Wang, J., Chen, Y., Cai, H., Zhang, Z., Liu, B., & Cui, S. (2018). An IoT-based real-time monitoring system for medication safety in smart hospitals. *Journal of Medical Systems*, 42(6), 1–10. doi: 10.1007/s10916-018-0938-6.

Wang, L., Chen, X., Yu, T., Liu, C., Sun, L., Wang, Q., & Wang, J. (2021). An IoT-based healthcare system for COPD self-monitoring and personalized therapy. *Journal of Ambient Intelligence and Humanized Computing*, 12(5), 4459–4472. doi: 10.1007/s12652-020-02980-1.

Wang, X., Zhou, X., Zhao, Y., Luo, L., Yin, Q., Zhang, Y., & Wang, L. (2020). An Internet of Things-based healthcare system for managing chronic heart failure: A randomized controlled trial. *Journal of Medical Systems*, 44(9), 174. doi: 10.1007/s10916-020-01663-1.

World Health Organization. (2018). Noncommunicable diseases. Retrieved from https://www.who.int/news-room/fact-sheets/detail/noncommunicable-diseases

Xie, B., Su, Z., & Zhang, W. (2018). Impact of wearable health technology on patient engagement: Systematic review and meta-analysis. *JMIR mHealth and uHealth*, 6(12), e242. doi: 10.2196/mhealth.9392.

Xie, B., Su, Z., Zhang, J., & Liu, K. (2018). IoT-based intelligent perception and cognition system for healthcare. *IEEE Journal of Biomedical and Health Informatics*, 23(1), 14–22. doi: 10.1109/JBHI.2018.2838139.

Xiong, L., Huang, W., Ni, J., Hu, J., & Liu, X. (2020). An IoT-based patient engagement solution for heart failure management. *Journal of Medical Systems*, 44(4), 90. doi: 10.1007/s10916-020-01577-0.

Yaraghi, N., Sharman, R., Gopal, R. D., & Ramesh, R. (2017). The business of health: The role of information and communication technology in health markets. *MIS Quarterly*, 41(2), 301–302. doi: 10.25300/misq/2017/41.2.17.

Chapter 18

Fusion Strategies for Image Processing–Based Multimodal Biometric System

Nitin S. Nagori, Kiran V. Ajetrao, and Ameya K. Naik

18.1 INTRODUCTION

Nowadays biometrics-based systems (Deriche, 2008; Mishra, 2010) are recognized as a standard for person authentication in many applications. The basic advantage of any biometric system is that it offers improved security and user convenience as compared to traditional knowledge-based (password) and token-based (identity card) systems. This is primarily due to the convincing ability of biometric technology to discriminate between a genuine person and a fraudulent imposter. In the initial years of biometric development, only unimodal (single modality) systems were used. However, over time, it was apparent that unimodal biometrics suffered from drawbacks such as difficulty in handling noisy data, lack of sufficient intraclass similarities/interclass variation, nonuniversality, and spoofing. As a result, biometric systems became less accurate and insecure, thereby not complying with the minimum security requirements of certain applications. To overcome these problems multimodal biometrics systems were introduced.

Multimodal biometrics deploys multiple instances of information for person identification and authentication. Multimodal biometrics (Deriche, 2008; Golfarelli et al., 1997) is advantageous in many ways. It may be used to solve issues such as biological traits deteriorating because of age. In such cases relying on only one single trait may lose the credibility of authentication. It is therefore recommended to use multiple modalities/traits, as multiple modalities ensure adequate population coverage. Multimodal biometrics can also resolve the issue of spoofing to some extent, as it would be very challenging for an imposter to simultaneously spoof or secure information about the various traits of a genuine user.

Instead of using features of different modalities/traits, multimodal systems can also use different identities of the same attribute. This approach results in better identification, specifically reducing false denials. With numerous advantages in sight, multimodal biometric systems have the potential to be widely adopted in a comprehensive range of applications, such as ATMs, banking security, online transactions, and e-passports.

DOI: 10.1201/9781003466949-18

Generally, the performance of any multimodal biometric system is accounted for in terms of false acceptance rate (FAR), false rejection rate (FRR), genuine acceptance rate (GAR), and equal error rate (ERR). The accuracy of the system can be calculated using the true positives and true negatives of the biometric system. A lower FAR and FRR will eventually result in better accuracy of the system.

There are several challenges (Mane and Jadhav, 2009; Ross, 2003) in implementing a reasonable biometric system, solutions to which have considerable scope for investigation and research. The following is a list of our significant contributions in this direction as presented in this chapter:

- The major factors that affect the performance of a multimodal system are reviewed.
- Appropriate strategies are investigated for choice of modality, biometric fusion, and mode of operation.
- An attempt is made to suggest feasible solutions to some of the vital issues related to a multimodal biometric system.
- The performance of the system is analyzed in terms of objective measures for further optimization. This would eventually enhance the overall accuracy of the system.

The organization of this chapter is as follows. Section 18.2 discusses a general multimodal biometric system. In this section, factors affecting the performance of a multimodal biometric system and its associated challenges are also presented. In the next section, design considerations and implementation trade-offs for a multibiometric system are deliberated. A typical case study involving face and fingerprint modalities is investigated in Section 18.4. This is followed by conclusions and scope for future investigation.

18.2 MULTIMODAL BIOMETRIC SYSTEM

18.2.1 General System

A block diagram of a general biometric system is shown in Figure 18.1.

Biometric modalities are captured by the biometric sensors and these modalities act as inputs for the feature extraction module. Next, features are extracted from different modalities after preprocessing. These features yield a compact and unique representation of modalities. These extracted features are then further given to the matching module for comparison. Extracted features are matched against the template(s), which is (are) stored in the database. Finally, the user is either accepted or rejected based on the decision in the matching module.

A multimodal system may be operated in serial mode or parallel mode. In the serial mode of operation, the output of one modality is used to cap

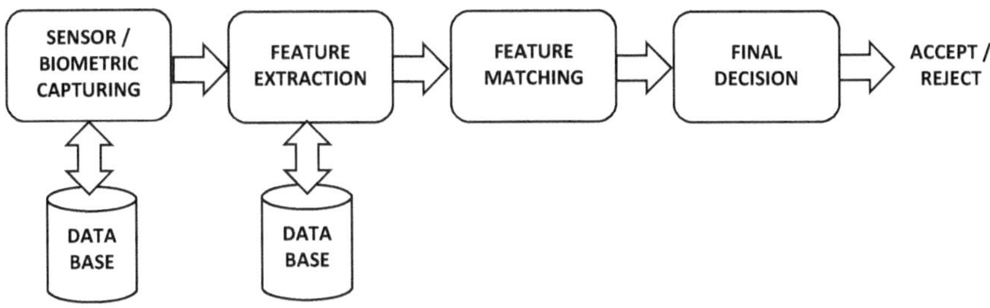

Figure 18.1 A general biometric system

the number of probable identities before testing the next modality. This may reduce the overall response time. A special case of serial mode is an indexed biometric system. There are various levels at which multiple biometric modalities can be combined to implement a multimodal system. The most practiced fusion levels are sensor level, feature level, match score level, and decision level. Each fusion level has its own significance in terms of information, desired output, and complexity.

Additionally, any multimodal biometric system largely operates in two phases, namely, the enrollment phase and the authentication phase. In the enrollment phase, the biometric traits of a user are captured using sensors and stored in the system database as a template for that user, which is further used for the authentication phase. The information obtained from the sensors may be stored directly or extracted features may be stored as a template. Whereas in the authentication phase, features are used to either verify or identify a person. Identification is one-to-many matching, whereas verification is one-to-one matching. Identification involves comparing captured data/features with templates corresponding to all users in a database, while verification involves comparing captured data with the template of the claimed identity only.

18.2.2 Factors Affecting the Performance of a Multimodal Biometric System

In general, the performance (Delac and Grgic, 2004; Kim et al., 2022; Choudhary and Naik, 2021) of any multimodal biometric system depends on the following factors. The same can be related to the issues stated earlier.

- Choice of combination of biometric traits: The number and types of biometric traits combined to authenticate a person need to be decided for optimum performance.
- Fusion level for multiple modalities: The choice of fusion level depends on the various factors required by the authentication system such as storage space, response time, and accuracy.

- Achieving optimal performance (Kim et al., 2022; Choudhary and Naik, 2021; Naik and Holambe, 2013, 2014, 2016): Optimization needs to be done for effective feature extraction methods, fusion levels, and matches to attain a balance across authentication performance, computational complexity, and storage resource requirement.
- Template security (Choudhary and Naik, 2021): Handling template security is crucial since biometrics is a permanent asset of any individual. Appropriate measures need to be used for the same.

18.2.3 Challenges with a Multimodal Biometric System

There are several challenges (Ross, 2003) for implementing a reasonable biometric system, solutions to which have considerable scope for investigation and research. A few of the issues relating to a multimodal biometric system can be listed as follows.

Issue 1: In case information obtained from the sensors is stored directly, it may require enormous space for storage. Also, the security and privacy of the information can be a matter of concern. In case features are extracted from the sensor information, it needs to be ensured that sufficient features are extracted before storage. In case lesser/insufficient features are stored, the issue of universality may arise resulting in false identifications.

Issue 2: In the case of identification, since it is a one-to-many matching system, the response time is quite large. Hence, algorithms need to be designed such that response time is less with minimum comparisons and acceptable accuracy. An indexing approach may be used in such a case.

Issue 3: The choice of appropriate modality is vital. For example, face images, although easy to capture may not yield sufficient accuracy. On the contrary, iris recognition requires specialized capturing devices but gives high performance. Moreover, the data from sensors are to be stored and mechanisms need to be designed that permit storage within the least storage space.

Issue 4: The choice of features and number of features are important parameters that directly affect the performance of the system. More features guarantee better performance of the system but at the cost of storage space and computation time.

Issue 5: The number of features used for comparison needs to be determined. More comparisons guarantee better identification but at the cost of response time. This parameter is of prime concern in real-time identification systems.

Issue 6: Decision-making is dependent on the chosen threshold value. This value has a direct impact on the FAR and FRR values. A low threshold value may result in a higher FAR, and a high threshold value may result in a higher FRR. An optimized value needs to be chosen.

Issue 7: In case the first modality used has lower accuracy, the same may have a negative impact on the overall accuracy of the system.

In the parallel mode of operation, information from different modalities is used simultaneously. The parallel mode results in higher accuracy as compared to unimodal and serial multimodal biometric systems.

Issue 8: Feature level fusion may accomplish the issue of using minimal storage space to some extent. Match score and decision level need substantial logic since individual biometric modalities have different performances that need to be considered during fusion.

18.2.4 Performance Evaluation of a Multimodal Biometric System

Although various parameters exist for measuring the performance of a multimodal biometric system, the following three parameters are considered to be the most important.

1. False accept rate (FAR)/false match rate (FMR) is the ratio of the total number of forgery attempts accepted by a biometric system to the total number of forgeries submitted to the system. This rate must be as low as possible.
2. False reject rate (FRR), or false non-match rate (FNMR), is the ratio of the total number of genuine attempts rejected by a biometric system to the total number of genuine attempts submitted to the system. This rate must be as low as possible.
3. Equal error rate (EER) is the point at which the false accept rate and false reject rate are equal. This parameter is important since it is difficult to achieve low FAR and FRR simultaneously. Hence, a tradeoff is required between FAR and FRR. This value should be as low as possible.

The performance of any biometric system can be summarized as shown in Figure 18.2. The overall accuracy can be calculated by measuring true acceptances or true rejections as compared to overall biometric attempts.

18.3 DESIGN CONSIDERATIONS AND IMPLEMENTATION TRADE-OFFS FOR MULTIBIOMETRIC SYSTEM

In line with the various issues as depicted in Section 18.2.3, the solution to many of these issues primarily requires the determination of the following factors:

SYSTEM RESPONSE → SYSTEM INPUT ↓	ACCEPT	REJECT
GENUINE	TRUE ACCEPT	FALSE REJECT
IMPOSTER	FALSE ACCEPT	TRUE REJECT

Figure 18.2 Performance evaluation of a biometric system

1. Choice of proper biometric modalities/traits
2. Template design and number of biometric features
3. Level of biometric fusion
4. Mode of operation and calculation of overall complexity and matching scores
5. Template security

The detailed investigation for the aforementioned parameters is as presented.

18.3.1 Choice of Proper Biometric Modalities/Traits

There exist numerous modalities that can be deployed for a multimodal biometric system. A detailed investigation has been done by researchers in terms of modalities, level of fusion, FAR, FRR, and overall accuracy. The same can be summarized in Table 18.1.

Design considerations. From Table 18.1, it is evident that the best performance can be achieved using the palm vein as one of the modalities. However, considering the ease of capturing for day-to-day applications, the same may not be a good choice. Reasonable performance can also be achieved using the iris as a modality. However, it suffers from the same drawback as that of the palm vein in terms of a specialized and costly capturing device. Additionally, it may be noted that a comparable performance can be achieved using the fingerprint and face as a biometric combination. The same can be used for most of the practical applications where ease of modality capture may be an issue. Nevertheless, iris and fingerprint combinations can be used for sophisticated applications where consistently higher accuracy is required.

Table 18.1 Comparison of Various Multimodal Biometric Systems

Reference	Biometric Modality		Fusion Level	FAR %	FRR %	Accuracy %
	Modality 1	Modality 2				
Muhammed et al., 2010	Face	Finger vein	Score	0.05	0.23	95
Muhammed et al., 2010	Face	Speech	Score	0.087	0.67	96
Krzyszof et al., 2007	Face	Speech	Decision	1.1	3.0	87
Rattani et al., 2007	Face	Fingerprint	Feature	1.98	3.18	98
Hong and Jain, 2008	Face	Palm print	Decision	1.0	1.8	92
Bokade and Sapkal, 2012	Face	Palm print	Feature	0.5	1.2	95
Nageshkumar et al., 2009	Face	Palm print	Score	2.4	0.8	97
Bahgat et al., 2013	Face	Palm vein	Feature	0.5	1.0	98
Mohamad et al., 2013	Fingerprint	Iris	Decision	2.0	2.0	98
Jagadessan and Duraisamy, 2010	Fingerprint	Iris	Feature	10	5.3	91
Dhameliya and Chaudri, 2013	Fingerprint	Palm print	Feature	0.2	1.1	87
Krishneswari and Arumugam, 2012	Fingerprint	Palm print	Feature	1.02	0.9	98
Cui and Yang, 2011	Fingerprint	Finger vein	Score	1.2	0.75	95
Vaidhya and Pawar, 2014	Palm print	Palm vein	Feature	0.029	1.0	99

18.3.2 Template Design and Number of Biometric Features

For most of the traits, the data captured by a biometric sensor is in the form of 2D data, i.e., image. Although higher resolution data can be made available by the biometric sensor, typical specifications of images used for automated biometric identification (using face, fingerprint, and iris modalities) are as shown in Table 18.2.

Generally, sensor (image) data is not stored in the raw format as it requires enormous storage space. Moreover, the number of instances of a single user also needs to be sufficient to ensure acceptable accuracy. Hence features are extracted from the data to create a template.

Design considerations. The features should be sufficient enough to reasonably represent the original data. This is necessary since a sufficient number of features must be available at any point in time to maintain distinctiveness between different users. Although statistical features are normally used, they may not provide complete representation since they offer global information in most cases. It is suggested to use spectral-based features since the same may also assist in compression of the data. Wavelet-based features based on the SPIHT (set partitioning in hierarchical trees) (Said and Pearlman, 1996) algorithm may be used. SPIHT supports progressive image transmission and hence offers flexibility in adjusting the number of features as per requirement and can regenerate the sensor data if required.

The storage space required for storing biometric templates can be reduced by using techniques such as image fusion. For image fusion, wavelet-based techniques with appropriate fusion logic can be used. Experimentations indicate that three levels of wavelet decomposition are optimum for fusion applications. However, care needs to be taken to ensure that information on any of the biometric modalities is not compromised during the fusion process.

Table 18.2 Specifications of Biometric Data for Face, Fingerprint, and Iris

Properties	*Face*	*Fingerprint*	*Iris*
Width	112	388	852
Height	92	374	480
Horizontal resolution	96	96	96
Vertical resolution	96	96	96
Bit depth	24	8	24
Storage for single sample	JPEG or PGM 120KB	TIFF uncompressed 142 KB	JPEG compressed format, 40 KB

For determining the appropriate number of instances and number of features per instance, the following pseudo code can be used. For a typical biometric system, FAR and FRR up to 0.1% are considered to be acceptable. Also, it is desired that the overall system response should be less than a second for real-time applications. The extracted features can also be used for biometric recognition using machine learning (ML)/artificial intelligence (AI) algorithms. Using biometric features for training yields better results than using biometric images directly for training the ML/AI systems.

Pseudo Code for Calculating Number of Instances/Samples per User

```
i=2
while i <=10 do
calculate FRR
if FRR < 0.001
if response_time < 1sec
number of instances = i
break
else
display ('RESPONSE TIME HIGHER')
break
end
else
i=i+1
end
end
number of instances=i
```

Pseudo Code for Calculating Feature Length per Instance

```
i=5
while i <=1000 do
calculate FAR
if FAR < 0.001
if response_time < 1sec
feature length = i
break
else
display ('RESPONSE TIME HIGHER')
break
end
else
i=i+1
end
end
feature length=i
```

18.3.3 Level of Biometric Fusion

Biometric fusion can be done primarily at the sensor level, feature level, or decision level. For sensor level fusion, the sensor data must be compatible with each other in terms of size and memory requirement. Sensor level fusion can be done with the face and fingerprint as the modalities. It is more appropriate to hide face data in fingerprint data. Fingerprint data can be used for the first level of identification and if required face information can be retrieved for the second level of identification. This approach also provides security to the biometric data.

Feature level fusion can be done by extracting features from multiple modalities and fusing them together. The most common approach to fusion is concatenation of individual features. The features before combination need to be normalized with respect to mean absolute deviation or maximum absolute value. Nevertheless, in the case of either sensor level or feature level fusion, spectral features are preferred. A better choice would be to use spatio-spectral features using transforms such as wavelet transform. Normalized score level or decision level fusion is preferred in case both modalities have performances on par with each other. The final decision can be taken based on various fusion rules, one of which is depicted in Table 18.3.

18.3.4 Mode of Operation and Calculation of Overall Complexity and Matching Scores

A multimodal biometric system can be implemented in serial, or parallel mode with each having advantages and disadvantages.

18.3.4.1 Serial Mode

In this mode, the identification process is first performed using one of the modalities followed by the other modality. It is always advisable to deploy a more accurate modality first since it has a direct impact on the overall recognition accuracy. However, it is also desired that the response time of the first modality is lesser since the first would most probably be a one-to-many match system. The second modality would mostly be a one-to-one/less number match and a slightly longer response time can be tolerated. The total time (maximum) required for the final system response can be calculated using the following equation:

$$T_s = t_1.n_1 + t_{2.}n_2 \qquad n_1 >> n_2 \tag{18.1}$$

where T_s is the (maximum) overall response time, n_1 is the number of templates in the first database, n_2 is the number of templates in the second

Table 18.3 Strategy for Combination of Results in a Multimodal Biometric System

Result of Modality 1 (R_1)	*Result of Modality 2 (R_2)*	*Strategy for Final Decision (FD)*
Match	Match	Match

Match
Non-match
	Non-match
	Match
		if $(w_1.CL_1 > w_2.CL_2)$ ***then***
		FD= R_1
		else
		FD= R_2
		end

Non-match	Non-match	Non-match

i. Where w_1 and w_2 are the weights assigned to modalities 1 and 2, respectively.

ii. CL_1 and CL_2 are the confidence levels associated with the modalities 1 and 2, respectively.

iii. In general, w_1 and w_2 can be determined on the basis of the average accuracy value provided by modalities 1 and 2, respectively.

iv. CL_1 and CL_2 can be determined by the deviation from the thresholds while making a decision for modalities 1 and 2, respectively.

database, t_1 is the time required for a single biometric comparison using the first modality, and t_2 is the time required for a single comparison using the second modality.

The total complexity in terms of the number of comparisons required would be $O = (n_1 + n_2) \approx n_1$. The overall probability of a perfect true match can be given as

$$P_{TM} = P(TM_1 / TM_2) = \frac{P(TM_1).P(TM_2 / TM_1)}{P(TM_2)}$$

where P_1 and P_2 probabilities of true matches for modality 1 and 2, respectively.

18.3.4.2 Parallel Mode

In parallel mode, both modalities perform the identification process simultaneously. The results obtained from both modalities are then combined to yield the final result. The total time (maximum) required for the final system response can be calculated as

$$T_p = \max(t_1.n_1, t_2.n_2) + t_m \tag{18.2}$$

where T_p is the overall system response time; t_1, t_2, n_1, and n_2 have meanings as defined earlier; and t_m is the additional time required to combine the results from both modalities.

The total complexity in terms of the number of comparisons required would be $O = (n_1 + n_2)$. The overall probability of a perfect true match can be given as $P_{TM} = P_1.P_2$, where P_1 and P_2 are the probabilities of true matches for modalities 1 and 2, respectively.

In either serial or parallel mode, the final decision can be taken based on the combination of individual results. Four cases can arise as depicted in Table 18.3 with the decision strategy as suggested.

In order to reduce the overall response time, especially in the case of serial mode of operation, the following strategies can be used (Figure 18.3).

In the prominent instance approach, the unknown template is first matched with the most prominent instance of each user. Once a reasonable match is found, the next matching is done using the second modality with all the instances of the previously matched user.

In the prominent feature approach, prominent features from all instances are matched first with the first modality rather than all the features. In case a reasonable number of prominent features match, matching can be done with the second modality.

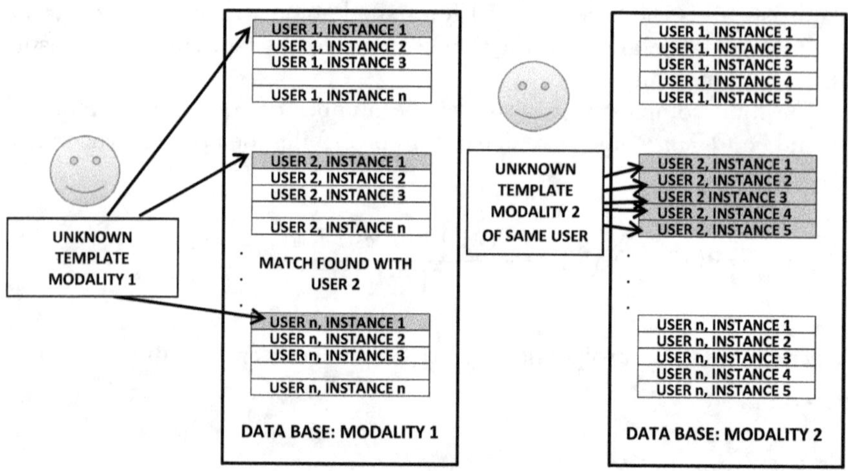

Figure 18.3a Strategy 1: Prominent instance approach

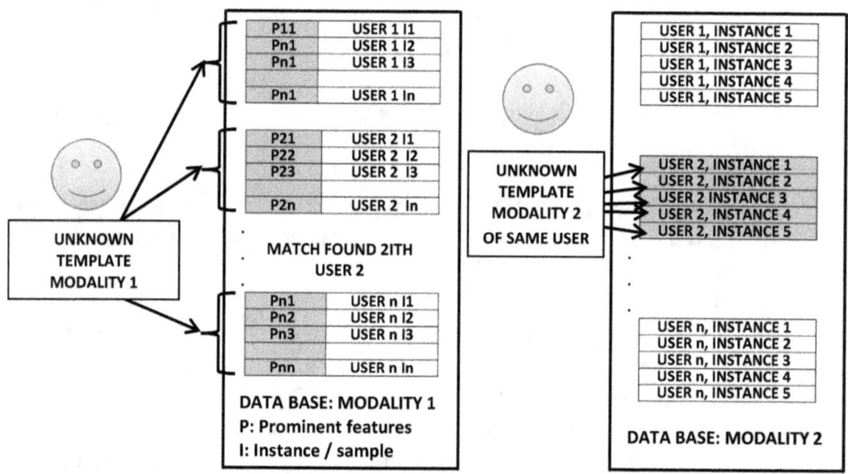

Figure 18.3b Strategy 2: Prominent feature approach

18.3.5 Template Security

The security of biometrics is at risk when it is either transmitted through a channel or stored in a database. Hence, to ensure the security of the biometric templates, the templates are either transformed or deformed. The templates are then stored or operated in the transformed form instead of the original format. There are several approaches for achieving the security of biometric templates.

In the first approach, data-hiding techniques can be used to hide/watermark one modality into another. For example, fingerprint data can be watermarked into face modality or vice versa. For watermarking, discrete wavelet transform (DWT) (Strang and Nguyen, 1996) along with quantization index modulation-based encryption can be used. A DWT level of at the most three is suggested since more levels of decomposition may not offer any significant advantage but may however increase the computation time. The final authentication is achieved using the match score function without the need for separate storage for two traits. If the prominent feature approach is to be used, then it is advisable to choose the higher accuracy biometric modality image as a cover image. This reduces the response time, as dewatermarking processes may not always be required.

In the second approach, feature-based transformation is applied to the original biometric data/template to obtain cancelable templates. Techniques such as random projection-based index of maximum hashing technique may be applied on features of two different instances for securing the stored templates. Instead of the maximum hashing technique, some other methods can also be used.

18.4 RESULTS AND DISCUSSION (CASE STUDY OF FACE- AND FINGERPRINT-BASED MULTIMODAL SYSTEM)

In this section, a case study of a multimodal biometric system using faces and fingerprints is investigated. The parameters and specifications used for both modalities are tabulated in Table 18.4. All the simulations are performed on 2.4 GHz octacore i5 (11th generation) intel processors supported with 16 GB RAM.

The performance of face modality is first analyzed for an unimodal system. The impact of increasing the feature length on system accuracy is observed. It can be seen from Figure 18.4 that although performance improves with an increase in feature length, the same is also attributed to an increase in response time (Table 18.5). Moreover, an accuracy of more than 90% can be achieved with a feature length of 37 with an original face image size of 112 × 92 pixels. With a reduction in face resolution, performance degradation is observed. A higher feature length would be required to achieve the same accuracy level.

Similar observations (Figure 18.5) are made for fingerprint modality as well. It can be seen that the accuracy level using the fingerprint modality is substantially higher than the face modality. Although the fingerprint image size is much higher (640 × 480) as compared to face images, the region of interest for fingerprint images is only 25% of the total image area. A

Table 18.4 Specifications for Face and Fingerprint as a Case Study

Property	*Face*	*Fingerprint*
Imager width	112	640
Image height	92	480
Horizontal resolution	96	96
Vertical resolution	96	96
Bit depth	24	8
Maximum number of instances per subject	10	10
Total number of subjects	20	20
Feature extraction method	PCA	Gabor
Distance measure	Euclidean	Euclidean
Multimodal fusion level	Decision/score	Decision/score

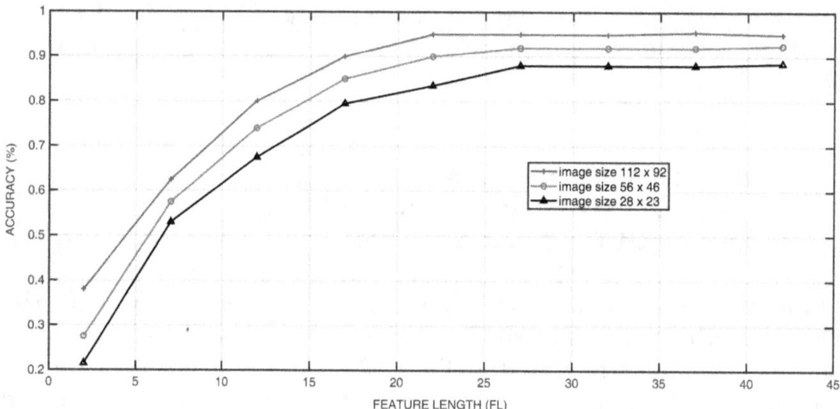

Figure 18.4 Performance of face modality with respect to feature length

Table 18.5 Response Time for Different Feature Lengths of Face Modality

Feature Length	2	7	12	17	22	27	32	37	42
Approximate response time in milliseconds (includes preprocessing time)	5	18	31	44	57	70	83	96	109

nearly 98% accuracy can be obtained with a feature length of 35 within a response time of approximately 92 milliseconds (Table 18.6).

It is well known that the performance of any biometric system improves with an increase in the number of samples (instances) per subject. This is investigated in Figure 18.6. It can be seen that although the performance improves with an increase in the number of instances per subject, the same

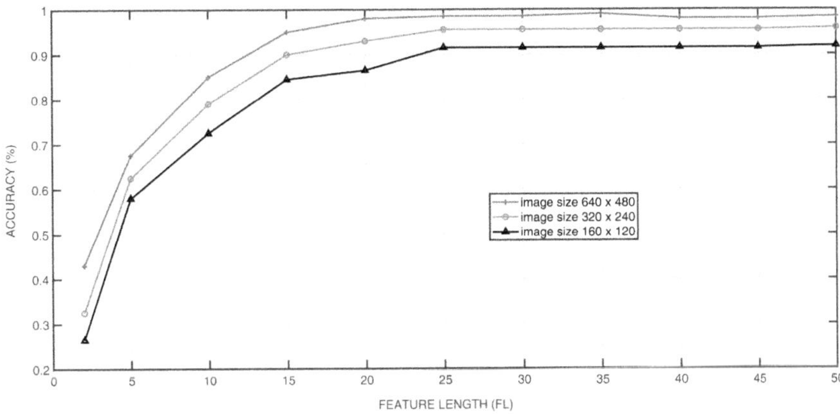

Figure 18.5 Performance of fingerprint modality with respect to feature length

Table 18.6 Response Time for Different Feature Lengths of Fingerprint Modality

Feature Length	*2*	*5*	*10*	*15*	*20*	*25*	*30*	*35*	*40*	*45*	*50*
Approximate response time in milliseconds (includes preprocessing time)	6	14	27	40	53	66	79	92	105	118	131

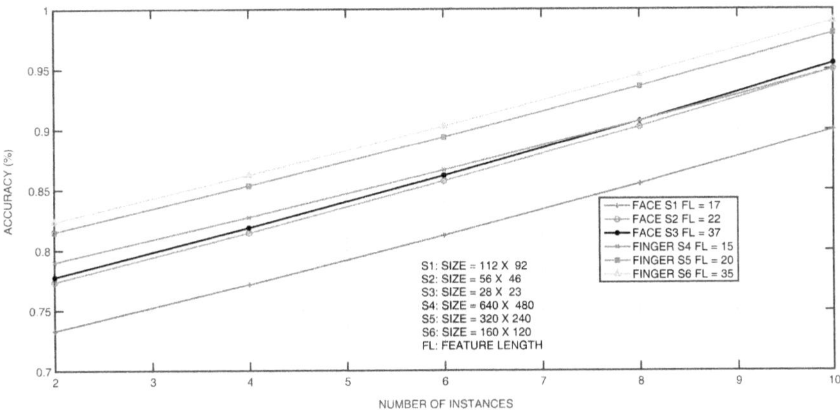

Figure 18.6 Performance of face and fingerprint modality with respect to number of instances

is not advisable beyond a certain limit. The reasons are more processing time and the amount of space required to store the templates. Rather a higher feature length may be a more appropriate approach for obtaining enhanced performance. Nevertheless, eight instances per subject may be sufficient in most practical applications.

Last we examine the performance considering a multimodal biometric system based on face and fingerprint modalities. It can be observed from Figure 18.7 that the multimodal approach offers significant improvement in performance. Since the fusion is done at the decision level, the total response time is the addition of processing individual modalities and the time taken to fuse the final scores. However, considering the enhancement in overall performance, it can be inferred that the combination of face and fingerprint can be a reasonable multimodal choice for most practical applications.

Face and fingerprint modality also has other advantages such as ease of capture, which is one of the most desirable features in most applications.

18.5 CONCLUSIONS AND FUTURE SCOPE

Various issues relating to the practical implementation of a biometric system are investigated. It can be inferred that a multimodal approach provides a reasonable solution to most of the problems faced by unimodal systems. It can also be concluded from simulations that for enhanced performance, a higher feature length may be a better choice as compared to increasing the number of instances. The response time can be reduced by using the prominent feature approach. More investigations can be done to determine the most prominent features of a biometric template. Moreover, the storage

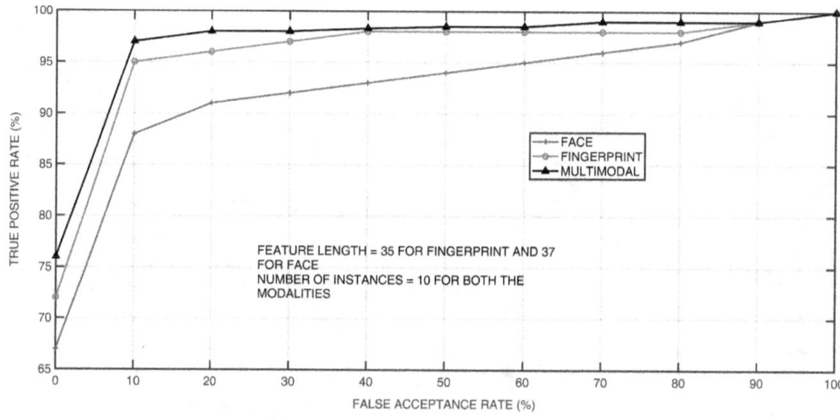

Figure 18.7 True positive rate versus false acceptance rate for face, fingerprint, and a multimodal biometric system

space required to store biometric templates can be reduced by using various fusion methods. In this direction, wavelet-based compression methods supporting progressive image transmission features may be further explored. Finally, various parameters affecting the performance of multimodal systems, if chosen appropriately, may lead to an optimum system in terms of enhanced recognition rates and response time. The same may find application in practical applications.

REFERENCES

Bahgat, S. F., Ghoniemy, S., & Alotabi, M. Proposed Multimodal Palm-Veins-Face Biometric Authentication. *International Journal of Advanced Computer Science and Applications* 2013, *4*(6), 92–96.

Bokade, G. U., & Sapkal, A. M. Feature Level Fusion of Palm and Face for Secure Recognition. *International Journal of Computer and Electrical Engineering* 2012, *4*(2), 157–160.

Choudhary, S, & Naik, A. K. Multimodal Biometric-Based Authentication with Secured Templates. *International Journal of Image and Graphics* 2021, *21*(2), 2150018.

Cui, F., & Yang, G. Score level Fusion of Fingerprint and Finger Vein Recognition. *Journal of Computer Information Systems* 2011, *16*, 5723–5731.

Delac, K., & Grgic, M. A Survey of Biometric Recognition Methods. *Proc. of 46th International Symposium on Electronics in Marine* (ELMAR). Zadar, **16–18 June** 2004, 184–193.

Deriche, M. Trends and Challenges in Mono and Multi Biometrics. *Proc. of Image Processing Theory, Tools and Application* (IPTA). Sousse, **23–26 Nov** 2008, 1–9.

Dhameliya , M. D., & Chaudri, J. P. A Multimodal Biometric Recognition System based on Fusion of Palmprint and Fingerprint. *International Journal of Engineering Trends* 2013, *4*(5), 596–600.

Golfarelli, M., Maio, D., & Maltoni D. On the Error-reject Tradeoff in Biometric Verification Systems. *IEEE Transactions on Pattern Analysis and Machine Intelligence*. 1997, *19*(7), 786–796.

Hong, L., & Jain, A. Integrating Faces and Fingerprints for Personal Identification for Personal Identification. *IEEE Transactions on Pattern Analysis and Machine Intelligence* 2008, *20*(12), 1295–1307.

Jagadessan, A., & Duraisamy, K. Secured Cryptographic Key Generation from Multimodal Biometrics: Feature Level Fusion of Fingerprint and Iris. *International Journal of Computer Science and Information Security* 2010, 7(2), 28–37.

Kim, J., Jung, Y. G., & Teoh, A. B. Multimodal Biometric Template Protection Based on a Cancellable Softmaxout Fusion Network. *Applied Sciences* 2022, *12*(4), 2023.

Krishneswari, K., & Arumugam, S. Multimodal Biometrics using Feature Fusion. *Journal of Computer Science* 2012, *8*(3), 431–435.

Krzyszof, K., Richard, J., Prodanov, P., & Drygajlo, A. Reliability- Based Decision Fusion in Multimodal Biometric Verification Systems. *EURASIP Journal on Advances in Signal Processing* 2007, *86572*, 1–9.

Mane, V. & Jadhav, D. Review of Multimodal Biometrics: Applications, Challenges and Research Areas. *International Journal of Biometrics and Bioinformatics (IJBB)* 2009, *3*(5), 90–95.

Mishra, A. Multimodal Biometrics it is: Need for Future System. *International Journal of Computer Application* 2010, *3*(4), 28–33.

Mohamad, A., Mohamadi, M., & Jafari, M. Multimodal Biometric System Fusion using Fingerprint and Iris with Fuzzy Logic. *International Journal of Soft Computing and Engineering* 2013, *2*(6), 504–510.

Muhammed, I. R., Rubiyah, Y., & Marzuki, K. Multimodal Face and Finger Veins Biometric Authentication. *Scientific Research and Essays* 2010, *5*(17), 2529–2534.

Nageshkumar, M., Mahesh, P. K., & Shanmuka Swami, M. N. A Efficient Multimodal Biometric Fusion using Palmprint and a Face Image. *International Journal of Computer Science* 2009, *2*(3), 49–53.

Naik, A. K., & Holambe, R. S. Design of Low-complexity High-performance Wavelet Filters for Image Analysis. *IEEE Transactions on Image Processing* 2013, *22*(5), 1848–1858.

Naik, A. K., & Holambe, R. S. New Approach to the Design of Low Complexity 9/7 tap Wavelet Filters with Maximum Vanishing Moments. *IEEE Transactions on Image Processing* 2014, *23*(12), 5722–5732.

Naik, A. K., & Holambe, R. S. Joint Encryption and Compression Scheme for Multimodal Telebiometric System. *Elsevier Neurocomputing* 2016, *191*, 69–81.

Rattani, A., & Kishu, D. R., & Bicego, M. Feature Level Fusion of Face and Fingerprint Biometrics. *1st IEEE International Conference on Biometrics: Theory, Applications and Systems*, **27–29 September** 2007, Crystal City, VA, USA, 1–6.

Ross, A., & Jain A. Information Fusion in Biometrics. *Journal of Pattern Recognition Letters* 2003, *24*, 2115–2125.

Said, A., & Pearlman, W. A. A New Fast and Efficient Image Codec based on Set Partitioning in Hierarchical Trees. *IEEE Transactions on Circuits and S ystems for Video Technology* 1996, *6*(3), 243–250.

Strang, G., & Nguyen, T. *Wavelets and Filter Banks*. Cambridge, MA: Wellesley-Cambridge 1996.

Vaidhya, D., & Pawar, S. Feature Level Fusion of Palmprint and Palm Vein for Personal Authentication based on Entropy Technique. *International Journal on Electronics and Communication Technology* 2014, *5*(*Sp. 1*), 53–57.

Index

access control, 62, 133, 249, 268, 270
accessibility and confidentiality issues, 59
adaptation to change, 44
algorithm, 3, 42, 43, 57, 87, 89–91, 110, 116–131, 175–192, 214–219, 225, 227–234, 252, 269, 300, 330
algorithmic details, 120
architecture, 79, 88, 91, 168, 211, 228, 247, 249–251, 265–266
artificial intelligence, 204, 292, 309, 331
attacks and prevention in IoT, 267
authentication, 56, 63, 98, 217, 270, 277, 323, 325, 326, 335
author's document production over time, 9
author's document publication in, 2022 12
author's impact, 10
authorization, 62, 63, 135
availability, 41, 57, 74, 89, 90, 116, 124, 146, 153, 156, 246
average citation per year, 7

background, 27
background of blockchain technology, 89
benefits of SWOT analysis, 42
Bibliographic Coupling, 20
blockchain, 55, 56, 59, 62, 87, 89, 91, 93, 100, 108, 109, 146, 162–169, 196–200, 243, 258–259, 279–280
blockchain and IoT overview, 279
blockchain and its principles, 280

chaincode, 283
challenges in mass adoption, 203
communication sector, 27, 33
competitive advantage, 43
conclusion, 22, 44, 64, 82, 110, 125, 142, 158, 172, 205, 220
conclusions and future work, 189
convergence of blockchain and IoT, 283
Corda, 250
crop identification, 232
cryptography issue, 58

data privacy and security, 287
data resources, 182
dataset acquisition, 121
decentralized (autonomous) organizations, 105
detection methodology, 57
development of IoT, 263
diabetic nephropathy, 175
diabetic prediction, 183
distributed and smart data storage, 104
distributed ledgers, 196, 199
distributed ledger technology (DLT), 147

end user's privacy, 58
enhanced resource allocation, 43
evolution of cryptocurrency, 201
examine the results of a specific technique, 170
experimental setup, 79
experiment discussion, 187

findings and discussion, 81, 156
framework, 212
functional specification of system, 216

hardware setup, 140
health and wellness monitoring, 80
healthcare, 29
healthcare sector, 39
health recordkeeping, 170
heterogeneity issue, 58
hyperledger, 198
hyperledger fabric, 247–260

identification of opportunities, 43
identifying fake information, 171
improved decision-making, 42
internet of things (IoT), 54–57, 59, 61–62, 68, 128, 133, 223, 226, 229, 258, 263–267, 270, 277, 280–286, 288, 290
internet of things and its applications, 281
interoperability, 28–30, 34, 39, 42, 55, 131, 147, 151, 164, 200, 201, 250, 258, 277, 287, 291, 299, 300, 309, 316
introduction, 1, 25, 54, 68, 116, 128, 146, 162, 196, 210, 223
introduction to industry, 4.0, 87
IoT cloud platform, 133
IoTA, 253
issues in IoT and the need for blockchain, 56

key enabling technologies, 72
keyword network visualization, 17

lack of generalizability, 219
limitations of blockchain, 172
limitations of machine learning algorithms, 219
literature review, 2
literature survey, 211

machine learning, 1, 116, 219, 223–226
machine learning and its use in agriculture, 223
main information, 7
maintaining hospital financial records, 171
major RPM components, 131
manufacturing sector, 27, 30
Merkle tree, 94, 95, 197
method and experiment methodology, 119
methodology, 186
most frequently used keywords, 19
most relevant affiliation, 12
multimodal biometric system, 324

necessity of blockchain in healthcare, 164
need for human intervention, 219

patient observation, 171
performance scrutiny, 7

Raspberry, 76, 139
references, 22, 51, 64, 82, 112, 126, 143, 159, 192, 206, 220
related work, 76, 129
related work and contributions, 178
research methodology, 5
results, 7, 142, 202
results and data analysis, 154
results and discussion, 122
risk mitigation, 43

screening, 7
search strategy, 6
securities, 100, 104, 151
security and openness, 170
sensing technology, 75
smart contracts and automated transactions, 102
smart healthcare, 56, 78, 129
source impact, 9
strategic planning, 42
SWOT analysis, 30

Three-Field Plot, 8
trial in medicine, 171
transportation sector, 28, 36

use of IoT in Agriculture and AI, 226

weed detection, 231

zero-day, 58

For Product Safety Concerns and Information please contact our EU representative GPSR@taylorandfrancis.com
Taylor & Francis Verlag GmbH, Kaufingerstraße 24, 80331 München, Germany

www.ingramcontent.com/pod-product-compliance
Lightning Source LLC
LaVergne TN
LVHW020610110826
845149LV00002B/434